Complex Systems and Population Health

Computer Systems and Population Health

Complex Systems and Population Health

A Primer

Edited by Yorghos Apostolopoulos,
Kristen Hassmiller Lich, and
Michael Kenneth Lemke

With Forewords from

David C. Krakauer, Sandro Galea,
and David Byrne

Renowned scholars in complex systems science, population health science,
and the social sciences, respectively.

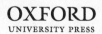

OXFORD
UNIVERSITY PRESS

OXFORD
UNIVERSITY PRESS

Oxford University Press is a department of the University of Oxford. It furthers
the University's objective of excellence in research, scholarship, and education
by publishing worldwide. Oxford is a registered trade mark of Oxford University
Press in the UK and certain other countries.

Published in the United States of America by Oxford University Press
198 Madison Avenue, New York, NY 10016, United States of America.

Library of Congress Cataloging-in-Publication Data
Names: Apostolopoulos, Yorghos, 1961– editor. | Hassmiller Lich, Kristen, editor. |
Lemke, Michael Kenneth, editor.
Title: Complex systems and population health : a primer /
edited by Yorghos Apostolopoulos, Kristen Hassmiller Lich, Michael Kenneth Lemke.
Description: New York, NY : Oxford University Press, [2020] |
Includes bibliographical references and index.
Identifiers: LCCN 2020001408 (print) | LCCN 2020001409 (ebook) |
ISBN 9780190880743 (paperback) | ISBN 9780190880767 (epub) |
ISBN 9780190880774
Subjects: MESH: Systems Analysis | Population Health | Models, Theoretical |
Computer Simulation | Social Theory
Classification: LCC RA418 (print) | LCC RA418 (ebook) | NLM WA 300.1 |
DDC 362.1—dc23
LC record available at https://lccn.loc.gov/2020001408
LC ebook record available at https://lccn.loc.gov/2020001409

9 8 7 6 5 4 3 2 1
Printed by Marquis, Canada

To Murray Gell-Mann (1929–2019)

Because without a science designed to take more than a "crude look at the whole" of population health challenges, we have little chance to advance the health of people most in need. ~ YA

To David Mendez, Rick Riolo, Carl Simon, Mark Newman, and Scott Page (University of Michigan)

Because without trailblazers teaching and building research portfolios using innovative methods, it might not have seemed possible (or nearly as fun). ~ KHL

To Donella Meadows (1941–2001)

Because without the accessible path laid out by her Thinking in Systems—my first steps into the world of complex systems—my scholarly journey would not have led me here. ~ MKL

CONTENTS

PART V TOWARD A NEW POPULATION HEALTH SCIENCE

FOREWORD

THE VALUE OF COMPLEXITY IN HEALTH

Any discipline or form of inquiry can be understood from three different perspectives: the historical, the methodological, and the domain of application.

When we speak of physics, we might be referring to the history of the scientific revolution producing an integration of empiricist philosophy, instrumentalism, and geometrical idealization. We might be referring to the methods of optical instrumentation and the accompanying use of approximate quantitative techniques such as conic sections and the calculus. Or we might be describing those ideas directed at the fundamental structure of the nonliving universe. All of these in totality are what we mean by physics.

Complexity science is no different. Its history is the attempt to articulate common principles and currencies governing the emergence of adaptive and robust states of matter spanning biological, social, and technological mechanisms with conceptual roots in materialism, vitalism, and evolutionism. Complexity methods occupy the union of nonlinear dynamics, information theory, the theory of computation, game theory, evolutionary theory, computer simulation, and nonequilibrium statistical mechanics. And the domain of complexity is that of networks of adaptive agents—nontrivially connected collectives of cells, organisms, and societies.

When introducing complexity, researchers typically reveal their own area of methodological expertise in their definitions, as such emphasizing the use of network theory, agent-based models, or scaling theory. These are simply methods that have proven useful in the domain of complexity and can be found used as profitably in domains of complication, such as physics, chemistry, and classical engineering. When speaking of complexity, it is essential to consider domain and method.

The domain of health from the complexity perspective is perhaps best thought of as robustness mechanisms operating in the arenas of organismal physiology, metabolism, and behavior. That is, health is the area of inquiry concerning properties of organisms that enable diverse action, fault-tolerance, adaptability, and evolvability. And we observe all of these in parallel and by analogy in ecosystems, economies, and cities.

The value of complexity science is knowledge transfer founded on structural analogies that underpin its domain of application—networks of adaptive agents. This creates surprising connections among fields, such that rigorous ideas from statistical physics like phase transitions can promote understanding of neural processing, insights from simulation can be used to monitor the spread of disease, and measures of network structure used to predict metabolic efficiency through scaling theory.

And perhaps most profoundly, a complexity perspective creates long-range connections among all of these constituents such that health becomes the robustness of the jointly adapted ecology of organisms, microbial communities, patterns of behavior, social organizations, and techniques of control and remediation.

Hitherto the methods of science have imposed simple causality on questions of health and disease. These are historical constraints of epistemology and not ontological reality. At a minimum, complexity science asks that we consider the larger systems of interactions that we describe as healthy. And at a maximum, complexity science pursues unification and methods that might articulate quantitatively networks of causality that span the many space and time scales required to truly understand and maintain adaptive function.

David C. Krakauer
President, William H. Miller Professor of Complex Systems
Santa Fe Institute, Santa Fe, New Mexico

FOREWORD

Understanding population health science depends on a full appreciation of the characteristics of populations. These characteristics include dependence on their history, interconnections, reciprocity of behaviors, discontinuities, and nonlinearities among others. Importantly, these are all characteristics of complex systems. Recognizing that populations are complex systems makes it then clear that the study of population health must reckon with complex systems approaches and perspectives to meet its aspirations. This book aims to help population health scientists do just that through providing a comprehensive primer on the use of complex systems methods in population health.

To my mind systems science approaches hold potential for the population health scientist on three fronts, all of which are well served by this primer.

First, and perhaps most important, systems science approaches help population health scientists and public health practitioners *think* in systems. Population health science has long been guilty, as have perhaps all other sciences, of overreduction of complex problems, of deterministic causal thinking whereby we search for a single cause that explains health outcomes in the hope that acting on that single cause can change health. And yet, aside from very few notable successes (with smoking being the canonical example), public health has long discovered the limitations of this approach. A reckoning with the chronic disease that account for the vast majority of burden of illness globally today and with the multiple levels of determinants from individual experiences to social policies that shape these diseases clearly require that we see populations as complex systems and adapt our scientific and implementation lenses accordingly.

Second, a systems science approach provides us with a set of analytic tools that can help tackle questions that are very much complex systems questions. Computational simulation modeling, micro-simulations, systems dynamics models, among other approaches, all have a place in population health science, providing approaches that are adept to tackle what are fundamentally complex systems problems. The astute scientist recognizes well that we should always use the simplest methods possible to answer any given question, but also that using approaches that do not rise to the challenge posed by the question at hand does us no service. The combination, in this book, of theory that suitably positions population health as a system of systems and pragmatic chapters that guide the reader about how to apply these approaches to difficult questions in population health stands to serve a generation of scientists well.

Third, a systems science approach helps population health science articulate the assumptions that influence and bias our work. A systems science approach, through its formal articulation of the logic that underlies all our questions of interest, pushes the population health scientist to road test their assumption and to pay attention to what otherwise may remain in the shadows. This moves us beyond considering our particular question of interest as the only question of import to a place where we recognize that our questions are grounded in complex realities and that our values and assumptions shape what we ask and the answers that then inform our practice.

A decade ago, systems science approaches and population health science were strangers to one another. In the past decade we have seen a broader embrace of the utility of systems thinking in population health science. This volume is an important addition to this recent work that has pushed for a transdisciplinary synthesis of systems thinking and population health science. It stands to further infuse complex systems theory, modeling methodology, and analytical tools into academic curricula, population health science, and public health practice. I look forward to a generation of scientists who are comfortably conversant in these approaches to the betterment of the public's health.

Sandro Galea
Dean, Robert A. Knox Professor of Public Health
Boston University, Boston, Massachusetts

FOREWORD

This collection is an interesting, innovative, and important contribution to the field of population health. I agree entirely with Apostolopoulos's conclusion that there is a real need for an epistemological overhaul that addresses what Page and Zelner in their chapter described as the complex adaptive systems of systems that constitute the relationship between population health, the wider socioeconomic/cultural systems of the world *and* at this point the impending climate crisis with all the implications that has for health across the world now and in the near future. That is what this book does, and it does it well. Let me take the liberty of reflecting and commenting on issues raised across the collection.

If we consider the issue of 'policy resistance', which Apostolopoulos identifies in his introduction, I agree absolutely that there is a very considerable policy resistance in health fields precisely because the reductionist analytical program has been so successful in so many areas of both clinical practice and, more important, in relation to the contribution of immunization programs to the reduction of the impact of infectious diseases. In other words, an epistemological program based on simple understanding, much of it predicated on the specific etiology understanding of the origins of disease—that is, on an ontology with epistemological consequences—has generated real health gains, although as McKeown (1980) demonstrated it was not that program that was fundamental to the health transformation. However, in policy areas other than health there has been no equivalent gain from mechanistic reasoning. Rittel and Weber's (1979) delineation of wicked problems, referenced here in the chapters by Goodson and Wolfson, has been very widely taken up in policy by practitioners. For a synthesis of this with complexity theory, see Ho's (2017) elegant lecture "Black Swans and Black Elephants." There is real opening here in engagement with policymakers without the biomechanical field of understanding. And is any of this new?—a question asked to tease out and to emphasize the importance of exploration alongside model building in the complexity program; see the Report of the Cholera Inquiry Commission (1854), which was addressed precisely to a health issue derived from globalization when an Asiatic disease arrived in England.

These points are indulgent notices, but the key thing is that this book is important and innovative and should be read by all concerned with using complexity to engage with health.

David Byrne
Professor of Sociology and Social Policy
Durham University, Durham, UK

- Cholera Inquiry Commission Report of the Commissioners Appointed to Inquire into the Causes Which Have Led to, or Have Aggravated the Late Outbreak of Cholera in the Towns of Newcastle-upon-Tyne, Gateshead, and Tynemouth. London, Eyre and Spottiswoode, 1854.
- Ho, Peter. (2011). Hunting black swans and taming black elephants: Governance in a complex world, 5 April 2017. https://www.csf.gov.sg/media-centre/speeches/hunting-black-swans-taming-black-elephants-governance-in-a-complex-world/
- McKeown, Thomas. (1980). *The Role of Medicine: Dream, Mirage, or Nemesis?* Princeton, NJ, Princeton University Press.
- Rittel, Horst W.J., Webber, Melvin M. (1973). "Dilemmas in a general theory of planning." *Policy Sciences* 4(2): 155–169.

CONTRIBUTORS

Fernando Alarid-Escudero, PhD
Drug Policy Program
Center for Research and Teaching in
Economics
Aguascalientes Area, Mexico

Pierpaolo Andriani, PhD
Kedge Business School
Marseille, France

Yorghos Apostolopoulos, PhD
Complexity and Computational
Population Health Group
Texas A&M University
College Station, Texas

Georgiy V. Bobashev, PhD
Center for Data Science, RTI
International, Research Triangle Park
Durham, North Carolina

Sally C. Brailsford, PhD
University of Southampton
Business School
Southampton, United Kingdom

Brian Castellani, PhD
Department of Sociology
Durham University
Durham, United Kingdom

Neal V. Dawson, MD
Case Western Reserve University
School of Medicine
Cleveland, Ohio

Dave C. Evenden, PhD
University of Southampton
Business School
Southampton, United Kingdom

Leah Frerichs, PhD
Gillings School of Global
Public Health
University of North Carolina
Chapel Hill, North Carolina

Lazaros K. Gallos, PhD
Center for Discrete Mathematics &
Theoretical Computer Science
Rutgers, The State University of
New Jersey
Piscataway, New Jersey

Patricia Goodson, PhD
Department of Health
and Kinesiology
Texas A&M University
College Station, Texas

Roman Gulati, PhD
Fred Hutchinson Cancer
Research Center
Seattle, Washington

Kristen Hassmiller Lich, PhD
Gillings School of Global
Public Health
University of North Carolina
Chapel Hill, North Carolina

Karen Hicklin, PhD
Gillings School of Global
Public Health
University of North Carolina
Chapel Hill, North Carolina

Gary B. Hirsch, SM
Independent Consultant/Learning
Environments
Wayland, Massachusetts

Lee D. Hoffer, PhD
Department of Anthropology
Case Western Reserve University
Cleveland, Ohio

Jack Homer, PhD
Homer Consulting
Barrytown, New York
and
Massachusetts Institute of Technology
Boston, Massachusetts

Jill Kuhlberg, PhD
Gillings School of Global
Public Health
University of North Carolina
Chapel Hill, North Carolina

Francois R. Lamy, PhD
Faculty of Social Sciences and
Humanities
Mahidol University, Salaya Campus
Nakhon Pathom, Thailand

Michael K. Lemke, PhD
Department of Social Sciences
University of Houston-Downtown
Houston, Texas

René J. F. Melis, PhD
Radboud University Medical Center
Nijmegen, Netherlands

Bobby Milstein, PhD
Rethink Health and Massachusetts
Institute of Technology
Boston, Massachusetts

James Moody, PhD
Department of Sociology
Duke University
Durham, North Carolina

Jordan Nelon, MPH
Department of Health
and Kinesiology
Texas A&M University
College Station, Texas

Marcel G. M. Olde Rikkert, MD, PhD
Radboud University Medical Center
Nijmegen, Netherlands

Nathaniel Osgood, PhD
Computational Epidemiology and
Public Health Informatics Lab,
Department of Computer Science
University of Saskatchewan
Saskatoon, Canada

Scott E. Page, PhD
Center for the Study of Complex
Systems
University of Michigan
Ann Arbor, Michigan

Dana K. Pasquale, PhD
Duke Network Analysis Center
Duke University
Durham, North Carolina

Megan S. Patterson, PhD
Department of Health
and Kinesiology
Texas A&M University
College Station, Texas

Carolyn M. Rutter, PhD
RAND Corporation
Washington, DC

Noemi Schuurman, PhD
Department of Methodology and
Statistics
Tilburg University
Tilburg, Netherlands

Natalie R. Smith, PhD
Gillings School of Global
Public Health
University of North Carolina
Chapel Hill, North Carolina

Joe Viana, PhD
The Health Services Research Unit
Akershus University Hospital
Lørenskog, Norway

Michael C. Wolfson, PhD
School of Epidemiology and
Public Health
University of Ottawa, Ottawa
Ontario, Canada

Jon Zelner, PhD
School of Public Health
University of Michigan
Ann Arbor, Michigan

PROLOGUE

While our research universities remain beacons of innovation, we have been witnessing alarming trends. Changing cultural values and resultant societal priorities also change academia, and not always for the better. Universities have begun to place uncharacteristically high emphasis on the pursuit of outputs often measured using arbitrary and questionable metrics for scholarship. Not only have these changes triggered adverse ramifications for the academic enterprise as a whole, but they have also begun to negatively affect exceptionally creative faculty members who pursue innovative avenues of research with potential for broad impact. In this simplified but accurate depiction of today's research expectations of academics, particularly true in the health sciences, the authorship of books that can inspire discovery and innovation is discouraged due to its perceived low return on investment. This is especially true for books that require significant, high-level intellectual effort and are deemed relatively insignificant endeavors for faculty evaluations. In this reality, taking on a book project in unchartered territory might be wise to avoid.

These are not random musings, but rather the dilemma I found myself in when I joined Texas A&M University in 2015. When preparing to teach a novel graduate seminar on complex systems and population health, I was faced with the complete absence of textbooks on which to build the course. While relevant scientific journal articles have always comprised the bulk of materials I use in my graduate seminars, I found the use of a foundational textbook particularly helpful for guiding novices—especially for a course planned to introduce new subject matter intended to challenge the prevailing paradigm. While not typically integrated into academic curricula, courses on complex systems thinking and complex systems methodologies in population health have been offered in diverse forms and fora for over a decade now. Despite this, my course preparation research did not yield even a single course focused on what I had in mind: a comprehensive examination of the capabilities of complex systems science in tackling some of the most intractable population health challenges of our time—all of them embedded in, shaped by, or consisting of complex systems. What I wanted to accomplish was much more than introducing students to the technical details of new analytical methods embedded within the prevailing paradigm of population health, currently under question. Despite my extensive search, I was unable to find a book that provided a unifying framework integrating complex systems science into population health science.

Thus, this long-overdue introductory book is intended to fill the enormous void in the English-language literature of the health and social sciences. About 25 years after the introduction of complex systems methods in population health, there still exists a dearth of books, and above all, there exists a lack of academic curricula built on a comprehensive amalgamation of current population health epistemologies with network and complex systems science perspectives. In its current form, this book is conceptualized as a traditional text for nontraditional topics; it is a systematic presentation of how complex systems science can advance theory, methodology, and analytical methods in population health in the context of extant epistemology. Because I deeply believe that an epistemological overhaul in population health science grounded in network and complex systems sciences is urgently needed, this book presents itself as the first step toward that direction. Population health science has been at a crossroads for quite some time now, and my hope is that this book contributes to the ongoing discourse on the role of complex systems science in population health education, curricula, scholarship, and action.

As is always the case with large-scale scholarly projects, this book is a collaborative effort of a great number of innovative scholars. It was a challenge to locate, commission, coordinate, and work with 32 high-caliber scholars from eight countries and originating from a range of sciences, disciplines, and professions; however, the high quality of their work has made the weighty review, revision, and editing process both enjoyable and enlightening. It is important to note that, given the chapter contributors' distinct perspectives and backgrounds, this volume represents diverse views and that my coeditors and I cannot be assumed to agree with all views expressed throughout the chapters. This book is better for it and would never have materialized without their collective and insightful contributions and "out of the box" thinking. My coeditors and I wholeheartedly thank our contributors.

I also owe a great debt of gratitude to my colleagues Kristen Hassmiller Lich and Michael Kenneth Lemke (my two coeditors), who wholeheartedly supported this demanding endeavor from its onset, when I presented first drafts of the book proposal to them two years ago. This unconventional book, which transcends usual academic boundaries and established paradigms, is the outcome of our joint intellectual effort.

I would be remiss if I did not thank our Oxford University Press editors, Chad Zimmerman and Chloe Layman, who believed in the potential of the project and have provided continued support and guidance. I would also like to thank my academic home, Texas A&M University, for providing me with a generous faculty development leave—contrary to prevalent academic trends—during the final and most demanding phases of this project.

Finally, I owe a tremendous debt of intellectual gratitude to the Santa Fe Institute. This unique think tank of complex systems innovators has remained my constant inspiration, learning platform, and virtual sounding board.

Yorghos Apostolopoulos
Summer 2019
Houston, Texas

PART I

Population Health Science in a Complex World

1

Bridging the Divide

Where Complex Systems Science Meets Population Health Science

YORGHOS APOSTOLOPOULOS

> Complexity starts when causality breaks down.
>
> Nigel Goldenfeld, excerpt from Editorial, *Nature Physics,* 2009

1.1. FROM HUNTING FOR CAUSES TO EXAMINING THE WHOLE

As an emerging scientific field in the 1870s, public health sought legitimacy by replicating the natural sciences. The pursuit of knowledge in this burgeoning field was founded on the presumption that public health problems are ordered systems and that their reduction to their individual parts, to be studied in isolation, would cumulatively lead to an understanding of the whole. Gradually, the *prevailing paradigm* in public health embraced key pillars of Newtonian science—reductionism, linear deterministic modeling, macroscopic laws of averages, homogeneous behavior of system parts, proximal causation, and equilibrium[1,2]—and later adopted counterfactual causal inference[3] and emphasized randomized controlled trials.[4] Today, researchers, policymakers, and practitioners continue to draw upon these principles while designing studies, analyzing data, making inferences, implementing and evaluating interventions, and devising policies—in their efforts to tackle pressing population health problems.

During this nearly one-and-a-half-century period, and despite the unparalleled progress in curbing diverse population health problems around the world, which coincided with the expansion of institutionalized public health,[5] there persists an

Yorghos Apostolopoulos, *Bridging the Divide* In: *Complex Systems and Population Health*. Edited by: Yorghos Apostolopoulos, Kristen Hassmiller Lich, and Michael Kenneth Lemke, Oxford University Press (2020). © Oxford University Press.
DOI: 10.1093/oso/9780190880743.003.0001

excess and uneven distribution of disease burden that is especially pronounced along socioeconomic, racial/ethnic, and geographic lines.[6] Notwithstanding varying levels of socioeconomic development, prevention impasses are marked by the ubiquitous *dynamic complexity* of population health and the enduring misunderstanding or mismanagement of it—not addressed by a prevalent epistemology designed for ordered problems. Some of the most obstinate population health challenges of our time, however, are neither ordered nor chaotic (polar opposites in the scientific landscape). They lie between these two boundaries, where *complex systems* abound, marked by dynamic complexity and intertwined causality.[7] Not only has dynamic complexity repeatedly defied well-intentioned efforts to develop long-lasting policy solutions, but it has also driven well-resourced interventions and anticipated outcomes to plateaus, relapses, or even unintended adverse consequences.[8]

It is this pervasive dynamic complexity of population health problems that regularly leads to *policy resistance*. When policy goals are misaligned with the goals of system "actors," then interventions are delayed, diluted, or defeated by "unforeseen" system reactions to the interventions themselves.[9] Even some of the best interventions that are designed to curtail persisting problems can exacerbate them when founded on overly simplified science (e.g., overuse of antibiotics, leading to spread of drug-resistant pathogens; road expansion programs increasing traffic, delays, and pollution).[10,11] Numerous such examples confirm that the prevailing paradigm requires substantial updating and that instead of an emphasis on isolated factors or events that keep defeating our policies, a meaningful recognition of the role of underlying causal structures of such problems would better serve the population health community in devising appropriate epistemological amendments to ameliorate the state of people's health as effectively and equitably as possible.

Within this overall inadequate prevention milieu, particularly for persistent population health challenges that disproportionately affect the most disadvantaged demographics,[12,13] the health community has begun to acknowledge that the prevailing epistemology cannot move population health promotion and protection forward[14]—there is no "silver bullet." Consequently, since the 1990s, the prevailing paradigm has been undergoing a thorough evaluation,[15,16] based on the belated recognition that "the network of relationships linking the human race to itself and to the rest of the biosphere is so complex that all aspects affect all others to an extraordinary degree."[17] Thus, the "study of the whole system, however crudely that has to be done," is essential "because no gluing together of partial studies of a complex nonlinear system can give a good idea of the behavior of the whole."[17] Simply put, because *all* major population health challenges of our time are either *complex systems themselves or are embedded in larger complex systems*—from cardiometabolic syndemics, unhealthful food systems, and the opioid crisis to the HIV pandemic, to mention just a few—*they should be studied as such.*

This incommensurability between the prevailing paradigm and the nature of population health problems has catalyzed calls for the introduction of complex systems thinking and associated methodologies to research and policy planning.[18]

Originating in a predominantly reductionist science, population health has gradually moved toward a fast-evolving epistemological discourse centered on how relationships among interdependent parts of population health components result in systemwide behavior that is oftentimes undesirable. Population health finds itself in the midst of a momentous transition: from being confined to proximal risk-factor epidemiology[19] and general linear reality[20] to steadily recognizing the benefits of taking a look at the whole of complex, nonlinear, and dynamic health problems, grounded in novel scientific advances, applicable to population health.

1.2. PROVIDING DEFINITIONAL CLARITY

Roughly about the time complex-systems analytical methods were being introduced to the field of public health, the emergence of "population health" prompted a debate over differences of the two and implications for the people's health. On the other hand, scientists who employ complex systems epistemologies regularly rely on disparate conceptions and interpretations of complexity. The following paragraphs delve into these two areas to provide clarity and a shared language.

1.2.1. Population Health and Population Health Science

Recurrent disease outbreaks along with the growing role of government in the people's health, mainly in industrialized nations, led to the formation of the American Public Health Association in 1872, followed by the establishment of the Johns Hopkins University School of Hygiene and Public Health in 1916 and the London School of Hygiene and Tropical Medicine in 1922. These developments spurred the creation of similar academic institutions around the world, thus precipitating an enormous growth phase for public health. Ever since, *public health* has aimed to protect and improve the health of communities through policy recommendations, health promotion and outreach, and research for disease and injury detection and prevention.[21]

A sluggish introduction to *population health* was initiated in the 1990s, first in the United Kingdom and Canada, followed by the United States,[22] amidst a growing appreciation for the role of social determinants in health[23] and the determinants of health of populations.[24,25] *Population health*—the prevalence, determinants, and distribution of disease and injury—highlights the importance of socioeconomic, environmental, and biological forces in shaping the health and well-being of people living in a geographic area or those of a demographic or other cohort.[26] This slow transition also triggered a discourse on the implications of these differences between the two, both epistemologically and for the people's health.[27] Further, it has also led to the onset of *population health science* and the formation of the Interdisciplinary Association for Population Health Science in 2015. As a more inclusive account of people's health, *population health science* examines those conditions that shape the distribution of disease and injury within and across populations and those mechanisms through which these conditions manifest as the people's health.[28]

In this book, we take an all-encompassing look at population health covering governmental, nongovernmental, and academic efforts and policies to improve public health, organizational and social conditions that define the people's health, health systems and budgets, health insurance, health protection and promotion, health services, and healthcare. In this holistic approach to population health, we emphasize how diverse macrostructural forces produce socioeconomic, geographic, and demographic inequities that ultimately induce excess disease and injury burden and health inequities at large. *It is this book's thesis that the absence of any of the foregoing jeopardizes the health, safety, and well-being of populations.*

1.2.2. Complexity and Complex Systems Science

Complex comes from the Latin *cum* and *plexere*, meaning "intertwined," while *complicated* originates from *cum* and *plicare*, meaning "folded together"—a useful distinction when it comes to the limitations of the prevalent paradigm in advancing population health. Complex systems relate to the atomic innovations of the 1940s, when Stanislaw Ulam and John von Neumann, at Los Alamos Laboratories, began to blur disciplinary demarcations by developing mathematical and computational models that eventually gave rise to what we today call *complex systems science.* The following chapters delve into various aspects of complexity, key complex systems properties, and how they can contribute to advancing both societal needs and the scientific frontier. This first chapter only dives into organized *dynamic complexity* because of its indispensability to understanding how even well-planned health policies are often defeated by health problems themselves.

In dynamically complex situations, such as cardiometabolic syndemics, for instance, effects are not immediately apparent when causes are introduced, but as several causes intensify over time, the effects become more obvious. While cardiometabolic syndemics are complex systems that are conditioned by feedbacks, time delays, accumulations, and nonlinearities, we make decisions using mental models that are typically static, linear, or incomplete (see Chapter 8 of this volume). Cardiometabolic syndemics exhibit ample *dynamic complexity*— or, unexpected behaviors (e.g., excess myocardial infraction rates among rural minority populations) resulting from interactions and interrelationships of system components over time.[10] Dynamic complexity obscures causal relationships and, as a result, compromises the efficacy of interventions due to *policy resistance.*[10] Policy resistance arises because cardiometabolic syndemics are continually changing, tightly coupled, nonlinear, self-organizing, adaptive, counterintuitive, governed by endogenous feedback, and characterized by trade-offs. Cardiometabolic syndemics are not clear for policy planners because connections of circular causality are not intuitively detected; as a result, it is difficult to model them or make predictions. Policy planners are often faced with surprises, such as adverse consequences of their decisions in various parts of the system, because even well-intentioned programs often generate unanticipated "side effects" (or resistance to policies). For instance, technological advances that have increased sedentariness and access to cheaper calorie-dense foods have had an aggregate impact on obesity—a critical precursor to increasing cardiometabolic risk. In this particular case, the adverse consequences have arisen from a mismatch between features of cardiometabolic syndemics and simplistic mental models that are employed to reach decisions. Where consequences of our actions spill out across space and time, we tend to focus on the local, proximal, micro, and short-term. We usually ignore interdependencies between parts of complex systems, and the delayed, distal consequences of our actions—signifying that our mental model boundaries are too narrow and time horizons, too short.

Along these lines, *complex systems science* focuses on system parts, relationships, and wholes; how these parts give rise to collective behavior; and how the system interacts with its environment. Complex systems science flows in and out of restricting disciplinary boundaries—a great match for population health science—and creates efficacious paths among scientists from different disciplines, thus accelerating the proliferation of knowledge. It also reduces gaps between science and action, thereby facilitating connections between research, policy, and practice by catalyzing new ways of managing problems where dynamic complexity exceeds the capacity of the prevailing paradigm. As it has been the case with the physical sciences, the intersection of complex systems science and population health science has the potential to flourish through an ongoing and reciprocal process of re/constructing rigorous mathematical and computational models through the constant improvement of data.

In this book, grounded in the work of scholars from diverse scientific backgrounds, the terms (complex) *systems thinking, complexity* (science), (complex) *systems*, and (complex) *systems science* are often used interchangeably, in various forms or combinations. We aim to marry complex systems science with population health science to generate beneficial results for both our science and the people's health.

1.3. THE INTERSECTION OF COMPLEX SYSTEMS SCIENCE AND POPULATION HEALTH SCIENCE

1.3.1. Book Rationale and Objectives

Over the past 25 years or so, population health science has been slowly discovering complex systems science, with the primary emphasis being on analytical methods thus far and what they could mean for research, scholarship, policy planning, and action, as well as for the health of all people. At the other disciplinary end, the natural sciences, which were founded on Newtonian principles similar to population health, have long evolved and organically integrated complex systems science epistemologies into their armory. Within the broad area of health-focused disciplines, biology, medicine, and psychology have adopted and expanded broad complex systems science–grounded methodological and analytical frameworks, including mathematical, computational, and network modeling, with astounding discoveries for population health. Sequencing the human genome, advancing understanding of cancer metastasis, and delineating psychiatric disorders are representative examples that illustrate the boundless potential of complex systems science in population health research.[29-31]

Population health science has embraced a more systematic introduction of complex systems science into population health science as a result of these groundbreaking paradigmatic shifts. Other contributing factors include ongoing advances in computational and data sciences, recognition of the limitations of the "silver-bullet" paradigm in tackling inherently dynamic and complex population health challenges, recognition of the irreplaceable whole in delineating intractable problems, and increasing realization that macrostructural domains are critical health determinants. For instance, unresolved impasses in curtailing cardiometabolic syndemics—which top all disease burden categories—require epistemologies capable of illuminating such complexities and potentially leading to efficacious and equitable interventions amid perplexing demographic, political, socioeconomic, and environmental shifts. As such, population health challenges are required to be studied as complex systems, grounded in relevant, comprehensive theory, research designs, and analytical methods. Mounting evidence denotes that the organic integration of social, health, natural, computational, mathematical, data, and statistical science perspectives—grounded within academic curricula in population health science and founded on complex systems science—can bring about multipronged changes to education and training and can lead to innovative research, scholarship, interventions, and policies.

However, despite this significant, but underrealized, promise of complex systems science, many barriers have slowed down its integration into population health science. One of the principal barriers has been the haphazard knowledge base from which academics, researchers, students, policymakers, and practitioners draw. Such knowledge typically either takes the form of journal articles disseminated by a plethora of scientific journals in population health, the broader health sciences (e.g., medicine), or health-related disciplines (e.g., psychology); is contained within specialized and usually nonhealth-related books and journals; or can be found in introductory, nonsystematic books on systems science and population health. As a result, growing numbers of academics, who are genuinely interested in incorporating complex systems science into their own population health research, instruction, and student mentoring; graduate students; and public and population health and healthcare professionals and policymakers are hard-pressed to identify a starting point. This frustration then dampens interest and stagnates the enormous potential of the field, leading to largely inconsequential knowledge. Ultimately, this void diminishes potential for innovative education in population health science, which, in turn, has adverse ramifications for the next generation of academics, students, researchers, and professionals, along with the direction and outcomes of their research, scholarship, public and population health policy, and, above all, population health at large. Notwithstanding this gap in the systematic knowledge base, funding agencies and policy think tanks around the world are overall steadfast in their pursuit of innovations in population health based on the advantages of complex systems science. As more universities increasingly offer relevant courses, a clear need exists for a comprehensive and systematic book on the intersection of complex systems science and population health science that is accessible to diverse audiences.

This volume seeks to fulfill this growing need in the health and social sciences by offering the knowledge base necessary to introduce a new population health science grounded in complex systems science. As such, this will be the first English-language, comprehensive book in population health science that meaningfully integrates complex systems science theory, methodology, diverse types of modeling, computational simulation, the physical and natural sciences, and real-world applications, while incorporating current population health theoretical, methodological, and analytical perspectives.

1.3.2. Book Organization and Themes

Within these scientific and applied frameworks, the 20 chapters of the book are divided into five parts along lines of theory, research design, methodology, and analytical techniques, bridging the gap between complex systems science and population health science. In this way, we intend to emphasize the importance of a unifying theory, methodology, and analytical approaches that organically blend the old, the current, and the new in population health science for the purpose of moving the field forward and eventually improving the health of all people as equitably and efficiently as possible.

Part I: Population Health Science in a Complex World begins with the prologue to describe the impetus of the book and is followed by this chapter (Chapter 1), which both contextualize the volume and describe its organization. It begins by delving into the limitations of the prevailing paradigm in population health science and the need for a transition from a typically risk factor–based science to a science that recognizes the whole, as well as the relationships between the parts, of pressing population health problems. Next, it walks readers through distinctions between public and population health on the one hand and key concepts of complexity on the other, while offering a shared understanding of population health science and complex systems science.

Part II: Complex Systems and Theory in Population Health Science introduces readers to the theoretical foundations of complex systems science with applications in population health science. Foundational concepts of complex systems such as self-organization and emergence; network structure, six degrees of separation, and scale-free, random, and small-world networks; phase transitions, tipping points, and resilience; and complex adaptive systems of systems and other complex system properties such as heterogeneity, nonlinearity, feedbacks, self-organized criticality, power laws, and path dependence are described in the context of population health. In conclusion, Chapters 2 through 6 delve into whether and, if so, how complex systems science can transform population health theory.

Part III: Complex Systems and Methodology in Population Health Science presents readers with the uniquely different ways in which empirical research in population health grounded in complex systems science can be designed and conducted in Chapters 7 through 10. It draws attention to the importance of model thinking and to the ways a multimodel-centric population health science can help make sense of perplexing problems. It explains how model thinking and formal modeling can improve our frequently inaccurate mental models in population health research by concurrently examining above- and below-the-surface causal forces. Next, it delves into the importance of community and stakeholder involvement in deconstructing population health problems and building models to make sense of persisting challenges. Last, it draws attention to the importance of recognizing and providing appropriate meaning to the existence of both normal and nonnormal distributions in population health research and taking care in how we describe or more simply represent outcomes shaped by complex systems.

Part IV: Complex Systems and Analytical Techniques in Population Health Science walks readers through overviews and case studies of key complex systems science–grounded analytical methods. There is an extensive representation of model-centered analytical techniques ranging from the physical and mathematical to the computational, network, and data sciences. Chapters 11 through 18 cover mathematical modeling, system dynamics, agent-based and hybrid simulation modeling, and model validation and offer computational modeling case studies for health policy analysis. In sum, while this section delves into specific applications, these chapters also emphasize the necessity of an organic reconciliation of mathematical, physical, statistical, computational, qualitative, and data sciences, both demonstrated and emerging, in population health science.

Finally, in Part V: Toward a New Population Health Science, we offer readers a glimpse of our vision for a new population health science, as the organic outcome of the nexus of the past, present, and evolving scientific perspectives and advances from population health science and complex systems science. Within a globalized, hyperinteractive world, Chapters 19 and 20 describe how we can transition toward a new population health science grounded in the frontier of science to better understand, anticipate, curtail, and manage major population health challenges of our time by harnessing their complexity.

1.3.3. How This Book Differs From Others

This book is intended to serve as a *programmatic primer* for a broad spectrum of stakeholders—from university professors and graduate students to an array of health and policy scientists, researchers, policymakers, health planners, local and state governmental public health workforce, and practitioners representing diverse academic and applied domains. On the academic side, these individuals come mainly from public health, population health science, and their many subdisciplines (e.g., epidemiology, occupational health, and safety), health services, healthcare management and administration, nursing, and allied health.

Furthermore, individuals from those social and behavioral sciences with a vested interest in health, such as sociology; clinical, community, health, industrial/organizational, and social psychology; anthropology; geography; management; and organizational behavior, among others, would be prospective readers of this volume. On the applied side, the audience of this book includes various public health departments, federal agencies, and nonprofit organizations focusing on health, health program evaluators, and health and safety units from corporate and other private organizations.

Because of its strong *instructional mission*, this book includes introductory materials, take-home messages, and resources for further reading for Parts II, III, and IV, as well as case studies throughout the volume and a concise glossary of terms at the conclusion, inviting newcomers to immerse themselves in this new, holistic direction of population health science. In addition to filling a vast void in population health literature and academic curricula, this book promises to open new paths in scientific thinking that are grounded in integrated new concepts and theories, epistemology, and methodology in population health science. These new paths hold promise to define research conceptualizations, designs, operations, analyses, policies, and interventions in the years to come. This book also hopes to provoke long-overdue discourse on the need for updated new curricula in population health science.

1.4. THE FUTURE OF POPULATION HEALTH SCIENCE

Amid tremendous cultural, demographic, socioeconomic, and political shifts in a hyperinteractive and globalized world, the scientific frontier is also rapidly evolving. The time is ripe and population health science seems to be ready to accelerate this more than two-decade-old epistemological transition. The emerging, organic intersection of complex systems science and population health science has the potential to rejuvenate population health science at the edge of the scientific frontier, which can only strengthen the ongoing quest for population health equity by curtailing structural and systemic socioeconomic disparities.

REFERENCES

1. Henrickson, L. and B. McKelvey (2002). Foundations of new social science: Institutional legitimacy from philosophy, complexity science, postmodernism, and agent-based modeling. *PNAS*, 99, 7288–7297.
2. McMichael, A.J. (1999). Prisoners of the proximate: Loosening the constraints on epidemiology in an age of change. *American Journal of Epidemiology*, 149, 887–897.
3. Glass, T.A., S.N. Goodman, M.A. Hernán, and J.M. Samet (2013). Causal inference in public health. *Annual Review of Public Health*, 34, 61–75.
4. Cockcroft, A. (2017). Randomized controlled trials and changing public health practice. *BMC Public Health*, 17(Suppl 1), 409. doi:10.1186/s12889-017-4287-7
5. Fielding, J.E. (1999). Public health in the twentieth century: Advances and challenges. *Annual Review of Public Health*, 20, xiii–xxx.

6. Sepulveda, J. and C. Murray (2014). The state of global health in 2014. *Science*, 345, 1275–1278.
7. Miller, J.H. and S.E. Page (2007). *Complex Adaptive Systems*. Princeton University Press.
8. El-Sayed, A.M. and S. Galea (eds.) (2017). *Systems Science and Population Health*. Oxford University Press.
9. Sterman, J.D. (2006). Learning from evidence in a complex world. *American Journal of Public Health*, 96, 505–514.
10. Sterman J.D. (2000). *Business Dynamics*. Irwin/McGraw-Hill.
11. Fong, I.W. and K. Drlica (eds.) (2003). *Reemergence of Established Pathogens in the 21st Century*. Kluwer/Plenum.
12. National Academies of Sciences, Engineering, and Medicine (2017). *Communities in Action: Pathways to Health Equity*. The National Academy Press.
13. Braveman, P.A., C. Cubbin, S. Egerter, D.R. Williams, and E. Pamuk (2010). Socioeconomic disparities in health in the U.S. What the patterns tell us. *American Journal of Public Health*, 100(Suppl 1), S186–S96.
14. Keyes, K. and S. Galea (2017). The limits of risk factors revisited: Is it time for a causal architecture approach? *Epidemiology*, 28, 1–5.
15. Kuller, L.H. (2013). Point: Is there a future for innovative epidemiology? *American Journal of Epidemiology*, 177, 279–280.
16. Ness, R.B., E.B. Andrews, J.A. Gaudino, et al. (2009). The future of epidemiology. *Academic Medicine*, 84, 1631–1637.
17. Gell-Mann, M. (1997). The Primer Project. International Society for the Systems Sciences seminar, October 12—November 10.
18. Salway, S. and J. Green (2017). Towards a critical complex systems approach to public health. *Critical Public Health*, 27, 523–524.
19. Rockhill, B. (2005). Theorizing about causes at the individual level while estimating effects at the population level: Implications for prevention. *Epidemiology*, 16, 124–129.
20. Abbott, A. (1988). Transcending general reality. *Sociological Theory*, 6, 169–186.
21. Centers for Disease Control and Prevention (2019). What is public health? Retrieved from https://www.cdcfoundation.org/what-public-health, June 25.
22. Kindig, D. and G. Stoddart (2003). What is population health? *American Journal of Public Health*, 93, 380–383.
23. Marmot, M. and R. Wilkinson (eds.) 2006. *Social Determinants of Health*. Oxford University Press.
24. Evans, R, M. Barer, and T. Marmor (1994). *Why Are Some People Healthy and Others Not? The Determinants of Health of Populations*. Aldine de Gruyter.
25. Young, T.K. (1998). *Population Health: Concepts and Methods*. Oxford University Press.
26. Interdisciplinary Association of Population Health Science (2019). What is population health? Retrieved from https://iaphs.org/what-is-population-health/, June 22.
27. Improving Population Health (2019). Population health basics. Retrieved from https://www.improvingpopulationhealth.org, June 28.
28. Keyes, K. and S. Galea (2016). *Population Health Science*. Oxford University Press.
29. Venter, J.C., M.D. Adams, E.W. Myers, et al. (2001). The sequence of the human genome. *Science*, 291, 1304–1351.

30. Michor, F., J. Liphardt, M. Ferrari, and J. Widom (2011). What does physics have to do with cancer? *Nature Reviews Cancer*, 11, 657–670.

31. Borsboom, D., A.O.J. Cramer, and A. Kalis (2019). Brain disorders? Not really: Why network structures block reductionism in psychopathology research. *Behavioral and Brain Sciences*, 42, e2. doi:10.1017/S0140525X17002266

PART II

Complex Systems and Theory in Population Health Science

Introductory Material: Preview and Objectives

PREVIEW

As stated in Chapter 1, because population health challenges operate as complex systems, and/or are determined by other complex systems, relevant theory, research designs, and analytical methods must be brought to bear. Part II, which spans across Chapters 2 through 6, delves into the first of these three domains by introducing readers to the theoretical foundations of complex systems science. These theoretical foundations are accompanied by applied examples from population health.

Chapter 2 provides the foundational concepts, properties, and theoretical frameworks that complex systems science is designed to understand and impact. Using cardiometabolic disease as an example of a pressing population health challenge, these frameworks are defined, described, and demonstrated in the context of cardiometabolic disease. The following concepts are defined and illustrated: systems, complexity, dynamic complexity, and complex systems; stable states, resilience, and critical transitions; nonlinearities; feedback loops; random and scale-free networks; and adaptation, self-organization, and emergence.

Chapters 3 through 5 build upon the foundational concepts laid out in Chapter 2. Moving from a simple notion of complex systems, Chapter 3 describes "complex adaptive systems of systems" (CASoS)—collections of connected complex systems. This chapter advocates for considering population health outcomes and disparities as stemming from CASoS and introduces a framework for feasibly understanding CASoS in the context of population health that iterates between broad system conceptualization, narrowing focus to each subsystem/constituent part (itself as a system), and deliberate aggregation—putting the pieces back together to understand how and why the CASoS behaves.

Chapter 4 expands on foundational network theories in the context of population health. The authors begin by introducing three key assumptions that underlie network science in population health: First, individuals (whether people or some other entity) constantly interact with each other and their environments in a way that is not random; second, interactions at multiple levels—from the cellular to the environmental—shape the experiences of individuals and affect population health; and third, these interactions can be represented as a set of networks through which diverse health-relevant outcomes such as infection, beliefs, and behaviors spread. This chapter focuses on the complex relationship between human social networks and behavioral patterns, which is often reciprocal, and how this relationship impacts population health outcomes.

Chapter 5 describes the promise of applying critical transitions, tipping points, and resilience in prognosis and treatment in health care and clinical psychology. First, the urgent need for complex systems theories in the study of disease is provided. Next, the specific and varied roles of complex systems theories and analytical methods are discussed, with a specific focus on resilience and tipping points in clinical practice. This is followed by a description of how the complexity and resilience of physiological and psychological systems can be studied. Finally, future applications of complex systems science in patient care and medical science are prognosticated.

Finally, Chapter 6 looks at the "big picture" of complex systems theory in population health research and practice by addressing two key questions. First, does current population health theory need revolutionizing? And, if so, can complex systems science spark that needed revolution? The author first defines what "theorizing" itself is and its inherent difficulties. This leads to the exploration of the aforementioned questions, and three specific ways that complex systems science may affect theory building and testing are then considered. The chapter concludes with potential implications of a "theory revolution" in population health science.

OBJECTIVES

The objectives of Part II are as follows:

1. Provide an overview of the foundational concepts, principles, and theories of the study of complex systems and complex adaptive systems of systems.
2. Describe complex adaptive systems in population health and advocate for the value of complex adaptive systems frameworks in understanding and advancing population health outcomes.
3. Explicate network science in population health by introducing traditional network analysis and exploring examples of interactions between macro-level networks, including connectionist and relational models.
4. Propose future directions for network analysis in population health research.
5. Explain how critical transitions, related tipping points, and resilience can be monitored in human physiological and psychological processes.
6. Introduce valid predictors of proximity to tipping points in population health (with examples from diseases such as depression, heart failure, and heart syncope).
7. Define theory and the practice of theory building, and outline the difficulties found in current population health theorizing.
8. Characterize the mechanisms through which complex systems science can influence, change, and advance current theorizing efforts in population health science.
9. Consider the implications of adopting complex systems science frameworks to theorizing for practice, policy development, and training of the future public health workforce.

Complex Systems in a Nutshell

Foundational Concepts for Population Health

MEGAN S. PATTERSON, MICHAEL K. LEMKE, AND
JORDAN NELON

2.1. INTRODUCTION

"It's complicated."

When someone asks you about a new romantic relationship, what it is like to
have a newborn, how the social dynamics are at work, politics, and just about any
other reality, your answer can probably be simplified and summed into the phrase,
"It's complicated." If you live, work, speak, interact, or socialize with other people,
chances are you have heard this phrase. It is a simple way of summarizing a situation that likely has many moving parts, including details about what happened
in the past, and might be hard to explain. While most people use this phrase in
common conversation, it does unveil a generally common understanding: Reality
is far from simple.

If reality is far from simple, then how do we understand it? This is the realm
where complex systems science lies.

This chapter will highlight what complex systems science is, why it interests us,
and how it can be used to understand reality. We will discuss how complex issues
often consist of networks of factors that interact to produce bottom–up emergent
phenomena. We will also discuss common properties across complex systems,
using cardiometabolic disease (and associated comorbidities) as a thematic population health example.

Megan S. Patterson, Michael K. Lemke, and Jordan Nelon, *Complex Systems in a Nutshell* In: *Complex Systems and
Population Health*. Edited by: Yorghos Apostolopoulos, Kristen Hassmiller Lich, and Michael Kenneth Lemke, Oxford University
Press (2020). © Oxford University Press. DOI: 10.1093/oso/9780190880743.003.0002

2.1.1. Complexity: What It Is and Why It Matters

To understand and appreciate complexity for what it is, it is helpful to contrast it with what it is not. Most scientific inquiry derives from a framework called *reductionism*.[1] Reductionism requires taking something complicated and breaking it down into its component parts, studying those parts in isolation, and aggregating what is learned to understand the whole.

The dominance of reductionist inquiry is seen throughout population health science. For example, the bulk of research and action related to *cardiometabolic disease*—a constellation of interlinked cardiovascular and metabolic diseases—bears many hallmarks of reductionism. Based on central tenets of analytical decomposition and linear thinking, the sole reliance on reductionist perspectives in academic and applied cardiometabolic work has led to theoretical explanations that are rooted in spatiotemporally proximal, rather than distal, cause–effect relationships. Theory is informed by reductionist-grounded methodology rooted in risk-factor epidemiology and analytical approaches grounded in linear statistical modeling, which together explore the "whole" (i.e., cardiometabolic disease) by reducing it into component parts and investigating those component parts independently to tease apart cause–effect relationships. However, the complex systems concepts that will be highlighted in this chapter define cardiometabolic disease and cannot be fully understood using such reductionism-grounded approaches, nor are they adequately captured in prevailing reductionism-based theory. More broadly, the dominance of reductionist perspectives in cardiometabolic disease research and action (and, indeed, throughout population health science) is increasingly confronted by a growing body of complex systems-science–grounded empirical work, of which a handful of examples will be described in the following discussion.

2.1.2. Complicated vs. Complex Systems

A *system* is an array of interconnected elements, bounded in space and time, that form a collective whole.[2] There are innumerable systems, and systems can be described in any number of ways, including whether they are *complicated* or *complex*. There is a difference between complicated and complex systems. Consider a jigsaw puzzle. Picture a 20-inch by 24-inch puzzle that is a picture of a cityscape. If our puzzle consisted of eight large pieces that all fit together, we might consider it a simple puzzle. However, if the same cityscape puzzle was made of 400 pieces, it would be more complicated. Or, if the puzzle was made up of 800 pieces, it would be more complicated still. By having more pieces, and dividing the whole picture into more and more individual parts, the puzzle is more complicated, and the final picture is harder to understand by looking at the individual parts—each of which must be studied for the whole to be reconstructed. Think about it—if you chose one puzzle piece at random from the 800-piece box, it is unlikely you would know what the whole picture would look like after all 800 pieces are assembled.

That said, whether there are 8, 400, or 800 pieces, the puzzle is only complicated, and not complex.

Why is the puzzle only a complicated system? First, it is important to realize that no matter the number of individual pieces (8, 400, 800), they never interact in a way that changes the outcome. For instance, if you remove one piece of the puzzle, you are left with the same overall picture, minus the puzzle-piece–sized hole in the finished product. This suggests that each puzzle piece makes independent contributions to the whole and does not impact the contribution of the rest of the pieces. Removing a piece of the puzzle does not instigate change or require the remaining pieces to adapt to the loss—they maintain their original purpose. Contrarily, in a complex system, removing (or adding) a single element alters system behavior far beyond what any individual element brings.

Let's consider two examples of complex systems that meet this definition. One example is a watch. If you wanted to learn about how to fix your grandfather's watch, it would help to reduce it into component parts and figure out how each part functions. But the interactions matter, too. One watch part triggers action in another part—and the sum of all the parts emerges into a functioning time-telling device. Unlike with the jigsaw puzzle, where you are likely to get a good sense of the whole with a few missing pieces, a watch is unlikely to function if any of its components are missing or malfunctioning. And new components, like a ball bearing, can wreak havoc on the watch's function.

Another example of a complex system is a family. We have more options for how to bound (draw the boundary around one's definition of) a family—it could be bounded by a house, blood/genetics, or love—and the boundary would likely vary based on culture/context. What are the component parts of a family? The answer likely depends on what you are trying to understand. With the watch, the function is clear: to tell time. With a family, it might be child rearing, social and economic support/stability, or other such outcomes that families typically support. Let's consider families that have a primary function of supporting the upbringing of healthy children. What are the component parts of such families? Perhaps children, parents, the house, family rules/values, financial resources, health insurance (or lack thereof), local educational resources, and more. These components interact, affecting child health over time. This family system is complex because the whole is greater than the sum of the parts. If a part is removed (e.g., a parent dies), the system adjusts. Interactions between the parts matter, as families evolve, learn, and adapt.

While we are making a clear distinction between complicated and complex, this distinction is not always so clear in practice. For example, Peter Senge defines *detail complexity* as a system in which outcomes arise from a large number of parts (e.g., components, variables).[3] This is the jigsaw puzzle with many pieces. As previously described, without the interaction of component parts, a system is not complex at all, but rather *complicated*.[1,4]

Both complicated and complex systems can have a multitude of parts that make it difficult to understand, but the primary difference lies in whether the system's overall, collective function is dependent on the interactions of elements within the system. In other words, it is the interactions and adaptation of various components of the system, and not just the additive characteristics of those components, that make a system complex. *Organized complexity*,[5] as defined by Warren Weaver, refers to systems with interdependencies between variables. Removing a single element from a complex system would alter the system altogether based on the interactions and connections between component parts. The watch is an example of organized complexity. In the same vein but with more emphasis on dynamics, *dynamic complexity* is defined as a characteristic of a system where the temporal interactions and interdependencies among elements in the system, rather than the large number and characteristics of elements that constitute the system, are most important in determining system structure and behavior, and the system changes over time. An example of a dynamically complex system is a family, adapting in response to changes. In the presence of dynamic complexity, cause and effect relationships are unclear and system behavior is often counterintuitive.[6]

In sum, most population health problems feature dynamic and/or organized complexity, even though they are most commonly studied using a complicated/ detail complexity framework. In much of the scientific work on cardiometabolic disease and other complex population health challenges, we dismiss the interdependence of variables and ignore or oversimplify dynamics, and instead we treat problems like jigsaw puzzles. However, to best model reality and find leverage points for population-level change, we must understand cardiometabolic disease (and other population health problems) as embedded in, shaped by, or consisting of *complex systems*, which are characterized by many parts that interact with one another across multiple scales to generate overall system behavior. The emergent behaviors that occur as a result of interactions and relationships between and among system parts over time are usually undetectable when only considering component parts one at a time. However, there are defining characteristics and properties that are common to most complex systems that help make them more easily understood.

2.2. CHARACTERISTICS, PROPERTIES, AND THEORIES OF COMPLEX SYSTEMS

To understand complex systems and how they shape cardiometabolic disease and other population health challenges, it is necessary to grasp their key characteristics, properties, and the theories that are central to the study of such systems. In this section we will introduce some of these characteristics, properties, and theories, many of which will be expounded on further in subsequent chapters in this book. Throughout this chapter, we will provide existing complex systems science work in the realm of cardiometabolic disease to illustrate and ground these concepts.

2.2.1. Properties Related to the Behavior of Complex Systems

The behaviors of complex systems are marked by distinct and interlinked properties and characteristics. Complex systems typically operate within one or more *stable states* (also described as *steady states* or *equilibria* [resting points]). Stable states are defined by relative constancy of *state variables*—variables that capture the state of the system—over time (e.g., presence/absence of disease in an individual or the number of people with/without a disease in a population; levels of demand and supply; who provides income in a household). The current stable state of a complex system is shaped by several forces, including historical forces that have shaped the system over time; in other words, complex systems have "memory," and because of this, current and future system states are informed by and dependent on the sequence of states preceding them.[7] These historical forces lead the system to go toward a specific steady state (for example whether a disease outbreak dies out, becomes endemic—and at what level, or has a more complex trajectory such as oscillation). *Path dependence* refers to situations when small historical events can become durable effects within the greater system, and once on this "path," it can be difficult, if not impossible, to switch to a new "path".[8,9] For example, in their review of genetic pathways to cardiovascular disease outcomes and risk factors, Rankinen, Trumo, and colleagues[10] found that abdominal obesity, insulin resistance, cholesterol, and hypertension have an estimated heritability between 40% and 90%, depending on the risk factor. Thus, the constellation of factors that predicate cardiometabolic syndrome are likely path dependent on genetic code.

Theoretically, there are multiple or even infinite stable states that a complex system may operate in, and external perturbations to the system may "push" a complex system into a new stable state. Complex systems can be characterized by their *resilience* to such perturbations, which describes to what degree complex systems can recover from destabilizing forces. To put this another way, resilience captures how strong of a "push" is needed for a system to shift into an alternate stable state. State transitions are known as *critical transitions*, or *tipping points*, which represent instances where a complex system loses its resilience to perturbations and shifts into a new stable state. Originating in the field of epidemiology, tipping points were identified as the "turning point" within disease spread, when the disease is no longer controllable, and will undoubtedly spread more widely.[11] A tipping point is often considered a critical point, or threshold, within a system where a small change yields additional and synergistic consequences.[11] Given the importance of critical transitions/tipping points in complex systems and their behaviors, an array of *early warning signals* have been identified that allow researchers to evaluate the resilience of a system and its relative likelihood of transitioning into a new stable state.[12,21] Several tipping points have been identified in cardiometabolic disease development; for example, tipping points flag the transition from a predisease stable state to a disease stable state for both type 1 and type 2 subtypes of diabetes; further, biomarkers serving as "warning signals" for diabetes progression and other population health outcomes have been discovered.[12]

Critical transitions and tipping points have conceptually been of great interest to public health professionals, as they present an important place for intervention. Across the array of population health systems, critical transitions may be undesirable, such as the aforementioned tipping points between predisease to disease stable states in type 1 diabetes. Alternately, a theoretical critical transition to a new steady state may be desirable in certain population health contexts; for example, the current healthcare system in the United States chronically underserves individuals of lower socioeconomic status, and a critical transition to a more equitable stable state in this system is advocated for by many researchers, activists, and policymakers. When viewed through this new lens, population health protection and promotion efforts can be reconceptualized across three contingencies, given the specific context of a given population health problem: (1) a critical transition is impending or already underway and cannot be prevented, but action can be undertaken to mitigate its negative effects; (2) an undesirable critical transition is impending, and we can take action to prevent it from taking place; and (3) a desirable critical transition is possible, and we can take action to encourage it and control its shift into a new desirable stable state.[13]

2.2.2. Complex System Properties Related to the Interaction and Sequence of System Factors

The interrelationships and interdependencies among system elements often give rise to *nonlinear* properties in complex systems. A linear relationship is one that describes a proportional cause and effect relationship, whereas nonlinearity is the product of multiple interacting parts that leads to the whole (i.e., system behavior) being more—or less—than the sum of its individual parts. In other words, in the presence of nonlinearity, cause and effect relationships are nonproportional. In the context of cardiometabolic disease, numerous factors have been established as important determinants in disease development, including nutrition,[14] physical activity and sedentary behaviors,[15,10] drug/alcohol use,[16,17,11,12] genetics,[18,13] socioeconomic status,[19] geographic location,[20] and many others. Multivariate/multivariable statistical risk models have been successfully developed to ascertain cardiometabolic disease risk using these factors, such as the Framingham risk score. However, these models cannot predict cardiometabolic disease development with as much precision for all subpopulations; for example, in a study of the ability of the Framingham risk score to estimate 10-year risk of coronary heart disease, it was found that, among subjects with low short-term but high lifetime coronary heart disease risk, the measure may not be reliable.[21] Although there may be many reasons for this finding, one may be that the interactions among key coronary heart disease factors nonlinearly influence disease progression, leading to decreased reliability of this measure in subjects over time.

Many complex systems are dynamic.[1,22] This just means that neither the component parts of the system or the outcomes in a system are fixed—they change over time. Change can be driven by many system characteristics and properties, especially the interactions and interdependencies among system elements, and change may occur at different time scales—sometimes quickly, sometimes slowly. System dynamics may also be driven by the presence and arrangement of variables within *feedback loops*.[2,22] A feedback loop exists when two or more variables mutually influence each other over time (e.g., a change in X triggers a change in Y, which triggers further change in X over time). Feedback loops can be positive or negative based on whether the feedback is a mechanism for maintaining stability in a system (negative) or triggering exponential change (positive). Negative feedback loops are also called balancing loops because they work to maintain stability by counteracting changes that could alter the system. Examples of negative feedback loops include temperature regulation, balance, or maintaining blood pressure in the body. A positive feedback loop is also called a reinforcing loop because it amplifies changes within a system, and as a result the system moves away from its current state.

Diabetes as a disease is an example of a "broken" negative (balancing) feedback loop that is incapable of restoring equilibrium in the body's metabolic system.[23,24] In a person without diabetes, blood sugar levels are controlled by insulin. When a nondiabetic person eats a meal, blood glucose levels rise, and as a result, insulin is secreted into the bloodstream. Insulin secretion is the result of a negative feedback loop that triggers the body to regulate levels of blood sugar when they rise after meals. When someone has diabetes, either their pancreas is incapable of making enough insulin to regulate blood sugar levels, or their cells stop responding to insulin altogether (or both). Either way, the body is incapable of responding when a diabetic's blood sugar gets too high, which impedes the body's ability to regulate blood sugar. More broadly, numerous feedback loops have been systematically identified, mapped, and investigated in several areas of cardiometabolic disease, including cardiovascular disease,[25] diabetes,[26] obesity, and cardiometabolic disease-related syndemic afflictions.[27,28]

Stable states, path dependence, resilience, critical transitions/tipping points, and feedback loops are properties that demonstrate how the arrangement of system factors and their interaction with one another shape the behaviors exhibited by complex systems. In addition to these properties, a system's collective behavior and robustness is also influenced by the overall structure of the system. Specifically, how the entire system is structured and patterned will largely determine outcomes. Just as the interconnected factors shape system outcomes, so do interconnected individuals in a social or other relational network. In the next section, we will introduce two common system-wide structures: random networks and scale-free networks. Characterizing system structure within a network can help us identify meaningful network properties that affect system behavior over time.

2.2.3. Complex Systems Properties Related to Overall Network Structure

Because they are defined as an interconnected set of elements, complex systems are often represented as networks.[29] Or, networks (e.g., friendship or sexual networks) might be an important component of a broader system. A *network* is a collection of elements (most often called nodes or components), connected by edges or links.[29,30] Components can be people, organizations, constructs, communities, molecules, and endless other things that make up the various parts of a system. Edges represent the interactions and connections between component parts. For example, using data from more than 300 million medical records, researchers[31] demonstrated variances in illness diagnosis and progression by constructing a network where components were comorbidities, and links indicated whether the two comorbidities were correlated. In this case, for example, hypertension was strongly correlated with diabetes mellitus and hyperosmolality; moderately correlated with urinary tract infection, acute cerebrovascular disease, headaches, cognitive deficits, congestive heart failure, and coma (among others); and slightly connected to hypertrophy of the prostate and malignant hypertensive heart disease. Based on the comorbidity network, researchers were able to ascertain risk profiles specific to gender and race/ethnicity.

Random networks imply that the likelihood of two parts of the system being connected is completely random. Random networks have a scale, meaning there is a set probability that any two nodes will create connections within a network.[29] Because random networks are scaled, individual component parts of the system have comparable degrees (the number of connections any factor of the system has to others), and the average degree serves as the scale for the network.[7,29] If links are created at random (independent and identically distributed), degree remains fairly homogenous across the network, and those component parts that have higher (or lower) than average degree are due to chance. Additionally, if connections are created at random, the network is not structured hierarchically— there are not a select few factors that serve as the connection point for the rest of the network. Thus, the average path length (the distance between two parts of the system) tends to be higher in random networks and traveling through the network would require passing through many component parts. However, most systems that have to do with humans are not random. Indeed, most connections are built around and branch off important or powerful parts of the system, and as a result are structured as scale-free networks.

Scale-free networks are more hierarchical in structure than random networks and follow what are called *power laws*. A power law describes a variable whose distribution is characterized by an extreme variation between two variables, where a small change in one variable can lead to a large change in another.[32] This translates into long and fat tails on a distribution curve. One of the most famous power laws coined by Vilfredo Pareto is the 80/20 rule. The 80/20 rule was originally computed to explain wealth distribution in Italy. The tail on the income distribution was so long/fat that roughly 20% of the population earned 80% of the money.

This law has since been demonstrated across many domains, including within sexual relationship networks, where a small number of individuals have extremely large numbers of sexual partners. Regarding cardiometabolic disease, the fat tail is also important; the few people receiving 20% of therapeutic strategies are responsible for 80% of health gains (e.g., lower blood pressure or cholesterol).[33] The premise of power laws is that a select few high-degree parts of the system have great impact on the entire system—in terms of spreading sexually transmitted diseases or realizing health benefits from screening and treatment.

Based on their structure, scale-free networks create what are called *small world networks*. With the presence of major "hubs," the average path length between two factors drastically reduces by providing shortcuts to various parts of the system. You may have heard of the "six degrees of separation" phenomenon. Despite having over 7.5 billion inhabitants on Earth, choose any two people and you will find an average path length of six between them, meaning they can be connected through a chain including five other social contacts. In other words, while most of the population is not connected to one another, we are all linked through strings of mutual connections. Having highly central and connected people serves to connect everyone together in a seemingly smaller world, despite billions of people in existence.

Ultimately, the network structure of a system can reveal a lot about overall behavior and how a system responds to change. When considering cardiometabolic disease, whether we are "zooming in" on one aspect (e.g., diabetes, social determinants of health, genetics, etc.) or "zooming out" to understand the entire system of comorbidities that translate to cardiometabolic disease, the underlying commonality is that how various factors are structured, and how they interact with one another, have large implications on population health outcomes.

2.2.4. Emergence

A common phrase describing complex systems is "the whole is more than the sum of its parts."[2p11] This phrase is analogous to *emergence*, which is the process by which the interactions among micro-level entities, and the interactions between micro-level entities and their environments, produce macro-level patterns that are novel and separate from what could have been created by summing each micro-level entity. A growing number of cardiometabolic disease domains have been described as consisting of emergent phenomena, and this has been facilitated by the proliferation of agent-based modeling, which has become an instrumental methodology for the study of emergent phenomena in complex systems. For example, researchers have employed agent-based modeling to study emergence (and other characteristics and properties of complex systems) within the obesity epidemic to better understand how various social and environmental influences shape population-level obesity trajectories.[27,34,35]

Those local (micro-level) behaviors that generate emergent patterns in complex systems are carried out by individuals that are often referred to as *agents*. Agents are goal-seeking, and they exhibit *adaptation* (e.g., adaptive behaviors) as they interact with other agents and their environments in their pursuit of their goals. Further, agents are not omniscient nor omnipotent; instead, they pursue their goals based on proximal interactions and information and local (micro-level) constraints and rules. As a result, complex systems do not have a central controller or coordinator. This is called *self-organization*, or the creation of a global-level coordination out of local-level interactions. Because each entity is limited to their own individual contexts, they are blind to the big picture, and are operating completely independent from a central controller or coordinator.[1,4,36] Consider our diabetes example from before. We have sensors in our bodies that simply evaluate whether there is too much glucose in our blood, with a goal of alerting the body when blood sugar levels are abnormal. Therefore, when the glucose is in a normal range, the body is at equilibrium and the sensors only monitor for changes. However, when glucose is too high, these sensors must signal the pancreas to release insulin, meeting their goal of alerting the body to abnormal blood sugar levels. There is no central controller instructing the sensor to alarm the pancreas of high glucose levels, but the independent, goal-seeking behaviors are interacting to create systemic change. The pancreas works independently of the digestive system, not monitoring when the body is consuming food or what is being eaten, but instead focuses innately on blood sugar levels. In this case, one component part of the system (the sensor) is independently trying to meet its goals, but by interacting with the pancreas based on those goals, a cascade of interactions can result in emergent phenomena, such as diabetes. When taken in isolation, these individual goal-seeking agents would be relatively simple. However, it is the collection of interactions among these goal-seeking individuals that result in adaptive, system-wide behavior.

An example of emergence from the cardiometabolic disease literature is centered on how social norms impact eating behaviors and obesity among school children.[37] By simulating micro-level agent behaviors (connections with other students; understanding of the social average body mass index; fruit and vegetable consumption), population health scientists configured how those micro-level behaviors translate to system-wide changes and outcomes of childhood obesity. Each agent in the system evaluated their status within their environment and adjusted to engage in socially acceptable behaviors according to what they believed was the social average body mass index. In this case, as agents interacted with one another, their perceptions of social norms evolved, and their fruit and vegetable consumption adapted accordingly. Their understanding of social norms changed as their relationships changed, and their recognition of social norms continually informed their own decisions and goals, which had a system-wide effect when interactions across all agents are accounted for within the system. Wang and colleagues concluded that high obesity prevalence will result in increases in children's body mass index because the socially acceptable body mass index will continue to rise, and behavioral patterns such as fruit and vegetable consumption will adjust to "fit" the socially acceptable body mass index.[37]

2.3. CONCLUSION

In 1972, physicist Philip W. Anderson coined the phrase, "More is different," arguing that breaking a system down into more and more component parts does not mean we understand it more fully; in fact, it is quite the opposite. With each component part, there are more interactions and variations in outcomes that are impossible to predict by simplifying, or understanding, the individual parts.[38] In this chapter, we illustrated that cardiometabolic disease is indeed a complex system. Based on properties such as stable states, path dependence, and nonlinearity, we can conclude that cardiometabolic disease incorporates numerous interacting component parts that produce a variety of population health outcomes (i.e., heart disease, stroke). Most research uses a reductionist approach to understand cardiometabolic disease by breaking it down into individual, additive factors, however, based on the "more is different" observation, we can assume that these factors do not "add up" to cardiometabolic disease but interact in a way that produces emergent phenomena unlikely detected from using a reductionist perspective.

Embracing key problems in population health as dynamically complex systems allows us to appreciate how "more is different" and integrate its broader meaning into population health research and action. Further, conceptualizing the various facets of population health—including cardiometabolic disease—through a complex systems lens requires an understanding of the key characteristics, properties, and theories that shape the underlying networks and network properties, interactions, and nonlinearities that give rise to emergent properties and broader system-wide behaviors. Many of these same characteristics, properties, and theories will be revisited and expounded upon throughout this book to cement the power of complex systems science in transforming population health research and action.

REFERENCES

1. Mitchell M. *Complexity: A Guided Tour*. Oxford, NY: Oxford University Press; 2009.
2. Meadows DH. *Thinking in Systems: A Primer*. White River Junction, VT: Chelsea Green Publishing; 2008.
3. Senge P. *The Fifth Discipline: The Art & Practice of The Learning Organization*. New York, NY: Doubleday; 1990. https://www.amazon.com/Fifth-Discipline-Practice-Learning-Organization/dp/0385517254. Accessed April 29, 2019.
4. Miller JH, Page SE. *Complex Adaptive Systems: An Introduction to Computational Models of Social Life*. Princeton, NJ: Princeton University Press; 2007. https://press.princeton.edu/titles/8429.html. Accessed April 29, 2019.
5. Weaver W. Science and complexity. *Am Sci*. 1948;36(4):536–544.
6. Newman LL. Human–Environment Interactions, Complex Systems Approaches for Dynamic Sustainable Development. In: Meyers RA, ed. *Encyclopedia of Complexity and Systems Science*. New York, NY: Springer New York; 2009:4631–4643. doi:10.1007/978-0-387-30440-3_273

7. Santa Fe Institute. Complexity Explorer. https://www.complexityexplorer.org/explore/glossary. Published 2019. Accessed April 29, 2019.

8. Arthur WB. *Urban Systems and Historical Path-Dependence*. Stanford, CA: Food Research Institute working paper 0012; 1988.

9. Arthur WB. *Increasing Returns and Path Dependence in the Economy*. Ann Arbor: University of Michigan Press; 1994.

10. Rankinen T, Sarzynski MA, Ghosh S, Bouchard C. Are there genetic paths common to obesity, cardiovascular disease outcomes, and cardiovascular risk factors? *Circ Res*. 2015;116(5):909–922. doi:10.1161/CIRCRESAHA.116.302888

11. Gladwell M. *The Tipping Point: How Little Things Can Make a Big Difference*. 1st Back Bay pbk. ed. Boston: Back Bay Books; 2002.

12. Trefois C, Antony PM, Goncalves J, Skupin A, Balling R. Critical transitions in chronic disease: Transferring concepts from ecology to systems medicine. *Curr Opin Biotechnol*. 2015;34:48–55. doi:10.1016/j.copbio.2014.11.020

13. Scheffer M, Carpenter SR, Lenton TM, et al. Anticipating critical transitions. *Science*. 2012;338(6105):344–348.

14. Kallio RE. Factors influencing the college choice decisions of graduate students. *Res High Educ*. 1995;36(1):109–124. doi:10.1007/BF02207769

15. Laaksonen DE, Lakka H-M, Salonen JT, Niskanen LK, Rauramaa R, Lakka TA. Low levels of leisure-time physical activity and cardiorespiratory fitness predict development of the metabolic syndrome. *Diabetes Care*. 2002;25(9):1612–1618. doi:10.2337/diacare.25.9.1612

16. Baik I, Shin C. Prospective study of alcohol consumption and metabolic syndrome. *Am J Clin Nutr*. 2008;87(5):1455–1463. doi:10.1093/ajcn/87.5.1455

17. Correll CU, Frederickson AM, Kane JM, Manu P. Metabolic syndrome and the risk of coronary heart disease in 367 patients treated with second-generation antipsychotic drugs. *J Clin Psychiatry*. 2006;67(04):575–583. doi:10.4088/JCP.v67n0408

18. Groop L. Genetics of the metabolic syndrome. *Br J Nutr*. 2000;83(S1):S39–S48. doi:10.1017/S0007114500000945

19. Manuck SB, Phillips JE, Gianaros PJ, Flory JD, Muldoon MF. Subjective socioeconomic status and presence of the metabolic syndrome in midlife community volunteers: *Psychosom Med*. 2010;72(1):35–45. doi:10.1097/PSY.0b013e3181c484dc

20. Friend A, Craig L, Turner S. The prevalence of metabolic syndrome in children: A systematic review of the literature. *Metab Syndr Relat Disord*. 2013;11(2):71–80. doi:10.1089/met.2012.0122

21. Lloyd-Jones DM, Wilson PWF, Larson MG, et al. Framingham risk score and prediction of lifetime risk for coronary heart disease. *Am J Cardiol*. 2004;94(1):20–24. doi:10.1016/j.amjcard.2004.03.023

22. Sterman J. *Business Dynamics: Systems Thinking and Modeling for a Complex World*. New York, NY: Irwin/McGraw-Hill; 2000.

23. Khan Academy. Homeostasis. Khan Academy. https://www.khanacademy.org/science/high-school-biology/hs-human-body-systems/hs-body-structure-and-homeostasis/a/homeostasis. Published 2019. Accessed April 15, 2019.

24. Learn By Doing, Inc. Positive and Negative Feedback Loops in Biology. ALBERT. https://www.albert.io/blog/positive-negative-feedback-loops-biology/. Published 2016. Accessed April 15, 2019.

25. Orenstein DR, Homer J, Milstein B, Wile K, Pratibhu P, Farris R. Modeling the local dynamics of cardiovascular health: Risk factors, context, and capacity. *Prev Chronic Dis.* 2008;5(2). https://www.ncbi.nlm.nih.gov/pmc/articles/PMC2396963/ . Accessed April 29, 2019.

26. Homer J, Jones A, Seville D, Essien J, Milstein B, Murphy D. The CDC's diabetes systems modeling project: Developing a new tool for chronic disease prevention and control. In: *22nd International Conference of the System Dynamics Society.* Albany, NY: System Dynamics Society; 2004:22.

27. Hammond RA. Complex systems modeling for obesity research. *Prev Chronic Dis.* 2009;6(3):A97.

28. Vandenbroeck IP, Goossens DJ, Clemens M. *Tackling Obesities: Future Choices—Obesity System Atlas.* Government Office for Science; 2007:46. https://assets.publishing.service.gov.uk/government/uploads/system/uploads/attachment_data/file/295153/07-1177-obesity-system-atlas.pdf.

29. Barabási AL. *Network Science.* Cambridge, UK: Cambridge University Press; 2015. http://networksciencebook.com/. Accessed April 29, 2019.

30. Valente TW. *Social Networks and Health: Models, Methods, and Applications.* New York, NY: Oxford University Press; 2010.

31. Hidalgo CA, Blumm N, Barabási A-L, Christakis NA. A dynamic network approach for the study of human phenotypes. *PLoS Comput Biol.* 2009;5(4). doi:10.1371/journal.pcbi.1000353

32. Farnam Street. Power Laws: How Nonlinear Relationships Amplify Results. Farnam Street. https://fs.blog/2017/11/power-laws/. Published 2017. Accessed April 15, 2019.

33. Fadini GP, de Kreutzenberg SV, Tiengo A, Avogaro A. Why to screen heart disease in diabetes. *Atherosclerosis.* 2009;204(1):11–15. doi:10.1016/j.atherosclerosis.2008.08.044

34. Zhang J, Tong L, Lamberson PJ, Durazo-Arvizu RA, Luke A, Shoham DA. Leveraging social influence to address overweight and obesity using agent-based models: The role of adolescent social networks. *Soc Sci Med.* 2015;125:203–213. doi:10.1016/j.socscimed.2014.05.049

35. Bourisly AK. An obesity agent based model: A new decision support system for the obesity epidemic. In: Tan G, Yeo GK, Turner SJ, Teo YM, eds. *AsiaSim 2013: 13th International Conference on Systems Simulation,* Heidelberg: Springer; 2013:37–48.

36. Agar M. Complexity theory: An exploration and overview based on John Holland's work. *Field Methods.* 1999;11(2):99–120.

37. Wang Y, Xue H, Chen H, Igusa T. Examining social norm impacts on obesity and eating behaviors among US school children based on agent-based model. 2014;14(923):1–11. doi:10.1186/1471-2458-14-923

38. Anderson PW. More is different. *Science.* 1972;177(4047):393–396. doi:10.1126/science.177.4047.393

3

Population Health as a Complex Adaptive System of Systems

SCOTT E. PAGE AND JON ZELNER

3.1. INTRODUCTION

Systems thinking reveals flaws in reductionist, cause-and-effect thinking and policymaking. A well-defined systems model can reveal why changing a single variable, even one that has been shown to have a causal effect, may not have substantial population-level impact because of system-level feedbacks.

In this chapter, we advocate considering population health outcomes and disparities as produced not by isolated complex systems but by *complex adaptive system of systems* (CASoS), that is, collections of connected complex systems.[1,2] We argue that our understanding of the entire system can be advanced by first considering each subsystem in isolation and then aggregating the lessons learned from each constituent system to explore their interactions. Further, we emphasize the relevance and implications of a CASoS framework for explaining health disparities, predicting disease outcomes, designing interventions, and taking action, and we illustrate these contributions through several cases that we consider at different levels of analytic depth. We conclude that efforts to improve population health outcomes would benefit from a CASoS approach, due to the inherent complexity of their interacting subsystems.

Over the past few decades, a growing number of researchers have begun to think of population health outcomes—and disparities—as outcomes of complex systems.[2] The fit should be clear. Population health outcomes—which are hard to predict and explain—are produced by systems of interacting diverse actors—the population at risk, medical professionals, governments, businesses, and so on. Advocates of a complex systems perspective also point to the fact that population

Scott E. Page and Jon Zelner, *Population Health as a Complex Adaptive System of Systems* In: *Complex Systems and Population Health*. Edited by:Yorghos Apostolopoulos, Kristen Hassmiller Lich, and Michael Kenneth Lemke, Oxford University Press (2020). © Oxford University Press. DOI: 10.1093/oso/9780190880743.003.0003 health outcomes arise from interactions at multiple scales, ranging from cel-lular reproduction to face-to-face human interactions to policies impacting entire populations. They also point out that each scale includes feedbacks and interactions.[1]

We believe that population health scholars should also adopt a CASoS perspec-tive: Population health operates at cellular, human, and social levels. At each level, the interactions involve diverse adaptive entities. In other words, at each level—genetic, personal, household, community—we find different *complex adaptive systems* (CAS) with distinct types of diversity, adaptions, and network structures. In addition, each scale adapts to the other scales. We have biological responses to individual adaptations to social pressures.

Therefore, in its entirety, systems that produce population health outcomes are more accurately characterized as CASoS than as individual complex systems. This claim is more than semantic. It suggests that our understanding of popu-lation health outcomes and disparities might be improved by considering com-plex systems in isolation and then recombining what we know to better grasp the implications.

The shift in perspective to thinking of population health outcomes as produced by a system of systems directs policymakers away from the search for simplistic, magic-bullet solutions to achieve reductions in obesity or improvements in mental health.[3] In a CAS, actions thought to produce one effect often result in its opposite or otherwise: For example, efforts to cut costs by reducing hospital staff can set off a chain of cascading failures that increase mortality and cost. This un-predictability of complex systems can be vexing to those responsible for managing them. Hence, attempts to manage population health, much like efforts to maintain ecologies and international political systems, require vigilance and humility.

3.2. COMPLEXITY AND COMPLEX ADAPTIVE SYSTEMS OF SYSTEMS

The notion of complexity itself defies neat characterization. Complexity, by defi-nition, must be nuanced.[4,5] Wolfram defines complexity as lying between ordered and random.[6] Others define complexity in terms of information content[7] and as phenomena that are difficult to explain, engineer, evolve, or predict.[8]

Regardless of the definition employed, whether it be a numerical measure of excess entropy or a qualitative assessment, complex phenomena share several properties. Their behavior is *nonstationary*, making prediction of future behavior difficult. And, for the most part, their outcomes are not normally distributed, with the distribution of event sizes often characterized by longer tails. For example, for many infectious diseases, the distribution of outbreaks consists primarily of small events punctuated by occasional large epidemics. The phenomena produced by complex systems, including transient patterns such as a wave of disease outbreaks and large events like epidemics, emerge from the interactions of the diverse, adaptive entities. Emergent phenomena can be thought of as macro-level patterns (the flocking of birds), properties (wetness), and functionalities (cognition) that exhibit functional properties that cannot exist at the micro level.[9] A single bird cannot flock. A single water molecule cannot be wet. A single neuron cannot think. All three phenomena emerge and do so without any central coordination. No field marshal organizes geese in formation. No physical lattice arranges the loose hydrogen and oxygen bonds. And, no "mindmaker" connects axons and dendrites to neuron bodies.

Population health outcomes such as waves of disease spreading across a geographic region also emerge. No central plan or simple process can explain the most pernicious population health challenges: For example, obesity trends across Organization for Economic Cooperation and Development countries reveal rising obesity in every country. But the magnitude of the problem and rate of change is heterogeneous across countries. In each case, the trend of rising obesity emerges from interactions at multiple levels ranging from genes to bacteria, to social interactions. Obesity is not caused by vending machines in school hallways, a lack of sidewalks, or from income inequality. Instead, those factors, along with many others, contribute to an unhealthy system of systems. Therefore, reversing these trends will not be accomplished by "one-size-fits-all" interventions targeting a single dimension of risk.

The first step in that system-level thinking consists of mapping out the various contributing forces. A causal map produced by the Foresight Group[a] identifies 10 contributing systems for obesity: media, social, psychological, economic, food, activity (exercise), infrastructure, developmental, biological, and medical. By identifying ten distinct systems, the Foresight Group characterizes the obesity epidemic not as a single CAS but as a CASoS.

A CAS can be usefully considered as a CASoS if two properties hold: (1) the system must be divisible into subsystems that can be analyzed in isolation, and (2) those subsystems must interact in nonobvious ways. Thus, a CASoS lies on the continuum between a collection of isolated CAS and a single CAS. In the former case, to borrow Plato's language, we can carve nature at its joints.

In evaluating the causes of the obesity epidemic, we can carve out distinct systems and reassemble them to draw insights. The economic factors—employment, access to food sources, and pressure on food providers to cater to preferences—comprise a system that can be analyzed in isolation to gain key insights. However, the analysis cannot start and end with economics. Economic factors interact with social influences such as peer pressure and eating habits (food). If we focus just on the economic system, we would infer that income subsidies plus creating access to healthy food—that is, eradicating food deserts—could create a virtuous loop. The logic goes as follows: Income subsidies create an incentive for businesses that offer healthier food options to enter a neighborhood. People then have an incentive to purchase healthier food. Those purchases, in turn, will pay for the jobs at the purveyors of the healthy food, resulting in a simple reinforcing loop shown in Figure 3.1.

a. https://assets.publishing.service.gov.uk/government/uploads/system/uploads/attachment_data/file/287937/07-1184x-tackling-obesities-future-choices-report.pdf

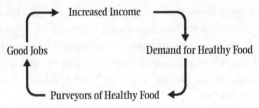

Figure 3.1 Economic factors and obesity (from Foresight Group Obesity Causal Map).

Within the economic system, we have identified, what appears to be a sound policy: income subsidies plus healthy food options.

If we view these policies through a CASoS framework, we have more reasons to be skeptical about their success. To predict the policy outcome, we must consider linkages to other systems. Two that immediately come to mind are infrastructure (how will people get to the purveyors of healthy food?) and social influences (how to we get people to change their eating patterns?). People may choose to eat higher cost, less healthy prepared foods offered by the new high-end "grocerant." On top of that, the price of various foods is a function of agricultural policies and international agreements that may artificially depress the price of unhealthy foods. In both cases, with more income, the result could be a diet even richer in salt and sugar.

Put simply, even if healthier food exists and people can afford it, they must have the means to get to the store, and the social support and encouragement to change their behavioral patterns away from salty and sweet foods. As this simple example makes clear, the same social system can support multiple behaviors—some beneficial, some harmful.[10] The presence of healthy food purveyors, increased incomes, and even transport infrastructure that increases accessibility introduce the *potential* for a good outcome. They do not guarantee it. Success will depend also on social support at multiple levels from the individual to the market.

The outcome that arises will depend on how people are connected and how they learn.[11,12] Insights into how to intervene in the learning process so as to be more likely to get the good outcome may be improved by also studying the social system. Here again, we see how a CASoS framework yields benefits.

Keep in mind that, although we had to think through the interactions between the economic system and other systems, we did not need to include every dimension and attribute of the other systems. We only needed to consider those that connected to the proposed economic changes. Thus, we can gain analytical and empirical traction from considering the subsystem of primary interest first and then connecting it to other complex systems within the larger CASoS.

How we can identify the subsystems in a CASoS? One approach is to use community detection algorithms.[13] One class of such algorithms removes links (chosen by their betweenness) until the graph becomes disconnected. Consider the social network in Figure 3.2. The network consists of distinct friendship communities. Yet, even in this graph, there exists sufficient overlap of those friendship clusters (the communities), that in tracking the flow of a disease through the network, we must allow for its spread between as well as within clusters.

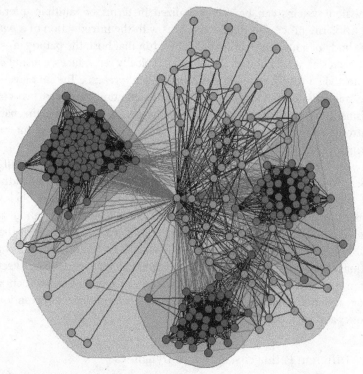

Figure 3.2 Communities in a social network.
SOURCE: Francisco Pochetti.

We advocate for conceptualizing interactions between CAS along a continuum. At one end are largely independent CAS with minimal overlaps. These subsystems may communicate, but they do so at well-defined boundaries. We define this as a *system of CAS*. As the interconnections between these CAS increase, we approach a threshold in which the system can be conceptualized as a CASoS, with each interacting component influencing the behavior of another at multiple points. However, as the number of interconnections between subsystems increases, the system again collapses into a single, large CAS without distinctly identifiable components.

In a CASoS, a few key nodes may account for the majority of connections between subsystems. In a social network, the people who connect distinct clusters are said to fill structural holes.[14] People who fill those holes have brokerage power.[15] In the Foresight obesity map, a node called *conscious control of accumulation* appears to fill a structural hole as it connects to various subsystems. That positioning suggests that changes to that node will be important to the success of any intervention or policy. Thus, when contemplating a policy intervention, we should consider how it affects that node.

3.3. A CASE STUDY: INFECTIOUS DISEASE TRANSMISSION

To further explicate the value of a CASoS framework, we now take a deeper dive into the case of infectious disease transmission. Most infectious disease transmission systems can be conceptualized in terms of multiple interacting, nested *CAS*. The process of infection begins with the introduction of a *pathogen* into the body of a human or animal *host*. Within that host, the pathogen—which may be bacterial, viral, parasitic, or fungal—typically reproduces, causing disease in the host via a set of processes described as *pathogenesis*. The first layer of the disease transmission CASoS consists of the interactions between two complex organisms, host and pathogen. However, the process by which the pathogen was introduced to the host often reflects contact patterns involving interactions occurring over complex, dynamic networks.

At a *micro* (local) level, contact may reflect the day-to-day interactions of family members in a household. At a *meso*, regional level, we find flux of individuals in and out of a city due to commuting patterns. And at a *macro*, global level, we find long-distance travel spanning continents. Finally, host and pathogen adapt via *evolution*. Because the life cycle of most pathogens is much shorter than that of their hosts, they can respond to changing social, environmental, and medical conditions. Bacteria may quickly acquire antibiotic resistance; insect vectors of infection may become resistant to insecticides—an interaction between *natural selection* and the social and political systems that produce interventions like antibiotics and insecticides.

3.3.1. Different Pathogens, Different Dynamics

We have established that the relationship between host and pathogen typically represents a CASoS style of interaction: Pathogenesis plays out in the cells of the host, with the pathogen subject to natural selection within the host. Nevertheless, the distinction between pathogen and host is clear. But what about the process of transmission? The infectiousness of a pathogen is typically summarized using what is known as the *basic reproduction number*, denoted by R_0.[16]

This value indicates the average number of new cases a single infectious individual would be expected to create in a population that is completely susceptible to infection. The value of R_0 depends on a variety of factors: How does the disease spread? By air, touch, or through sexual contact? How long is a person infectious? How often do people wash their hands? How clean is the water supply? How efficient is the ventilation system?

A disease that spreads easily will have a high R_0. If $R_0 > 1$, that is, if the average individual infects more than one other person, we should expect to see an outbreak, epidemic, or pandemic. However, if $R_0 < 1$, the infection will fizzle out and we will be unlikely to see an outbreak or epidemic. This parameter is often implicitly assumed to be primarily biological in nature, reflecting the inherent infectiousness of the pathogen. In truth, however, it represents a complex interaction of host and pathogen that is *mediated* by a system of social relationships structuring transmission.

When we understand such transmission systems only in terms of their average infectiousness (i.e., R_0), it is hard to see the critical interactions between these factors. But when we start thinking about *distributions* of infectiousness across individuals, we are able to understand why for the same R_0 we can get very different dynamics: rare, explosive outbreaks when the distribution of infectiousness is overdispersed, and predictable, frequent ones when everyone is near the population mean.[17] Just by allowing infectiousness to vary across individuals we have adopted a CASoS mindset that accommodates variation arising from interacting biological and social systems.

Another way of understanding infectious disease CASoS is via spatial analysis: The classic image of a highly infectious pathogen, with a large value of R_0, which could be as high as 15, 20, or more, is an airborne pathogen. We often think of pathogens fitting this description, like pandemic influenza, measles, or the 2019 Novel Coronavirus, as blowing through cities with minimal regard for spatial boundaries. And it may be the case that, within a single city, we might expect an outbreak of a highly infectious airborne pathogen to behave like a CAS defined by positive feedback (exponential growth in the number of infectious individuals in the early days of the outbreak) and negative feedback (epidemic slowing as the pool of susceptible individuals to infect is exhausted and individuals adopt protective behaviors). But when we zoom out, we see that this is actually a CASoS defined regionally by links between cities connected by commuting, and by international air travel that may rapidly transport pathogens around the world.

However, social networks also must be understood as conduits of information and influence that can have either salutary or negative effects on infection risk. Because of this, infectious disease outbreaks may often represent *complex contagions*[18] in which the flow of information and pathogens are mutually reinforcing. Consider the rise of antivaccine sentiment and behavior in the wake of a now-discredited study suggesting that the measles–mumps–rubella vaccine causes autism. The spread of this fallacious information over social networks created spatial pockets of susceptibility to childhood infections, such as measles and whooping cough, which were either eliminated or on the wane in the United States and other high-income countries. This process can work in reverse as well: For example, a recent analysis using social media data showed that a trend of rising antivaccine sentiment in California, leading to reduced childhood immunization rates, quickly reversed in the wake of large measles outbreak at Disneyland.[19] This reflects CASoS dynamics in which the processes of social and biological "transmission" are not only intertwined, but also recognizable as separate systems.

At a *meso* level, complex political, policy, and scientific systems both drive and respond to the behavior of the individuals composing the transmission system. For example, in the early stages of an influenza pandemic, supplies of vaccinations and antivirals are likely to be limited. To be effective, they must be targeted on both the individuals most susceptible to infection, and most likely to generate new infections, so-called *superspreaders*.[17] Developing a vaccination in response to an emerging infectious disease requires the mobilization of a complex scientific and manufacturing apparatus. The 2014 West African Ebola epidemic spurred the development of a novel Ebola vaccination, the efficacy of which was then evaluated during the ongoing epidemic. Similarly, the development of vaccinations against both seasonal and pandemic influenza requires significant and continuous scientific effort to *adapt* to the emergence of novel flu variants against which there is limited or nonexistent population immunity. Finally, the delivery of vaccinations often requires a complex logistical system in which vaccines are maintained at a consistent temperature at every step in the process, known as the "cold chain." Coordinating the interactions of all of these levels are local, state, national, and international population health authorities, which are themselves outgrowths of political systems. The sum of these parts is a *biosocial* CASoS representing interactions between governmental and civil organizations, individual hosts, and pathogens.

3.3.2. How Do CASoS Generate Health Disparities?

Careful observation of interacting social and biological systems led the social medicine pioneer Rene Dubos to describe *Mycobacterium tuberculosis*, as a "necessary, but not sufficient, condition" for the emergence of tuberculosis (TB) disease.[20] Dubos described the case of a lacquer sprayer working in a factory where he was exposed to harsh chemicals and abrasives that facilitated infection upon exposure, with the risk of such exposure reflecting class boundaries. In this system, Dubos argued that a reductive understanding of *Mycobacterium tuberculosis* as the cause of infection obscured critical social causes of disease and of socioeconomic and occupational disparities in TB infection and mortality.

The implications of these mechanisms are made clear by a detailed history of racial inequality in TB infection risk in Baltimore in the early 20th century, which documents the relationship between racial residential segregation and vast disparities in TB infection risk between African Americans and whites in that city.[21] In this work, the historian Samuel Kelton Roberts argued that Jim Crow era policies enforcing residential segregation forced blacks into overcrowded, poorly ventilated housing, as well as high-risk occupations that increased their exposure to TB and susceptibility to infection upon exposure. In addition, the poverty and deprivation that accompanied residential segregation and rampant, legalized discrimination increased rates of malnutrition and susceptibility to other infections, such as pneumonia, which increased the risk of death from TB. Recent work suggests that during this period the risk of TB infection posed by each infectious case was more than 10 times great for African Americans living in northern cities than for whites living in the same places.[22] Taken together, these findings suggest that disparities in infection risk and mortality are often the product of a CASoS representing the interconnection of a social system orchestrating and maintaining inequalities and a pathogen that capitalized on the environmental and biological conditions generated by this socioeconomic inequity.

Although social inequality and segregation may induce differences in risk between advantaged and disadvantaged population groups, spillover effects from one to the other are inevitable. At the level of a city, if we ignore variation in risk between neighborhoods or social groups, we may see "boring" dynamics: a continuous trickle of cases or variation over time that resembles white noise. But

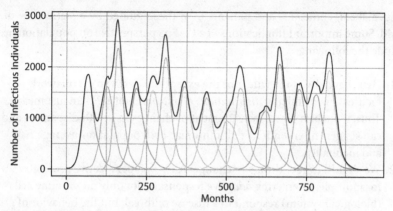

Figure 3.3 Schematic of a CASoS of loosely connected infectious disease outbreaks (colored lines) that produce a single epidemic (dark line).
SOURCE: Jon Zelner.

when we zoom in and look at the distribution of infection in space or across demographic groups, using tools like geographic information systems and molecular genotyping, we may see a bunch of overlapping epidemics representing transmission within specific social and demographic groups. For example, racial and economic residential segregation may have led to separation in TB transmission between African Americans and whites in Baltimore. Each of these subepidemics was a CAS, but their overlaps likely connected them into a CASoS in which transmission in one subpopulation fed infection into the other.

Figure 3.3 provides a schematic representation of this idea: The solid line is a time series of infectious disease cases you might observe as belonging to a unified system. But if we are able to look at the *genotype* of each case, we see a series of loosely connected subepidemics. If we project this into physical space, we might see these playing out in individual neighborhoods, reflecting variable rates of transmission over community social networks. Analyses of TB transmission in the present day in high-burden contexts in Peru and Brazil suggest that the *hotspot* neighborhoods play an important role in regional epidemics, with high rates of transmission in disadvantaged groups living in overcrowded conditions sustaining transmission in wealthier, more advantaged areas.[23,24] These patterns reflect layered CASoS interactions, beginning with host-level variation in susceptibility to infection and disease and scaling up to the social conditions that induce disparities at the neighborhood level, and the patterns of within- and between-city migration that allow pathogens to move between subpopulations.

3.4. THE ADVANTAGES OF CASOS THINKING IN POPULATION HEALTH

Treating population health as the product of a CASoS can be productive because it provides a set of *attitudes* and *expectations* that are more likely to be useful to policymakers, clinicians, and patients than those guided by a static view of the world. Some important implications of a CASoS perspective on population health include the following:

1. **Heterogeneity is the rule, not the exception:** A CASoS framework focuses on optimizing *distributions of outcomes* rather than just means. Thus, it enables direct measurement of changes in health disparities and can suggest interventions that minimize *both* population-average risk and inequality.

2. **We should expect things to change:** A CASoS perspective accounts for multiple, interacting *adaptive* responses: Not only do immune cells (biological system) respond to a disease outbreak but the behavior of people (the social system) in response to infection risk can change the trajectory of an epidemic.

3. **Don't believe everything that you read:** The precision and accuracy of information produced by the medical community (the information system) influences responses and needs to be taken into account. An analyst taking a CASoS perspective understands that data are often generated by a CASoS reflecting the robustness of public health surveillance in a given place and that this information may impact awareness, fear, and behavior with respect to a given health condition in the population. The predictive accuracy of Google queries on the timing of influenza epidemics degraded rapidly once Google searches for flu symptoms began to return suggestions that the individual might have influenza, resulting in massive spikes in search queries even when the true burden of flu was not increasing rapidly.[25]

4. **Sometimes you need to address one system to impact another:** Even interventions that appear to be free can have significant economic costs that prevent people from taking advantage of them. For example, in Peru, researchers found that individuals who were poorer were less likely to take advantage of free treatment for drug-resistant TB, because of both lost wages associated with being isolated to prevent transmission and because of the social stigma associated with such a diagnosis. However, providing income support to buffer the economic effects of seeking treatment resulted in a significant reduction in disparities in care-seeking.[26] In other words, when everything is intertwined, one approach is to find a lever that operates on all of them in unison.[27]

For progress to be made, we must entertain multiple ways of thinking about population health that take us beyond a single input/single outcome framework to one that allows us to address key connections between social, economic, and biological inputs and feedbacks between diverse biological outcomes. We should use many models.[28] These additional models oblige us to lean new analytic tools, including agent-based modeling[29] and network analysis. Agent-based models in particular are important because they represent a set of habits of the mind that are critical for understanding the CASoS we interact with daily.

But with all this said, it is critically important to note that a CASoS perspective does not imply conceptual and analytical models of ever-increasing complexity, the inevitable conclusion of which is the useless world-sized map cautioned against in the short story "On Exactitude in Science."[30] Instead, we advocate for focusing first on finding the "joints" at which we can make distinctions between subsystems, making careful abstractions that capture the most meaningful behaviors of each component system, and then stitching them back together to understand the implications of their interactions.

REFERENCES

1. Diez-Roux AV. Complex systems thinking and current impasses in health disparities research. *Am J Public Health.* 2011;101(9):1627–1634.

2. El-Sayed AM, Galea S. *Systems science and population health.* Oxford, UK: Oxford University Press; 2017.

3. Colander D, Kupers R. *Complexity and the art of public policy: Solving society's problems from the bottom up.* Princeton, NJ: Princeton University Press; 2016.

4. Byrne D, Callaghan G. *Complexity theory and the social sciences: The state of the art.* New York, NY: Routledge; 2013.

5. Castellani B, Hafferty FW. *Sociology and complexity science: A new field of inquiry.* New York, NY: Springer; 2009.

6. Wolfram S. *A new kind of science.* Champaign, IL: Wolfram Media; 2002.

7. Prokopenko M, Boschetti F, Ryan AJ. An information-theoretic primer on complexity, self-organization, and emergence. *Complexity.* 2009;15(1):11–28.

8. Page SE. *Diversity and complexity.* Princeton, NJ: Princeton University Press; 2010.

9. Anderson PW. More is different. *Science.* 1972;177(4047):393–396.

10. Durlauf SN, Ioannides YM. Social interactions. *Annu Rev Econ.* 2010;2(1):451–478.

11. Vriend NJ. An illustration of the essential difference between individual and social learning, and its consequences for computational analyses. *J Econ Dynam Control.* 2000;24(1):1–19.

12. Golman R, Page SE. Basins of attraction and equilibrium selection under different learning rules. *J Evol Econ.* 2010;20(1):1–49.

13. Newman MEJ, Girvan M. Finding and evaluating community structure in networks. *Phys Rev E.* 2004;69(2):026113.

14. Burt RS. *Structural holes: The social structure of competition.* Cambridge, MA: Harvard University Press; 2009.

15. Burt RS. *Brokerage and closure: An introduction to social capital.* New York, NY: Oxford University Press; 2005.

16. Keeling MJ, Rohani P. *Modeling infectious diseases in humans and animals.* Princeton, NJ: Princeton University Press; 2007.

17. Lloyd-Smith JO, Schreiber SJ, Kopp PE, Getz WM. Superspreading and the effect of individual variation on disease emergence. *Nature.* 2005;438(7066):355–359.

18. Centola D, Macy M. Complex contagions and the weakness of long ties. *Am J Sociol.* 2007;113(3):702–734.

19. Pananos AD, Bury TM, Wang C, et al. Critical dynamics in population vaccinating behavior. *Proc N Acad Sci.* 2017;114(52):13762–13767.
20. Dubos RJ, Schaedler RW. Effects of cellular constituents of Mycobacteria on the resistance of mice to heterologous infections: I. Protective effects. *J Exper Med.* 1957;106(5):703–717.
21. Roberts S. Where our melanotic citizens predominate: Locating African Americans and finding the "lung block" in tuberculosis research in Baltimore, Maryland, 1880-1920. In: Boi P, Broeck S, eds. *CrossRoutes—The meanings of "race" for the 21st century.* Piscataway, NJ: Transaction; 2003:91–112.
22. Zelner JL, Muller C, Feigenbaum JJ. Racial inequality in the annual risk of Tuberculosis infection in the United States, 1910-1933. *Epidemiol Infect.* 2017;145(9):1797–1804.
23. Dowdy DW, Israel G, Vellozo V, et al. Quality of life among people treated for tuberculosis and human immunodeficiency virus in Rio de Janeiro, Brazil. *Int J Tubercul Lung Dis.* 2013;17(3):345–347.
24. Zelner JL, Murray M, Becerra M, et al. Protective effects of household-based TB interventions are robust to neighbourhood-level variation in exposure risk in Lima, Peru: A model-based analysis. *Int J Epidemiol.* 2017;47(1):185–192.
25. Lazer D, Kennedy R, King G, Vespignani A. The parable of Google Flu: Traps in big data analysis. *Science.* 2014;343(6176):1203–1205.
26. Wingfield T. Mitigating the financial effects of tuberculosis requires more than expansion of services. *Lancet Glob Health.* 2017;5(11):e1056–e1057.
27. Link BG, Phelan J. Social conditions as fundamental causes of disease. *J Health Soc Behav.* 1995:80–94. Extra Issue: Forty Years of Medical Sociology: The State of the Art and Directions for the Future .
28. Page SE. *The model thinker.* New York, NY: Basic Books; 2018.
29. Epstein JM. *Generative social science: Studies in agent-based computational modeling.* Princeton, NJ: Princeton University Press; 2006.
30. Borges JL. On exactitude in science. In: Hurley A, trans. *Collective fictions.* New York, NY: Penguin; 1999.

4

Complex Network Dynamics in Population Health

JAMES MOODY AND DANA K. PASQUALE

4.1. BACKGROUND

A core element of the social determinants of health framework[1] is that the embeddedness within social networks shapes population health, and a growing body of literature examines how complex extended social networks affect both individual and population health. Over the last 40 years, the number of publications on social networks and health has grown dramatically, with similar trends in National Institutes of Health funding. Given the rapid growth and widespread use, how do we best make sense of networks in population health? Here we begin by reviewing the basic theoretical underpinnings of how networks should affect behavior, including population health, and then review key results. We then conclude with a discussion of open questions.

The scope of network research is wide, so here we focus on complete networks—the system(s) of relations connecting people beyond just their immediate set of friends. For the most part, we are interested in people as network vertices, though there is significant work in health treating health organizations as nodes.[2,3] There are two general ways that networks affect population health. *Connectionist* models focusing on diffusion and infection spread are the archetype for these models, though similar mechanisms have been effective for behavior. Information or influence can just as easily flow through the network, as in studies tracing the effect of peer exposure on population health.[4,5] The second approach is *positional*, focusing on how patterns of relations reflect social roles. For example, work on adolescent popularity trajectories suggests that when adolescents face losing social

James Moody and Dana K. Pasquale, *Complex Network Dynamics in Population Health* In: *Complex Systems and Population Health*. Edited by: Yorghos Apostolopoulos, Kristen Hassmiller Lich, and Michael Kenneth Lemke, Oxford University Press (2020). © Oxford University Press. DOI: 10.1093/oso/9780190880743.003.0004 status they engage in more risky health behaviors in an effort to regain status[6] or that adolescents embedded in networks where their friends are not friends with each other have heightened risk for suicidal ideation.[7] While connectionist models are most common, positional approaches promise new ways to think about network effect on population health.

4.2. NETWORK CONNECTIVITY AND ROBUST DIFFUSION

Since people are embedded in health-transmitting relations, insights from network complexity and graph theory can inform our understanding of population health. For example, random graph theory[8] tells us that small changes in behavior can have significant macro-structural effects on the network. When the population has less than 1 partner on average (degree <1), we expect no outbreak; while increasing average degree from >1 to ≤2 creates a steep gradient, and average degree >2 will lead to nearly complete connectivity. This is significant because infections flow along these paths, which increases the potential for connected nodes to be reached by an infection. Importantly, moving a distribution from one side or the other of this phase transition point can occur despite no behavior change on the part of most members of the population.

This well-known result has significant implications for population health. For example, Morris and Dean demonstrated that sexual contact networks in and around New York City in the 1980s and 1990s were near the phase transition.[9] If behavior remained constant, disease would likely die out, but a small increase in connections would be sufficient to create endemic HIV. Similar simulations have examined risk in China[10] and across a much wider array of behavioral distributions.[11] Similar models have been applied to the global transmission of influenza making use of connectivity patterns within airline networks[12] or among social support and kin.[13]

Generalizations of epidemic threshold models focus on robust connectivity. An early result from this work suggests that highly skewed distributions of numbers of partners creates connectivity that requires targeted interventions to be successful in efficiently reducing infections.[14] This insight has important ramifications for immunization models, where we might have significant cost and efficiency savings by targeting high-connectivity nodes compared to generalized immunization strategies. Similarly, if our goal is to intervene efficiently, selecting nodes with the greatest likelihood of reaching many others can be optimized.[15]

Centrality, which is the relative position of a node in the network and the benefits of that position, generalizes this idea—centrality captures node heterogeneity in a dimension of a network's topology (for review, see Borgatti and Everett[16]). Simulation models generally show that infection risk correlates with centrality, though the result is dependent on the fraction of nodes already infected and ease of transmission.[17] When the epidemiological reproductive rate—R_0—is low, centrality matters more.[18] Real-world empirical studies are often fraught with data completeness issues, but we generally find that high centrality vertices are more likely to be exposed to infection.[19,20] We can further extend notions of connectivity to multiple connectivity,[21] where nodes are linked by multiple independent paths. For example, in bi-connected components (where every pair is linked by at least two paths), there is never a node that can thwart diffusion. Simulation results suggest a complex dependence on the mean and variance of the degree distribution that can lead to counterintuitive policy implications.[11]

Multiple paths reconnecting vertices within a network quickly takes us to modular network structures, where networks can be effectively partitioned into subsets where most of the relations fall within clusters, which can have a profound impact on diffusion[22] (see Figure 4.1). In networks with strong community structure, diffusion is rapid within communities, but diffusion across communities depends on how modular the structure is: When cross-community connections are rare, diffusion may die out before it jumps to a new group, which leads to spreading behavior that is clumpy temporally.

Network community structure is particularly important for social reinforcement processes. So-called complex contagion models[23] assume that something is adopted only if multiple neighbors have already adopted it. Particularly for social diffusion of health-relevant behavior, social reinforcement helps identify a sense of importance or generalized acceptance that increases pressure to adopt. For example, recent work suggests that adolescent healthy mood spreads via complex contagion,[24] as does preference to avoid vaccines,[25] which can lead to clustering of nonvaccine-related disease contagion.[26] The notion that people respond to

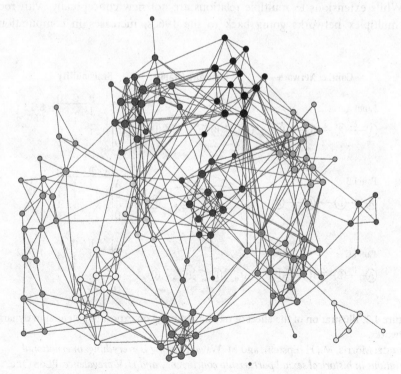

Figure 4.1 Community structure in adolescent networks.

the signal size of the number of alters who engage in health-relevant behavior provides a dose–response nuance to general diffusion models and has appeared in health topics as diverse as gunshot violence,[27] attempted suicide,[28] cannabis vaping,[29] and sentiments toward health screening.[30]

Recent work extends these formalisms to dynamic networks and networks with multiple types of relations and/or populations. Relationship timing constrains diffusion, since people can only pass infection down a set of relations that unfold in the future. As such, modeling that pools relations across wide temporal ranges can overstate the connectivity of the network. This temporal constraint is sketched in Figure 4.2.

While pairs of nodes connected are the same across panels, the timing (indicated by values on the edges) differs and thus so does the ultimate exposure. The structural limit on how infection can pass over dynamic edges gives insight into why concurrency (Figure 4.2C) can have dramatic effects on diffusion.[31] While serial monogamy (Figure 4.2A and 4.2B) generates asymmetric exposure through indirect links (e.g., B can reach D, but not vice versa), concurrency generates symmetric exposure opening new pathways for disease to spread,[32] which can have dramatic long-range implications. Timing interacts with structure, of course, and simulation results suggest that timing features are more critical in sparse networks, where there are fewer paths between nodes, than in highly cohesive networks, where there may be multiple redundant paths between nodes.[33] This is because the paths which are opened through concurrency have more of an impact in sparse networks.

While extensions to multiple relations are not new conceptually, with roots in multiplex networks going back to the 1960s, increases in computational

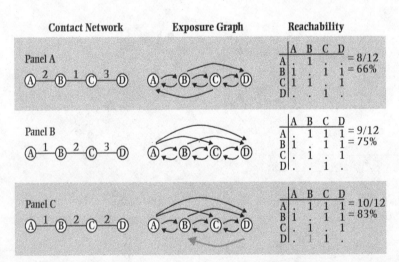

Figure 4.2 Illustration of the effect of relational timing on exposure potential in dynamic networks.

SOURCE: Morris, M., H. Epstein, and M. Wawer, *Timing is everything: international variations in historical sexual partnership concurrency and HIV prevalence.* PLoS One, 2010. 5(11): p. e14092. Reproduced with permission from Elsevier.

power and new approaches in complex systems modeling have made important inroads recently with multilayer networks (for a general review, see Kivela et al.[34]). Multilayer networks provide a general way to represent networks composed of different populations, relational types or times. For example, the network in Figure 4.3 has three layers, but note that the third layer is composed of organizations, while the first two layers depict relations of different types across a set of individuals. Links within layers represent the standard networks we have been discussing thus far, while links across edges indicate some sort of joint membership or identity. Tools for modeling these networks then consist of exploiting walks within and between layers. In the temporal case, for example, identity links between nodes might be directed from layer t to layer $t+1$, and thus diffusion is restricted to flow forward in time and concurrency would be represented by connected components within layers. Most diffusion and immunization studies on multilayer networks have been theoretical treatments that focus on relative spread within and between layers or diffusion processes that influence each other through synergism or antagonism, such as with competing pathogens.[35]

Positional approaches in population health are rarer and often build on Burt's question on the relative role of structural equivalence compared to contagion in adoption.[36] Actors may adopt a practice either because they learn it from their contacts or because the pressures and incentives of a position channel behavior in a particular way. Fujimoto and Valente[37] test this question for adolescent smoking and find strong support for structural equivalence, meaning that teens in similar network positions have similar smoking outcomes. Most other work focuses on the population health effects of a particular network pattern (rather than general equivalence). So, for example, we see much work on popularity and health[38] as well as the converse effects of isolation.[39] Others ask how being a bridge, or someone that connect groups, affects health.[40] For adolescent girls, having friends who are not friends with each other strongly predicts suicidal ideation.[7]

Since networks emerge from both contextual and endogenous factors, parsing the causal effects of networks on population health is fundamentally challenging[41] as it is difficult to know if the features that shape networks are also the features that shape health. Experimental and quasi-experimental designs offer the best hope for causal identification, followed by observational techniques that leverage

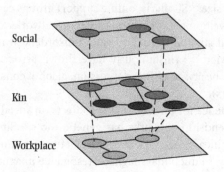

Figure 4.3 Example of multilayer network.

temporal variation on network and behavior change simultaneously.[42] Much like debates on nature versus nurture, questions over network "selection or influence" are usually answered "both." The balance of historical evidence across a range of designs and instruments suggest that peer influence is clearly positive and significant, though the magnitude might vary widely across settings.

4.3. DOMAIN SPANNING: SOCIAL, BIOLOGICAL, AND PHYSICAL INTERACTION NETWORKS AND POPULATION HEALTH

Here we expand briefly on the potential to think about how networks span different population health domains—spanning between social, biological, and physical interaction networks.

4.3.1. Social and Biological

The epidemiological links between social contact and disease spread are the most obvious connection between biological and social analysis levels, since biological infection travels via contagion through close social networks. However, these connections can have dynamics that might not be obvious from simple susceptible-infectious-susceptible or susceptible-infectious-recovered style models, as biological processes feedback on the dynamics of the social networks, which in turn shape spreading dynamics. For example, in work linking social interaction and HIV risk, Schneider et al.[43] find that social ties link people disassortatively by sexual activity while sexual contact networks tend to be assortatively mixed. This social mismatch highlights the roles of "enablers" who made engaging in particularly risky behavior more acceptable. Social network correlates of behavior, stigma, and general social situation likely moderate causal effects of social networks on sexually transmitted infection, but position in the network seems predictive of HIV status.[44]

Linking networks to population health has been exploited in multiple interventions and across many different domains aside from disease transmission. For example, there is good evidence that mental health interventions aimed at decreasing social isolation are effective, promoting better mental health and increasing network size.[45] Similarly, online support groups can be a way to prime neural network development.[46] Others find that networks can be exploited to help bullying, social stigma, sleep, and eating disorders to name just a few.[47–49] Christakis and Fowler[4,50,51] (in)famously have shown associations between network position and obesity, smoking, depression, alcohol consumption, and loneliness (among others).

There is also evidence for direct biological effects on social networks, showing that position in friendship networks has genetic roots.[52] Similarly, recent work finds there are significant feedback processes between brain structures and social network activity.[53] Functional magnetic resonance imaging studies show that network micro activity—namely, reciprocity and popularity—are well predicted by brain activity, independent of social exposure, similarity, and other behavioral correlates.[54] In general, the structure of social networks seems strongly related to brain connectivity network.[55] The flip side of this effect seems also possible, as social network size seems to predict brain size in monkeys[56] and humans with larger amygdalas have larger social networks.[57]

4.3.2. Social and Physical

The physical environment also constrains social networks, even in the digital age.[58] At the intersection of networks, health, and the physical environment, shared proximity leads to networks that generally affect health. For example, Lienert[59] finds that five-year survival rates among co-present patients receiving chemotherapy are correlated and proportional to the amount of time as neighbors in the cancer ward; while the causal mechanism is difficult to determine, it likely involves patients sharing information about how to cope with and recognize symptoms or general effects of social support.

The health system itself can have dramatic geospatial network effects as well, which is nicely illustrated in Figure 4.4. Hospitals often share patients across intensive care units to balance work and resources, leading to a network of hospitals that links the entire nation.[60] These networks may form a substrate upon which antibiotic resistant infection spreads,[61] as well as providing administrative challenges as hospitals at a destination location respond to choices rooted in the source hospital.

Social networks, and particularly social media, have proven interesting proxies for physical network processes. For example, monitoring mentions of physical symptoms on Twitter and similar platforms can be used to track the geographic

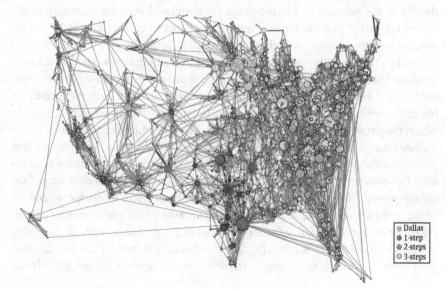

Figure 4.4 Hospital ICU transfer network.

spread of influenza,[62] predict asthma emergency department admissions,[63] and estimate air quality and its health effects.[64] Similarly, researchers have used online activity logs as a general proxy for disease monitoring.[65] Social network sites are also useful to bring people together who might not be geographically present, but who share common traumatic or health experiences for social support. The widespread success of the #MeToo movement has made such effects clear for sexual assault and harassment.

4.3.3. Biological and Physical

The least developed of these domains are network effects linking biological processes with physical and spatial embeddings. The clearest examples here are the geographic spread of large-scale infection. That each season's flu epidemic starts in China and works its way around the globe is a classic example, as are water borne diseases such as cholera. Since social networks tend to be rooted in geography, it is not surprising that we find a strong physical correlate with disease spread; however, the ways in which these features cross-link is not always obvious. For example, we see consistently higher sexually transmitted disease rates along interstate highways, which then link geographic centers (but not the rural spaces between the hubs) via long-distance trucking routes.[66] Geographic core areas of sexually transmitted infection endemicity have been noted, even as distinct from areas affected by an epidemic.[67]

If instead we consider how biological network structure is limited by physical structure, recent work on the spatial layout of neurons in brains makes use of the limits imposed by physical edge width. Unlike other networks where the edges exist in dimensionless space and can cross or occupy the same location, in neural networks the edges are the nerve fibers connecting the neurons. The size and density of the neurons and nerve fibers are correlated with the geometry of the neural network.[68] In other types of networks where physical systems influence biological systems, parasites which require multiple hosts often represent biological networks existing within extremely specific physical networks. Neither schistosomiasis (*Schistosoma* spp./blood flukes) nor guinea worm disease (*Dracunculus medinensis*) are directly transmitted between hosts. Instead, both have complex life cycles with aquatic intermediate hosts (snails or water fleas, respectively) in which the parasite develops to the point that it can infect its definitive host, which includes humans in both cases. Schistosomiasis results when *Schistosoma* spp. penetrates the skin of the host after bathing or entering a water source infected with free-swimming cercariae.[69] Dracunculiasis occurs when infected water fleas are consumed. The parasites are constrained by the physical landscape; alteration of the water source (or definitive host behavior around the water source) can increase or decrease human infection.[70] Agricultural practices, such as damming rivers, which creates slower-moving water and better habitats for the intermediate snail host,[71] or use of night soil as fertilizer[72] both increase human prevalence.

Network analysis has recently been applied to this field to study the sharing of parasites between host species.[73]

4.4. OPEN PROBLEMS AND FUTURE WORK

Networks provide a fertile analytical framework for thinking about complex dynamics across multiple domains of population health as the review above demonstrates. Looking forward, we think the field would benefit greatly by expanding along the following dimensions.

First, we need continued investment in realistic extensions of simple diffusion models. This includes not only new models for different generalizations of the base problem, but also clear evaluations of when such complications are actually necessary. There are many cases, for example, where known-to-be-unrealistic models do surprisingly well.[74] Explicit work on transmission variability via phenomena such as complex contagion or differential susceptibility/exposure is a promising direction. Similarly work that can disentangle such effects from real population dynamics—not just closed population edge timing, but also long-term turnover—are a necessary element for empirical realism. Finally, being able to estimate diffusion risk from sampled data (ideally, from the sorts of surveillance data already collected) would be a huge boon.

Second, while there is rich theory on positional approaches, there has been little work linking positions to population health. The original insights for these models are deeply rooted in role theory from structural anthropology.[75] In traditional models, the role/role-complement pair (parent–child, teacher–student) always entails a relational exchange (parents feed children, teachers give students homework). The network insight is to reverse this: If we can identify common exchanges, we can induce relevant roles. This is a powerful way to leverage interactions to discover deep features of social and health systems.

Third, networks can be leveraged to directly inform policy and improve population health. Much of the research in this area focuses on influence or diffusion of information within organizational or healthcare networks[76] or among individuals setting health policy.[77,78] However, researchers are also exploring whether social media can be harnessed to improve patient experience.[79] The goal of this research is to increase efficiency among existing organizations by coordinating their activities and then improve linkage between these organizations and the community.[80]

Finally, the biological and physical foundations of social relations focus on how biological or physical constraints shape social networks. This is reasonable, as social networks are often seen as much more fluid, and thus somewhat epiphenomenal. However, over the long term, we expect significant feedbacks, though to date these are largely unexplored. Longitudinal studies of social ties and neural networks in tandem, particularly as related to our new and evolving consumption of social media, will help us understand the feedbacks and associated mental and physical health outcomes.

REFERENCES

1. Solar, O. and A. Irwin, *A conceptual framework for action on the social determinants of health.* 2010, World Health Organization: Social Determinants of Health Discussion Paper 2

2. Provan, K.G. and H. Milward, *Do networks really work? A framework for evaluating public-sector organizational networks.* Public Admin Rev, 1999. 61(4): p. 414-423

3. Harris, J.K., et al., *Seeing the forest and the trees: using network analysis to develop an organizational blueprint of state tobacco control systems.* Soc Sci Med, 2008. 67(11): p. 1669–1678.

4. Christakis, N.A. and J.H. Fowler, *The spread of obesity in a large social network over 32 years.* N Engl J Med, 2007. 357(4): p. 370–379.

5. Aral, S. and C. Nicolaides, *Exercise contagion in a global social network.* Nature Comm, 2017. 8: p. 14753.

6. Moody, J., et al., *Popularity Trajectories and Substance Use in early Adolescence.* Soc Networks, 2011. 33(2): p. 101–112.

7. Bearman, P.S. and J. Moody, *Suicide and friendships among American adolescents.* Am J Public Health, 2004. 94(1): p. 89–95.

8. Harary, F., *The maximum connectivity of a graph.* Proc Natl Acad Sci U S A, 1962. 48(7): p. 1142–1146.

9. Morris, M., J. Zavisca, and L. Dean, *Social and Sexual Networks: Their Role in the Spread of HIV/AIDS among Young Gay Men.* AIDS Education and Prevention, 1995. 7(5): p. 24–35.

10. Merli, M.G., et al., *Heterosexual mixing in Shanghai: Are heterosexual contact mixing patterns in China compatible with an HIV/AIDS epidemic?* Demography, 2015. 52: p. 919–942.

11. Moody, J., J. Adams, and M. Morris, *Epidemic potential by sexual activity distributions.* Netw Sci (Camb Univ Press), 2017. 5(4): p. 461–475.

12. Marcelino, J. and M. Kaiser, *Reducing influenza spreading over the airline network.* PLoS Curr, 2009. 1: p. Rrn1005.

13. Zhou, Z., A.M. Verdery, and R. Margolis, *No spouse, no son, no daughter, no kin in contemporary China: prevalence, correlates, and differences in economic support.* J Gerontol B Psychol Sci Soc Sci, 2019. 74(8): p. 1453–1462.

14. Dezso, Z. and A.L. Barabasi, *Halting viruses in scale-free networks.* Phys Rev E Stat Nonlin Soft Matter Phys, 2002. 65(5 Pt 2): p. 055103.

15. Valente, T.W., Network interventions. Science, 2012. 337(6090): p. 49–53.

16. Borgatti, S.P. and M.G. Everett, *A graph-theoretic perspective on centrality.* Soc Netw, 2006. 28: p. 466–484.

17. Juher, D., et al., *Network-centric interventions to contain the syphilis epidemic in San Francisco.* Sci Rep, 2017. 7(1): p. 6464.

18. Ide, K., R. Zamami, and A. Namatame, *Diffusion centrality in interconnected networks.* Procedia Computer Science, 2013. 24: p. 227–238.

19. Havens, J.R., et al., *Individual and network factors associated with prevalent hepatitis C infection among rural Appalachian injection drug users.* Am J Public Health, 2013. 103(1): p. e44–52.

20. Gyarmathy, V.A., et al., *Social network structure and HIV infection among injecting drug users in Lithuania: gatekeepers as bridges of infection.* AIDS Behav, 2014. 18(3): p. 505–510.

21. Moody, J. and D.R. White, *Structural cohesion and embeddedness: a hierarchical concept of social groups.* Am Sociol Rev, 2003. **68**(1): p. 103–127.

22. Stegehuis, C., R. van der Hofstad, and J.S. van Leeuwaarden, *Epidemic spreading on complex networks with community structures.* Sci Rep, 2016. **6**: p. 29748.

23. Centola, D. and M. Macy, *Complex contagion and the weakness of long ties.* Am J Sociol, 2007. **113**(3): p. 702–734.

24. Hill, E.M., F.E. Griffiths, and T. House, *Spreading of healthy mood in adolescent social networks.* Proc Biol Sci, 2015. **282**(1813): p. 20151180.

25. Campbell, E. and M. Salathe, *Complex social contagion makes networks more vulnerable to disease outbreaks.* Sci Rep, 2013. **3**: p. 1905.

26. Salathe, M. and S. Khandelwal, *Assessing vaccination sentiments with online social media: implications for infectious disease dynamics and control.* PLoS Comput Biol, 2011. **7**(10): p. e1002199.

27. Green, B., T. Horel, and A.V. Papachristos, *Modeling contagion through social networks to explain and predict gunshot violence in Chicago, 2006 to 2014.* JAMA Intern Med, 2017. **177**(3): p. 326–333.

28. Zimmerman, G.M., et al., *The power of (mis)perception: rethinking suicide contagion in youth friendship networks.* Soc Sci Med, 2016. **157**: p. 31–38.

29. Cassidy, R.N., et al., *Initiation of vaporizing cannabis: individual and social network predictors in a longitudinal study of young adults.* Drug Alcohol Depend, 2018. **188**: p. 334–340.

30. Metwally, O., et al., *Using social media to characterize public sentiment toward medical interventions commonly used for cancer screening: an observational study.* J Med Internet Res, 2017. **19**(6): p. e200.

31. Morris, M., H. Epstein, and M. Wawer, *Timing is everything: international variations in historical sexual partnership concurrency and HIV prevalence.* PLoS One, 2010. **5**(11): p. e14092.

32. Moody, J., *The importance of relationship timing for diffusion.* Social Forces, 2002. **81**(1): p. 25–56.

33. Moody, J. and R.A. Benton, *Interdependent effects of cohesion and concurrency for epidemic potential.* Ann Epidemiol, 2016. **26**(4): p. 241–248.

34. Kivela, M., et al., *Multilayer networks.* J Complex Netw, 2014. **2**(3): p. 203–271.

35. Funk, S. and V.A. Jansen, *Interacting epidemics on overlay networks.* Phys Rev E Stat Nonlin Soft Matter Phys, 2010. **81**(3 Pt 2): p. 036118.

36. Burt, R.S., *Social contagion and innovation: cohesion versus structural equivalence.* Am J Sociol, 1987. **92**: p. 1287–1335.

37. Fujimoto, K. and T.W. Valente, *Social network influences on adolescent substance use: disentangling structural equivalence from cohesion.* Soc Sci Med, 2012. **74**(12): p. 1952–1960.

38. Narr, R.K., et al., *Close friendship strength and broader peer group desirability as differential predictors of adult mental health.* Child Dev, 2019. **90**(1): p. 298–313.

39. Copeland, M., et al., *Different kinds of lonely: dimensions of isolation and substance use in adolescence.* J Youth Adolesc, 2018. **47**(8): p. 1755–1770.

40. Borowski, S., et al., *Adolescent controversial status brokers: a double-edged sword.* Sch Psychol Q, 2017. **32**(1): p. 50–61.

41. Shalizi, C.R. and A.C. Thomas, *Homophily and contagion are generically confounded in observational social network studies.* Sociol Methods Res, 2011. **40**(2): p. 211–239.

42. Snijders, T.A.B., C.E.G. Steglich, and M. Schweinberger, *Modeling the co-evolution of networks and behavior*, in *Longitudinal models in the behavioral and related sciences*, K.V. Montfort, H. Oud, and A. Satorra, Editors. 2007, Lawrence Erlbaum: Mahwah, NJ. p. 41–71.

43. Schneider, J.A., et al., *Network mixing and network influences most linked to HIV infection and risk behavior in the HIV epidemic among black men who have sex with men.* Am J Public Health, 2013. **103**(1): p. e28–36.

44. Skaathun, B., et al., *Network viral load: a critical metric for HIV elimination.* J Acquir Immune Defic Syndr, 2018. **77**(2): p. 167–174.

45. Anderson, K., N. Laxhman, and S. Priebe, *Can mental health interventions change social networks? A systematic review.* BMC Psychiatry, 2015. **15**: p. 297.

46. Sendula-Jengic, V., M. Sendula-Pavelic, and J. Hodak, *Mind in the gap between neural and social networks—cyberspace and virtual reality in psychiatry and healthcare.* Psychiatr Danub, 2016. **28**(2): p. 100–103.

47. Bannink, R., et al., *Cyber and traditional bullying victimization as a risk factor for mental health problems and suicidal ideation in adolescents.* PLoS One, 2014. **9**(4): p. e94026.

48. Donoghue, C. and L.J. Meltzer, *Sleep it off: bullying and sleep disturbances in adolescents.* J Adolesc, 2018. **68**: p. 87–93.

49. Marco, J.H. and M.P. Tormo-Irun, *Cyber victimization is associated with eating disorder psychopathology in adolescents.* Front Psychol, 2018. **9**: p. 987.

50. Christakis, N.A. and J.H. Fowler, *The collective dynamics of smoking in a large social network.* N Engl J Med, 2008. **358**: p. 2249–2258.

51. Fowler, J.H. and N.A. Christakis, *Dynamic spread of happiness in a large social network: longitudinal analysis over 20 years in the Framingham Heart Study.* Brit Med J, 2008. **337**: p. a2338.

52. Fowler, J.H., J.E. Settle, and N.A. Christakis, *Correlated genotypes in friendship networks.* Proc Natl Acad Sci U S A, 2011. **108**(5): p. 1993–1997.

53. Falk, E.B. and D.S. Bassett, *Brain and social networks: fundamental building blocks of human experience.* Trends Cogn Sci, 2017. **21**(9): p. P674–690.

54. Zerubavel, N., et al., *Neural precursors of future liking and affective reciprocity.* Proc Natl Acad Sci U S A, 2018. **115**(17): p. 4375–4380.

55. Schmalzle, R., et al., *Brain connectivity dynamics during social interaction reflect social network structure.* Proc Natl Acad Sci U S A, 2017. **114**(20): p. 5153–5158.

56. Sallet, J., et al., *Social network size affects neural circuits in macaques.* Science, 2011. **334**(6056): p. 697–700.

57. Bickart, K.C., et al., *Amygdala volume and social network size in humans.* Nat Neurosci, 2011. **14**(2): p. 163–164.

58. Butts, C.T. and R.M. Acton, *Spatial Modeling of Social Networks*, in *The SAGE Handbook of GIS and Society*, T.L. Nyerges, H. Coucelis, and R. McMaster, Editors. 2011, SAGE: Thousand Oaks, CA. p. 222–250.

59. Lienert, J., et al., *Social influence on 5-year survival in a longitudinal chemotherapy ward co-presence network.* Netw Sci (Camb Univ Press), 2017. **5**(3): p. 308–327.

60. Iwashyna, T.J., et al., *The structure of critical care transfer networks.* Med Care, 2009. **47**(7): p. 787–793.

61. Karkada, U.H., et al., *Limiting the spread of highly resistant hospital-acquired microorganisms via critical care transfers: a simulation study.* Intensive Care Med, 2011. **37**(10): p. 1633–1640.

62. Broniatowski, D.A., M.J. Paul, and M. Dredze, *National and local influenza surveillance through Twitter: an analysis of the 2012-2013 influenza epidemic.* PLoS One, 2013. **8**(12): p. e83672.

63. Ram, S., et al., *Predicting asthma-related emergency department visits using big data.* IEEE J Biomed Health Inform, 2015. **19**(4): p. 1216–1223.

64. Wang, S., M.J. Paul, and M. Dredze, *Social media as a sensor of air quality and public response in China.* J Med Internet Res, 2015. **17**(3): p. e22.

65. Generous, N., et al., *Global disease monitoring and forecasting with Wikipedia.* PLoS Comput Biol, 2014. **10**(11): p. e1003892.

66. Cook, R.L., et al., *What's driving an epidemic? The spread of syphilis along an interstate highway in rural North Carolina.* Am J Public Health, 1999. **89**(3): p. 369–373.

67. Gesink, D.C., et al., *Sexually transmitted disease core theory: roles of person, place, and time.* Am J Epidemiol, 2011. **174**(1): p. 81–89.

68. Dehmamy, N., S. Milanlouei, and A.-L. Barabási, *A structural transition in physical networks.* Nature, 2018. **563**(7733): p. 676–680.

69. Inobaya, M.T., et al., *Prevention and control of schistosomiasis: a current perspective.* Res Rep Trop Med, 2014. **2014**(5): p. 65–75.

70. Evan Secor, W., *Water-based interventions for schistosomiasis control.* Pathog Glob Health, 2014. **108**(5): p. 246–254.

71. Abdel-Wahab, M.F., et al., *Changing pattern of schistosomiasis in Egypt 1935-79.* Lancet, 1979. **2**(8136): p. 242–244.

72. Carlton, E.J., et al., *Associations between schistosomiasis and the use of human waste as an agricultural fertilizer in China.* PLoS Negl Trop Dis, 2015. **9**(1): p. e0003444.

73. Pilosof, S., et al., *Potential parasite transmission in multi-host networks based on parasite sharing.* PLoS One, 2015. **10**(3): p. e0117909.

74. Melnik, S., et al., *The unreasonable effectiveness of tree-based theory for networks with clustering.* Phys Rev E Stat Nonlin Soft Matter Phys, 2011. **83**(3 Pt 2): p. 036112.

75. Nadel, S.F., *The Theory of Social Structure.* 1957, Glencoe, Ill: Free Press.

76. Blanchet, K. and P. James, *How to do (or not to do) . . . a social network analysis in health systems research.* Health Policy Plan, 2012. **27**(5): p. 438–446.

77. Contandriopoulos, D., et al., *Structural analysis of health-relevant policy-making information exchange networks in Canada.* Implement Sci, 2017. **12**(1): p. 116.

78. Wang, G.-X., *Policy network mapping of the universal health care reform in Taiwan: an application of social network analysis.* J Asian Pub Pol, 2013. **6**(3): p. 313–334.

79. Yaliraki, S. and A. Darzi. *Community detection, roles and information flows in social networks for the analysis of public opinion and patient engagement in public health policy.* Social network analysis for health policy n.d.; Available from: https://www.imperial.ac.uk/mathematics-precision-healthcare/research/social-network-analysis-for-health-policy/.

80. Leppin, A.L., et al., *Applying social network analysis to evaluate implementation of a multisector population health collaborative that uses a bridging hub organization.* Front Public Health, 2018. **6**: p. 315.

5

Phase Transitions and Resilience in Physical and Psychological Health

MARCEL G. M. OLDE RIKKERT, NOEMI SCHUURMAN, AND RENÉ J. F. MELIS

5.1. INTRODUCTION

To explain the usefulness of complexity science in medicine and clinical psychology, we will start with answering the golden *why*. Why do we need complex systems theory in studying diseases? Thereafter, we will discuss *how* this complexity thinking affects medicine, and *what* specific tools from complexity science can be applied. Both will be detailed in an in-depth description of our understanding of resilience and the dynamics of tipping points (TPs) that are often met in clinical practice. This will be followed by a methodological description of how the complexity and resilience of human physiological and psychological systems can be studied and quantified in medicine and psychology. We will end this chapter picturing the horizon of the next stage of application of complexity science in patient care and medical science.

5.1.1 The Why of Complex Systems for Complex Patients

The adjective "complex" for patients describes them in abstract ways as a multicomponent system (1), with many (feedback) interactions (2), that are at least partly nonlinear (3), history and environment dependent (4), and of different temporal and spatial scales (5).[1] The components can be organs, but also components in the environment (e.g., the patient's family) that impact the patient's physical and psychological health. In the following sections, we will discuss examples in which the complexity lens in medicine and psychology is helpful

Marcel G. M. Olde Rikkert, Noemi Schuurman, and René J. F. Melis, *Phase Transitions and Resilience in Physical and Psychological Health* In: *Complex Systems and Population Health*. Edited by: Yorghos Apostolopoulos, Kristen Hassmiller Lich, and Michael Kenneth Lemke, Oxford University Press (2020). © Oxford University Press.
DOI: 10.1093/oso/9780190880743.003.0005

in understanding and forecasting critical transitions between different disease states.

5.1.2. Complexity in Older Persons

Many examples of transitions and cascades of change can be seen in older people, who repeatedly have to adapt to changing conditions due to social change (e.g., retirement, loss of spouse) or incident chronic diseases (e.g., heart failure, dementia) against the background of the physiology of aging that involves diminishing physical and cognitive reserve capacity. The underlying multimorbidity dominantly presents in almost all older persons, and their multiform interactions (between the multiple disease causes, the symptoms, the medicines, and the other treatment components such as exercise and diet) reflect the multiple-agent condition in humans.[2] In these clinical scenarios, it is widely recognized that the linearly organized medical practice, fueled by the science of single disease management, is insufficient to understand, study, and handle such complex multimorbidity conditions.[3,4]

Many other patient problems may also profit from enriching the classical medical and psychological knowledge base by using a complexity science perspective. This holds true within the single disease domain, be it for complex chronic diseases such as depression, diabetes, or Alzheimer's disease or for infectious diseases such as HIV. All show similar complex phenomena in pathophysiology: They have multiple etiological and interacting components, multiple factors determining nonlinear spread, multiple organs involved in different historical time lines, and thus different consecutive stages and emerging stage-transitions in their patient's journeys.[5,6] This warrants a complexity science perspective in healthcare sciences as well as in psychological and medical sciences.

5.1.3 How Complexity Thinking Affects Medicine

The paths to improved understanding of many human diseases, including cancer, diabetes, chronic inflammatory diseases, and neurodegenerative disorders, lie in understanding the changed functioning (and malfunctioning) of interactions between biological components.[7] Often malfunctioning of a single organ (or organ part) does not cause serious problems due to redundancy in the physiological networks, but the combined effects of multiple malfunctioning components of an interacting network of organs are substantial and life threatening. For example, hippocampal and prefrontal cortex atrophy are often seen together with white matter lesions as malfunctioning components or nodes, of which only the summed pathophysiology in the neuronal network causes cognition and functional performance to deteriorate in daily living so that dementia must be diagnosed. An understanding of how individual (sub)components function is helpful, but not enough to understand the whole disease severity and the individually emerging disease presentations. This means that reducing the research focus to smaller and smaller components, which is the traditional scientific approach, has limits in understanding individual patients and the huge variation present in clinical practice. Precision medicine, with a focus on genetic, proteomic and metabolomic phenotyping, will not be able to forecast treatment effects in complex diseases that are further determined by relevant interactions at a higher level of scale (e.g., increasing amyloid-beta knowledge in Alzheimer's disease did not result in a single trial with positive effects on cognition and daily functioning nor in accurate predictions of Alzheimer disease trajectories). This requires multiscale modeling and predictors at a higher level, integrating not only molecular, cellular, and organ but also individual and group pathophysiological factors (e.g., also white matter lesions, sleep quality, loneliness, and caregiver support probably highly determine Alzheimer treatment effect and prognosis).[8]

5.1.4 Tools for Investigating HUMAN complexity

There are three modes of investigation of human physiology when working within complexity science: *theoretical, computational, and experimental*. These modes increasingly include quantitative, realistic, and even predictive models, bringing together statistical data analysis, modeling efforts, analytical approaches, and laboratory experiments.

As evidenced by the growing literature on complexity and TPs in medicine and psychology,[9,10] these constructs are already being applied in medical research and clinical practice. This may lead to an exciting time where our current, more static concepts of chronic diseases are likely to change, in favor of highly dynamic concepts with multiple scales taken into account in understanding and influencing health and disease.[10]

Complexity science perspectives in medicine and psychology demand attitudes quite different from those in physics, chemistry, and mathematics, where one may successfully search for fundamental laws, true for all conditions. Biological complex systems are different, as they also experience evolution, degeneration, and loss of entropy by added energy and human behavior, in contrast with the second law of thermodynamics that predicts stability of entropy in closed systems in equilibrium state and increase of entropy in open natural processes. Thus, there probably are no general laws for complexity in the domain of human physiology. Nevertheless, we may sharpen our reasoning on human complexity in health and disease by learning how complexity science tools were applied and helped to explain complex behaviors in other solid matter, biological and social systems. In the following section, we will discuss some of these tools, including (indicators of) TPs and resilience in the context of medicine and clinical psychology.

5.2. TIPPING POINTS, TRANSITIONS, AND RESILIENCE

It is becoming increasingly evident that many complex systems have critical thresholds, or TPs, during which the system shifts abruptly from one state to another. In clinical practice we often meet such unpredicted TPs, which therefore probably are the most undisputed phenomena that fit better with complexity than with deterministic theory. Well-known examples of TPs include acute transition toward delirium episodes, heart failure crises, recurrent falls, migraine attacks, epileptic seizures, and other acute severity states. In the psychological domain, the TPs in bipolar disorder are also studied using complexity science methods. The common denominator of complex systems in which these TPs for acute and theoretically reversible changes are observed is that they all rely on one or more positive feedback mechanisms. These can accelerate change and propel the system over the TP and into a different and less preferable, but stable, diseased state.

Within dynamic systems theory, the mathematical catastrophe model helps to understand how changes in a patients' systemic resilience act as risk markers of increased likelihood of passing TPs. In this model, TPs are known as catastrophic bifurcations. These bifurcations can be easily imagined for the equilibrium state of an older patient that can respond with either recovery or severe complications to stressors such as surgery or chemotherapy. Although some older patients (the "systems") with sufficient *resilience* may respond well, change can also be dramatic in patients with low resilience, causing a complication to pass a TP. The situation in which critical transitions occur, for example, toward delirium, a syncope (fall due to insufficient cerebral perfusion), or a stroke, can be modeled by an equilibrium curve that is acutely "folded." Notably, when a patient is close to such a "fold," or TP bifurcation, a minor stressor can already push his system across the safe boundary. Although declining systemic resilience may seemingly have little effect on older (or intensive care) patients when they are not meeting (anymore) stressors, they may be in a situation where even small (additional) stressors may push these patients over a TP, which shows lack of resilience. The concept of systemic resilience is therefore closely connected to the TP theory. However, it is in fact not obvious that a single overarching resilience property for the whole system exists that might determine the risk of passing through and recovering from TPs for the most important disease states in older adults. In principle, the acute severity states in different organs may have their own specific resilience. It is not yet known whether systemic resilience can be validly assessed.

Historically, resilience in humans was first defined as the system's ability to cope with stress and preserve functioning.[17] Since then, systemic resilience has been predominantly studied in the stress recovery system of the hypothalamic–pituitary–adrenal axis. Later, resilience was studied in-depth in medicine in the domains of psychology and psychiatry, where it was defined as the capacity to recover following psychosocial stressors.[18] A growing series of empirical studies in living systems returned to the original stress-concept of resilience and showed that this may be quantified by several mathematical measures of slowing recovery of complex systems from stressors, both artificial (e.g., heat, chemicals) and natural (e.g., climate change).[9] This was confirmed by controlled laboratory experiments, initially with cyanobacteria and algae.[10,11]

5.2.1. Resilience Indicators in Clinical Psychology

Although the study of complex systems in psychology is young, research on resilience and resilience indicators has made remarkable progress in recent years, especially in the context of emotional regulation research and research on psychopathology networks. Psychopathology network researchers conceptualize psychological disorders as a disordered state of a network of symptoms that directly affect each other and themselves over time.[12-14] Emotion regulation research focuses on the dynamics of emotions and particularly the (mal)adaptive responses of people's emotion processes to internal and external stimuli.[15]

Both fields are related in the sense that complex psychological dynamic systems are the central focus, and this system may become disordered at some point in time. The resilience of the systems determines (in part) the likelihood of unwanted outcomes occurring. For example, a lack of resilience in emotion processes is considered to play a key role in psychological maladjustment, including the development of psychological disorders.[15] In psychopathology networks, people who have symptom networks that are characterized by low resilience are prone to develop psychological disorders.[12,13]

In both emotion regulation and psychopathology network research, a lack of resilience is present when individuals are relatively strongly affected by, and show relatively weak recovery from, the effects of momentary perturbations on the psychological variables (emotions or symptoms) under study.[16] These perturbations can be either negative (e.g., stressors ranging from missing a train, to breaking up with one's partner) or positive (e.g., viewing beautiful art or getting a promotion at work). People with low resilience will have longer-lasting effects of perturbations on their emotions or symptoms, and because there is little recovery, the effects of multiple (even small) perturbations can more easily build up to problematic levels. Key indicators of a lack of resilience of the dynamic system that have been used in psychology are similar dynamical indicators of resilience as used in medical research: strong autocorrelations in the time series for the variables of interest (e.g., emotions or symptoms), strong cross-correlations (interrelations over time) between these variables, and high variability of these variables over time.

For example, a person with a strongly connected network of depression symptoms (see Figure 5.1) will, for example, after experiencing chronic stress (e.g., exacerbated by a strong autoregression for stress or worrying), more easily develop a depressed mood, then worry more, which may lead to sleep problems, subsequently fatigue, and then concentration problems, issues at work and self-reproach, and even more feelings of worthlessness (see Figure 5.1C).[12] On the other hand, someone for whom the effects of stress on mood, of worrying and fatigue on sleep problems and concentration, or of failure on their sense of self-worth are weak will be more resilient against developing a major depressive disorder (see Figure 5.1D).

Autocorrelation has arguably had the most attention within the context of emotion regulation, where it is used as a measure of "emotional inertia" or resistance to change in emotions,[16,17] although it is also an important part of dynamic (psychopathology) networks.[13] The autocorrelation (or autoregression coefficients) for a particular psychological variable (e.g., mood or a symptom) is obtained through time series modeling, and may be negative or positive (ranging from –1 to 1). Positive autocorrelations indicate that a relatively low score now (e.g., for mood) will partly carry over to the scores at later times. Positive autocorrelations are expected to occur for a plethora of psychological variables, especially those pertaining to mood, given that these are considered to typically show some stability over time. Negative autocorrelations indicate that a low score at this moment is followed by a high score at later times, and vice versa. This is something that is rarely seen for psychological variables but may occur for disordered psychological processes of intake (e.g., eating disorders). The stronger the autocorrelations, the stronger the carryover, and the easier it will be to predict future states of the variable from a past state. Importantly, this also means that the variables will recover relatively slowly from perturbations, because their effects are carried over for some period of time (see Figure 5.1A). Multiple perturbations will also more easily add up over time as a result of this. Hence, strong autocorrelation is used as an indication of low resilience. In contrast, when autocorrelations are weak, this indicates that each moment is a "new moment," with little or no

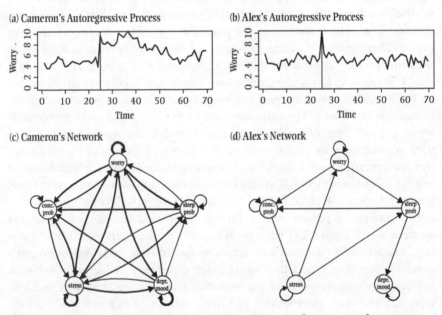

Figure 5.1 Panels A and B: Simulated autoregressive process for worrying for (hypothetical) individuals "Cameron," with an autocorrelation of 0.7 (A), and individual "Alex," with an autocorrelation of 0.1 (B). Both individuals experience a strong stressor at time point 25, but Cameron recovers much more slowly than Alex, because Cameron's process has more moment-to-moment carry-over. Panels C and D: Psychopathology networks for individuals Cameron (C) and Alex (D). Cameron's network is more densely connected than Alex's network, which has less, and weaker, autoregressive and cross-lagged associations.

carryover from previous moments, and as such the relatively resilient system can "recover" very rapidly from perturbations (see Figure 5.1B).

Multiple studies in psychology show evidence that emotional inertia is a risk factor for psychological maladjustment. For example, the level of people's emotional inertia has been found to be correlated to neuroticism, low self-esteem, lower overall positive affect, and higher negative affect; having a major depressive disorder; and even the onset of major depressive disorder two years later.[15,17]

Strong cross-correlations (or cross-lagged effects), which are correlations between variables over time, are also considered indicative of a lower resilience of psychological systems. If variables are strongly interconnected, the effects of perturbations on one variable in the system easily spread to other variables and, hence, can alter the system on a larger scale than may be expected based on just the original perturbation. As such, and especially when strong cross-correlations are combined with strong autocorrelations, consequences of small perturbations can be severe. This idea is central to psychopathology networks, which consist of networks of interrelated symptoms of psychological disorders.[12-14]

High variability in variables over time is also considered an indication of a lack of resilience to perturbations, such as when someone is overly reactive to what could be considered small stressors.[15] However, researchers report some concern in the robustness of using variability as an indicator for resilience, because high variability may also result due to actual strong perturbations instead of overreactions, low variability may also be maladaptive (e.g., when someone is so impervious to perturbations that emotions lose their adaptive function),[15] and a lower variance may also result due to either very low or very high mean levels of symptoms or emotions (ceiling or floor effects).[16,18]

As discussed previously, changes in resilience may indicate tipping points for sudden transitions in complex systems. Changes in resilience indicators, such as increasing autocorrelations, variances, and cross-correlations, thus may be used as early warning signals for sudden transitions from a normal healthy state to a disordered state.[16,19] Recent work in the context of psychopathology networks provides evidence in line with this, mainly in the context of the development of major depressive disorder (MDD). For example, van de Leemput et al.[16] found that people who showed sudden transitions from normal to depressive states, or vice versa, also had stronger autocorrelations, correlations between emotion scores, and higher variability in these scores before this transition, than people that did not show such transitions. Furthermore, in a case study, a person who had experienced repeated relapse into MDD was taken of their antidepressants during a healthy state (double blind), which eventually resulted in a sudden transition back into depression, and early warning signals were observed before this transition.[19]

Note that not all depression states are the result of a sudden transition, as gradual development is also observed among patients and is consistent with complex systems theory. What kind of change will occur in practice will most likely depend on the circumstances. For example, Cramer et al.[14] showed through simulations of MDD as a complex system people with dense networks may develop depression gradually, while people with strongly connected networks may be prone to sudden transitions to depression. Others presented time series models to study the nature of bipolar disorder and found in their empirical examples that one patient's disorder was better described by gradual transitions between manic and depressive states, while others showed sudden transitions.[20]

5.2.2. Resilience Indicators in Medicine

Personalized healthcare requires a balanced judgment based on the present disease states and the resilience of an individual person to resist or recover from alteration on one or more of these disease severity states. However, whereas a huge knowledge base is available about diseases, we know very little on how people resist, recover from, and adapt to disease. The same is true for how people will respond to or recover from treatment and surgery. This implies that, in medicine, we often have more knowledge on the perturbation (the external factor challenging the equilibrium of the system; i.e., the disease or treatment) than we have on the capacity of the system (the person involved) to deal with this perturbation. In disaster and public health-based theory, resilience is the trajectory a system follows in time while being perturbated. In public health, we want to predict prior to the perturbation the system will respond and how to design systems to maximize their resilience (ability to resist and readily rebound from) perturbations. This is equally true for clinical medicine. It assumes that the response of the system is followed in time (the so-called resilience trajectory) to quantify the resistance and recovery of the system after the perturbation. However, out the same negligence of resilience in clinical medicine, resilience trajectories are not often followed in a systematic way and with objective measures. This leaves clinicians to their clinical intuitions when predicting and following resilience for health challenges or treatments.

This may not be as problematic when enough resilience can be assumed. However, it is problematic and may cause iatrogenic damage when a person has multimorbidity or frailty. A lack of objective resilience indicators makes it difficult to provide personalized healthcare, and timely management of delayed recovery is often not possible. With the increasing availability of (sensor-based) time series on health indicators, the advent of new (dynamic) indicators of resilience now offers a means to quantify, monitor and understand resistance and recovery in medicine.

5.2.3. Indicators of Resilience

Possible measures to serve as indicators of resilience in medicine can be similarly as in the abovementioned field of psychology derived from dynamical systems theory, which first suggests "that the recovery rate after small experimental perturbation can be used as an indicator of how close a system is to bifurcation point."[7p1120] Indeed, in the literature, a number of striking similarities between warning signals for impending acute transitions across a range of chronic episodic disorders have been described, each characterized by longer recovery times following a stressor.[6-8] For example, elongation of the recovery period following an acute heart failure episode acts as risk marker for quick relapse of heart failure (Table 5.1), longer recovery time of repolarization in cardiac muscle cells (longer QTc interval) increases the risk of ventricular fibrillation, and longer neuronal recovery times in epilepsy and migraine predict subsequent seizures and headache attacks. On the other hand, very short periods of state change, also called "flickering," may also signal a later more permanent change (e.g., flickering periods of paroxysmal atrial fibrillation, before chronic atrial fibrillation or only more lasting recovery from substance abuse after several short attempts of quitting but with quick relapse, before it sticks).

In clinical practice, these principles may serve to develop bedside tests to measure the physical resilience of a patient by the development of tests based on the stimulus–response paradigm. These tests apply a standardized, but safe (in the sense that it doesn't carry the risk to elicit the actual critical transition),

Table 5.1 RECOVERY TIMES AS AN INDICATOR OF RESILIENCE AND PROGNOSIS FOR RECOVERY AFTER PASSING TIPPING POINTS IN THE COURSE OF A RANGE OF CHRONIC DISEASES.[6]

Discipline	Disease	Recovery time	Disease state predicted by longer recovery time
Cardiology	Arrhythmia	QTc elongation time	Torsade de Pointe arrhythmia
G-enterology	Colitis	Clearing time clostridium dif.	Clostridium D. overgrowth
Geriatrics	Falls	Centre of mass recovery time	Falls, loss of balance
Hematology	Acute leukemia	Lymphocyte recovery time	Relapse of disease
Immunology	Breast cancer	Lymphocyte recovery time	Relapse of disease
Neurology	Epilepsy	Depolarization recovery time	Epileptic state
Oncology	Neck cancer	Lesion regression time	Relapse state
Psychiatry	Depression	Positive mood recovery time	Depressed state
Public Health	Smoking	Craving decay over time	Relapse of smoking
Pulmonology	Tube-ventilation	Ventilation recovery time	Ventilation weaning failure

Source: Olde Rikkert MG, Dakos V, Buchman TG, et al. Slowing down of recovery as generic risk marker for acute severity transitions in chronic diseases. Crit Care Med. 2016;44:601–606. doi:10.1097/CCM.0000000000001564

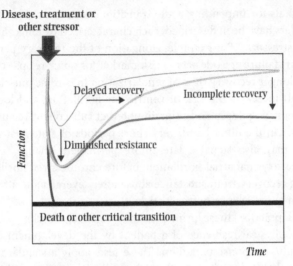

Figure 5.2 Relation between resistance and recovery as part of overall dynamical resilience of a person following a stressor or disease.

perturbation, and the response of the system perturbated is followed both for how much the system is perturbated (resistance) and for the recovery time (Figure 5.2).

Empirical evidence for the feasibility and validity of such stimulus–response paradigm based tests is available as is illustrated by impaired systolic blood pressure recovery after standing up under test conditions, which was predictive of this person's survival in the following period.[21] A second class of measures may be offered by characteristic changes in the patterns of fluctuations of a system in the response of the system to the natural perturbations it is permanently subject to. This response may also change when a system's resilience is changing. The specific changes hypothesized are an increase in variance and temporal autocorrelation within time series as well as an increased cross-correlation in two or more time series describing aspects of the functioning of the system of interest. In this respect, we followed the self-perceived physical, mental and social well-being of 20 persons living in a nursing home for 100 days, and this provided empirical evidence of the validity of these Dynamical Indicators of Resilience (DIORs) in discriminating persons with different levels of frailty.[2] In a group of high-functional older persons (i.e., the opposite of frailty) the DIORs (especially variance) also discriminated persons at different levels of successful aging persistently over one-year follow-up.[8] These DIORs may prove valuable as dynamical resilience indicators in other time series of biological systems as well.

5.3. FUTURE CLINICAL APPLICATIONS

Applying complexity science methods, if clinically verified, may lead to major scientific breakthroughs in psychology and medicine, as this could lead to new individualized forecasting tools to be used in a wide range of diseases and clusters of symptoms. The toolbox of time series analyses techniques and DIORs could go "viral" in a range of medical disciplines, as many medical researchers, psychologists and physicians regularly encounter TP dynamics.

However, first we must tackle the major challenge of moving complexity science applications beyond group level validity and realize improved predictions based on individual time series that may positively guide individual older patients toward improved outcomes. This may seem far away; however, studies on continuous glucose, wearable sensors, and electro-encephalographic monitoring already suggest that this complexity science approach enables improved forecasting and have successfully prevented hypoglycemic episodes, as well as epileptic seizures by a more reliable warning system for upcoming seizures.[21-24] In psychology, individual time series of mood and experienced emotion already can help explain major changes in mood in patients with bipolar disorders.[16,25]

Whether and how these tools will be implemented in clinical practice on a global scale is hard to predict, but complexity science tools may show up as emergent support tools in our more and more complex patient populations, and likewise in our complex medical system. Further, some of these tools are already in use in clinical practice, such as in intensive care units as wearable devices to alarm periods during which patients have higher risks on epileptic insults.[22] This can lead to changes in medication or lifestyle to guide patients toward a more resilient state, which may be considered as concrete successes of complexity science in medicine.

5.4. CONCLUSIONS

After a period of reductionism in medical and psychological sciences and clinical forecasting, focusing on in-depth and detailed characterization of individual diseases, molecular, cellular, and organ functions at a single time point, we can now make a move toward linking these subparts in human physiology and psychology. This integrative change is greatly supported by the availability of complexity science tools for time series and network analyses, and the clinical availability of technical devices ("wearables") to follow bodily and psychological signals reliably over time. This creates new data sets, not just consisting of large amounts of data (as in "big data"), but foremost of "complex data" with numerous interdependencies in the data structure. These data are interrelated as large series of data are acquired per person, which therefore have multiple cross- and auto-correlations. The current growth of complexity science with methodology to intelligently and reproducibly analyze such data is timely and pushes the frontier of insight in the complex problems of both the outside skin and the inside skin world greatly forward.

This results in many complex clinical and research questions and hypotheses to be answered and tested, complex data to be analyzed, and innovations to be developed using dynamic network knowledge and dynamic forecasting signals from clinical practice. Iterative cycles of knowledge acquisition and implementation according to complexity science may finally integrate specialized subparts of human knowledge again and therefore may also bridge the gaps between the many super-specialists and their disciplines involved in this process. Therefore, the application of complexity science in medicine, psychology and the humanities has the potential to open new horizons of interdisciplinary (team) research on the complex big clinical problems, such as how to manage the quickly increasing chronic and multimorbid disease burden and how to improve resilience for the stressors of modern life that we now globally face.

REFERENCES

1. Prigogine I. Sengers I. Order out of chaos. 2017, Verso New York. (Original publication 1978)
2. Gijzel SMW, van de Leemput IA, Scheffer M, et al. Dynamical resilience indicators in time series of self-rated health correspond to frailty levels in older adults. J Gerontol A Biol Sci Med Sci. 2017;72:991–996. doi:10.1093/gerona/glx065.
3. MacMahon S. Multimorbidity a priority for global health research. 2018, London.
4. Editor Lancet. Making more of multimorbidity: an emerging priority. Lancet. 2018;28;391:1637. doi:10.1016/S0140-6736(18)30941-3
5. Richters A, Nieuwboer MS, Olde Rikkert MGM, et al. Longitudinal multiple case study on effectiveness of network-based dementia care towards more integration, quality of care, and collaboration in primary care. PLoS One. 2018;13:e0198811. doi:10.1371/journal.pone.0198811.
6. Olde Rikkert MG, Dakos V, Buchman TG, et al. Slowing down of recovery as generic risk marker for acute severity transitions in chronic diseases. Crit Care Med. 2016;44:601–606. doi:10.1097/CCM.0000000000001564
7. Gijzel SMW, van de Leemput IA, Scheffer M, et al. Dynamical indicators of resilience in postural balance time series are related to successful aging in high-functioning older adults. J Gerontol A Biol Sci Med Sci. 2018;74:1119–1126. doi:10.1093/gerona/gly170
8. Canli T, Yu L, Yu X, Zhao H, et al. Loneliness 5 years ante-mortem is associated with disease-related differential gene expression in postmortem dorsolateral prefrontal cortex. Transl Psychiatry. 2018;10:2. doi:10.1038/s41398-017-0086-2.
9. van Nes EH, Arani BMS, Staal A, van der Bolt B, Flores BM, Bathiany S, Scheffer M. What do you mean, "tipping point"? Trends Ecol Evol. 2016;31:902–904. doi:10.1016/j.tree.2016.09.011
10. Scheffer, M. Carpenter SR, Lenton TM, et al. Anticipating critical transitions. Science. 2012;338:344–348. doi:10.1126/science.1225244
11. Veraart AJ, Faassen EJ, Dakos V, van Nes EH, Lürling M, Scheffer M. Recovery rates reflect distance to a tipping point in a living system. Nature. 2011;481:357–359. doi:10.1038/nature10723
12. Borsboom D, Cramer A. Network analysis: an integrative approach to the structure of psychopathology. Annu Rev Clin Psychol. 2013;9:91–121.
13. Bringmann, L, et al. A network approach to psychopathology: new insights into clinical longitudinal data. PloS One. 2013;8:e60188.
14. Cramer A. et al. Major depression as a complex dynamic system. PLoS One. 2016;11:e0167490.

15. Kuppens, Peter, Nicholas B. et al. Emotional inertia and psychological maladjustment. Psychol Sci. 2010;21:984–991.

16. van de Leemput, IA, Wichers, M. Cramer AOJ, et al. Critical slowing down as early warning for the onset and termination of depression. Proc Natl Acad Sci U S A. 2014:111:E879.

17. Suls J, Green P, Hillis S. Emotional reactivity to everyday problems, affective inertia, and neuroticism. Person Soc Psychol Bull. 1998;24:127–136.

18. Bos E, De Jonge P. Critical slowing down in depression is a great idea that still needs empirical proof. Proc Natl Acad Sci U S A. 2014;111:E878–E878.

19. Wichers M., et al. Critical slowing down as a personalized early warning signal for depression. Psychother Psychosom. 2016;85:114–116.

20. Hamaker E, Grasman R, Kamphuis JH. Modeling BAS dysregulation in bipolar disorder: Illustrating the potential of time series analysis. Assessment. 2016;23:436–446.

21. Lagro J, Schoon Y, Heerts I, et al. Impaired systolic blood pressure recovery directly after standing predicts mortality in older falls clinic patients. J Gerontol A Biol Sci Med Sci. 2014;69:471–478. doi:10.1093/gerona/glt111.

22. Cook MJ, O'Brien TJ, Berkovic SF, et al. Prediction of seizure likelihood with a long-term, implanted seizure advisory system in patients with drug-resistant epilepsy: a first-in-man study. Lancet Neurol. 2013;12:563–571. doi:10.1016/S1474-4422(13)70075.

23. Abraham MB, Davey R, O'Grady MJ, et al. Effectiveness of a predictive algorithm in the prevention of exercise-induced hypoglycemia in type 1 diabetes. Diabetes Technol Ther. 2016;8(9):543–550.

24. van Beers CA, DeVries JH. Continuous glucose monitoring: impact on hypoglycemia. J Diabetes Sci Technol. 2016;10(6):1251–1258.

25. David SJ, Marshall AJ, Evanovich EK, et al. Intraindividual dynamic network analysis—implications for clinical assessment. J Psychopathol Behav Assess. 2018;40:235–248. doi:10.1007/s10862-017-9632-8.

6

How Complex Systems Science Can Revolutionize Population Health Theory

PATRICIA GOODSON

> Most of our assumptions have outlived their uselessness.
>
> —*Marshall McLuhan*

6.1. INTRODUCTION

This chapter's title is "loaded": It presupposes complex systems science (CSS) *can*, in fact, deeply transform population health theory and all that readers (you) need to learn is *how* this happens. Yet, because unexamined assumptions can be dangerous, I argue for a more fruitful approach and ask instead: "*Can* CSS indeed revolutionize population health theory?" If the answer is "yes," only then should we determine "how."

Another supposition, however, also underlies the title: the change CSS could engender is nothing short of "revolutionary." Notice the question is not whether CSS can *contribute to, influence,* or *amend* population health theory. The title goes for the jugular: *revolutionize*—meaning, "change . . . radically or fundamentally."[1] By asking how CSS can *revolutionize* population health theory, we presuppose current theory requires changing—and *drastic* change, no less.

Therefore, before examining *how* CSS might ignite a theory revolution, we need to ask both questions: "Does current population health theory *need* revolutionizing?" If so, "*Can* CSS spark the revolution?"

Patricia Goodson, *How Complex Systems Science Can Revolutionize Population Health Theory* In: *Complex Systems and Population Health.* Edited by: Yorghos Apostolopoulos, Kristen Hassmiller Lich, and Michael Kenneth Lemke, Oxford University Press (2020). © Oxford University Press. DOI: 10.1093/oso/9780190880743.003.0006

To answer these, I define "theorizing," first, and outline several difficulties encountered in current theorizing. This brief incursion will help decide whether population health theory needs reform and, if it does, whether CSS can spark change. Subsequently, I discuss three ways in which CSS may affect current theory building/testing and conclude with examples alongside a quick reference to implications of a "theory revolution."

6.2. THEORY AND THEORIZING

Theory constitutes a phenomenon found only in human language. It is "no more than a linguistic device used to organize a complex empirical world."[2p496] *How* people use language to organize that world varies, but scientists build narratives explaining cause-and-effect relationships among factors and phenomena. Put simply, *theories are stories* crafted to make sense of experience. Scientific theories describe, explain, and predict phenomena.[3 p8,2p496]

In a previous text, I explored what theory *does* and how theory and practice are intimately connected.[3p9] There I concluded *theorizing is practice,* because building theory means engaging in the practical task of "mak[ing] the world *understandable.*"[4p65]

This *theorizing practice* is essential to applied fields such as population health. Why? Because it is through making sense of and trying to fully understand well-being and healthy living that scientists, practitioners, policymakers, educators, and laypeople create ways to improve and promote health.

Throughout its history, public health scholars have borrowed narratives produced in various disciplines—Psychology, Sociology, Economics, Biology, Genetics, Epidemiology, and Resource Management/Development, among others—to explain people's experiences with health, morbidity, and access to care. But theories and models designed to address phenomena *unique* to population health also have emerged. As examples, we recall the Health Belief Model, the PRECEDE–PROCEDE model, Socio-Ecological Models, Life-Course theories/models, gene–environment interaction models, and health services/healthcare theories.[5p552,6-9]

6.3. DIFFICULTIES EMBEDDED IN CURRENT POPULATION HEALTH THEORIZING

Despite their utility, these theories have become inadequate for explaining matters in the 20th and 21st centuries. Although space in this chapter is limited for delving into the inadequacies of most population theories—see Chapters 1, 19, and 20 of this volume for more—here I list three salient difficulties.

First, most theories focus primarily on causal factors within a *single level of explanation.*[3p245] The preferred one is the individual or intrapersonal factors level, where explanations for well-being reside in people's behaviors, cognitions, emotions, and abilities. This focus neglects causal forces from other levels and ignores the *interactions* among factors from (or across) various levels (e.g., a person's self-efficacy and the environmental barriers that moderate it). In the same manner, when scientists from disciplines such as Sociology, Social Epidemiology, or Community Psychology study structural factors (e.g., institutional racism or poverty), they tend to ignore variables found at the individual level, such as people's cognitive or biological features. Beckfield and Krieger noted, when reviewing 45 empirical studies "on the political production of health inequity,"[10p168] that "the empirical literature to date has focused on a relatively narrow range of political determinants of health inequities."[10p168]

Second, most population health theories employ reductionist "lenses" or paradigms.[3] Although focusing on a single explanatory level is already a type of reductionism, here I use *reductionism* as the view that the best way to understand a phenomenon *as a whole* is to reduce it to its main components, and then study each component in depth.[11] One example of this narrow perspective is the disproportionate focus on *rationality* as the predominant mechanism governing health behaviors. Most current theories explaining health behaviors are value-expectancy or rational choice theories[12] claiming human actions result from one critical mechanism: intentionally and rationally weighing pros and cons. Reductionism is also exemplified in theories focusing on structural factors shaping human health, which home in on social structures, exclusively—neglecting effects from the built environment or from the dynamic interactions among social, physical, and virtual environments.[10]

A third major difficulty most contemporary population health theories exhibit—even when they attempt to be multidimensional—is the *privileging of linearity*[3p123] whereby the dynamic, reciprocal and continual "movements" over time among factors and their nested systems are absent. At its most basic, linearity presupposes that more of one factor leads to more (or less) of another factor, that outputs from a system can be predicted from the sum of its inputs (a feature termed *superposition*), and that these outputs correlate, proportionately, with the inputs feeding them (the *proportionality* notion[13]). Other linearity principles we see employed in population health are hierarchy (control is centralized in a system), false dichotomies (social factors standing in contrast to genetic factors), independence of events (orthogonality and no multicollinearity in statistics), and unidirectionality (forces or factors influencing health outcomes in a single direction: the factor affects the outcome, and not vice versa).[6p53,13p1]

A closer look at 21st-century developments reveals public health has had a hard time dealing with deep-seated problems that resist simplistic, linear, or reductionist solutions such as health disparities or inequities, emerging or recurring epidemics, and widespread, chronic immune system dysfunctions (resulting in various cancers, AIDS, and auto-immune illnesses). Existing population health theories have struggled with these "wicked" or intractable problems involving complex dynamic interactions among structural and global factors such as political regimes, wars, climate change, widespread poverty, and human rights.[14]

6.4. MECHANISMS THROUGH WHICH COMPLEX SYSTEMS SCIENCE CAN AFFECT CURRENT POPULATION HEALTH THEORY

A CSS approach offers valuable alternatives to the prevailing theories explaining population health,[15] and there are three mechanisms[16] through which scholars can employ CSS to affect, influence, change and, yes, even *revolutionize* current population health theorizing:

1. *Juxtaposing* constructs from linear and complex systems theories.
2. *Integrating* CSS methods into current linear theories.
3. *Questioning current theories' assumptions* and reframing the problem(s).

6.4.1. Juxtaposing Constructs from Linear and Complex Systems Theories

Population health scholars have been juxtaposing or using constructs from both linear and complex systems theories in tandem, for a long time. Although most health theories can be characterized as single-level, reductionist, and linear, some do incorporate *constructs or concepts* from complexity theories that attempt to reflect change over time, multilevel interactions among factors, cyclical events, or other dynamic factors.

"Stage Models," such as the Transtheoretical Model of Change and the Precaution Adoption Process Model, for example, assume "behavior change is a process that unfolds *over time* through a sequence of stages."[17p97] These models acknowledge the dynamic role time plays in shaping behavior and describe changes by contrasting different phases. Yet, even though these theories embed dynamic concepts, they lack mechanisms to capture the *change process* itself. The best these theories can muster is to take "before-and-after" snapshots of specific behaviors, describing the "before" as one stage and the "after," as another. Moreover, this "before-and-after" approach focuses only on a couple outcome variables and disregards the reciprocal interactions among those variables, as well as among outcome and input variables in their system. The linearity lens, therefore, remains the backdrop against which these more dynamic constructs are interpreted, resulting, ultimately, in a nondynamic depiction.

When deploying the notions of *systems* and *socioecological determinants* of health, scholars also are juxtaposing complexity-related constructs (e.g., social norms' influence on individual behavior) with linear factors and perspectives (e.g., an individual's perception of those norms). Yet, even when doing so, most theorizing about systems and multilevel factors rely on linear assumptions as well as on linear measures and statistical analyses (e.g., employing a General Linear Model[18] to test associations between perceived social norms and individual behavior).

6.4.2. Integrating CSS Methods into Current Linear Theories

That people are embedded within dynamic systems is not a new notion; research and interventions in public health's early history accounted for it (e.g., the practice of quarantine during infectious outbreaks as a way to avoid spread or contagion). In the mid-20th century, however, innovations and improvements in statistics and computing power prompted better analytic tools to frame and examine these interactions. Studies of social networks and the relationships therein, for instance, as well as the effects these relationships have upon the network's components and on the network as a whole, began to emerge in various disciplines.[19] Network analysis soon became invaluable for understanding health-related issues such as obesity, smoking, drug use, romantic ties among adolescents, transmissible infections, and other topics[20-23] (for more on Networks, see Chapters 2, 4, and 11 of this volume).

Although network analysis began a movement to reframe various population health problems, many researchers adopt the analysis as a mere methodological tool or as another way to explore health problems still tethered to the "same old" linearity assumptions as previously described. These researchers ask, for instance, "Can adolescents' friendship networks affect their health?" Notice how linear and unidirectional the question is. Rarely do they ask, "Do adolescents' health affect their friendship networks?" In other words, many population health researchers have added network analyses to their methods toolbox but employ this tool the same way they use all others: in a linear, unidirectional manner. After employing network analyses, researchers often use the results to support linear interventions at the individual level, but rarely to design network-level programs.[24] For these reasons, population health scientists using Social Network Analysis still struggle with the question, "Do networks simply provide a tool to be used to measure concepts suggested by theory or does taking a network perspective change the nature of the theory being investigated?"[19p238]

I mention Social Network Analysis here as merely one CSS method incorporated into linear perspectives of population health; the case can be made for other complexity methods/tools, as well (e.g., System Dynamics Modeling)—so much so that prominent scholars such as Lawrence W. Green have pointedly questioned CSS's utility: "Do systems thinking and modeling really [provide an alternative to assessing evidence-based practice in public health]? Or are their initial modeling, network analysis, and simulation based on idealized or abstract versions of the realities of practice?"[25p408]

Put simply, when incorporating complexity approaches as methods or tools, the tools might be new, but the traditional framing of the issues remains, as the theories explaining them go unchanged. Entrenched within a linear viewpoint, population health researchers who attempt to integrate complexity-associated methods develop new ways to answer the "same old" questions, by collecting data in new formats (and quantities—notice the trend towards Big Data[26]) and presenting results with more alluring visuals. Integrating new analytical tools to examine traditionally framed problems, however, has had limited impact, as published reviews highlight.[27]

As will become clear in later chapters of this book, CSS methods can, therefore, encourage population health scholars to ask new questions and develop new theories—for example, about bidirectional influence over time (social networks), ways stakeholder responses to change can make problems worse (system dynamics), the nature of tipping points (system resilience), reasons for fat-tailed distributions (power laws), or how micro-behavior can produce macro phenomenon (agent-based modeling).

6.4.3. Questioning Current Theories' Assumptions and Reframing the Problem(s)

At this level, I would argue, CSS can be *revolutionary*. As a replacement for prevalent linear views, complex systems theories can, indeed, spark a "revolution" in population health. Why? Because—as this entire book demonstrates—not only does a CSS perspective carry, and account for, factors related to movement, adaptation, interdependence, change, feedback loops, and time, the perspective also *redefines* the problem. In other words, precisely because it explains dynamic factors and their interrelationships inside complex systems, a complex systems approach transcends the usual ways of identifying a problem, reframes it, and "sees" it as a different/new problem—one shaped by the dynamics and interactions within the complex system(s) that "house" the problem.[28,29]

Recall when I referred to theory *as practice*? Practicing theory, or theorizing, involves concrete actions such as (1) asking questions that lead to understanding a phenomenon and its causes more clearly or in-depth; (2) questioning prevailing assumptions and a theory's status quo; (3) seeking the most plausible and meaningful answer(s); and (4) building a narrative or logic structure for the questions and their answers.[3p9] CSS can revolutionize population health theory by *challenging* and *questioning* the assumptions anchoring existing theories, by transcending the narratives built to understand population health, and by crafting new narratives to replace ineffective ones.[a]

Theories are, themselves, complex dynamic *systems of meaning*, embedded within other complex systems (e.g., disciplines, academia, science, research centers, and higher education institutions). As with any other complex system, theories also have *boundaries*: the assumptions upon which they operate. According to Bacharach, "a theory may be viewed as a system of constructs and variables in which the constructs are related to each other by propositions and the variables are related to each other by hypotheses. The *whole system is bounded by the theorist's assumptions*."[2p496](emphasis added)

---

a. It is important to note that some scholars propose another way in which CSS can revolutionize population health theory—through "computational modeling." In this view, modeling a system "from the bottom up" is to theorize about it. Yet scholars who defend "computation *as* theory" (such as Miller and Page[4]) also acknowledge lack of consensus over this idea.

For any theoretical advancement to occur, therefore, a theory's assumptions or boundaries must be identified, questioned and, if found lacking, replaced or redefined "if a theory is to be properly used or tested, the theorist's implicit *assumptions which form the boundaries of the theory* must be understood.[30p51](em phasis added)

The noun *boundary* is, indeed, an interesting choice: *boundary* carries the notions of borders, limits, parameters, while the verb *bind* conveys restriction, confinement, and obligation (as in *duty-bound*). All theories have borders and delimitations—those points beyond which they dare not venture without turning into speculation—and all theories obligate users to operate within their limits.

CSS, therefore, can revolutionize population health theory not by juxtaposing new narratives to those currently available, nor by integrating dynamic systems methods into non-linear theories. Only through *problematizing* existing boundaries and questioning the assumptions underlying linear theories can new and "more interesting and influential" theories take hold. Alvesson and Sandberg argue, "... problematization—in the sense of questioning the assumptions underlying existing theory in some significant ways—is fundamental to the construction of innovative research questions and, thus, to the development of interesting and influential theories.[30p2]

In summary, CSS has the potential to problematize the way scholars currently understand specific concepts or phenomena and, in so doing, can engender a shift in thinking, a different understanding of these concepts/phenomena.

Yet, *how* do complex systems perspectives question current theories' assumptions in population health and re-frame phenomena? The answer is best given through examples. This book is a rich resource for these, but as support for my argument in this chapter, I describe two instances (chosen more or less randomly) in which scholars have examined the assumptions underlying current theories/approaches, challenged them, and proposed new ways to frame specific health issues.

6.5. EXAMPLES

One can find excellent examples of questioning current theories' assumptions and recommending CSS perspectives, in Nancy Krieger's writings. In one article, where she argues for "advancing theories useful for the 21st century" in Epidemiology,[31] Krieger proposes reframing the relationship between *pregnancy* and *breast cancer*. Even though available evidence points to a nonlinear relationship between these factors (i.e., "pregnancy decreases risk of breast cancer over the lifetime if it occurs early, but thereafter increases risk, especially after age 35"[31p672]), most research focuses either on factors affecting the age at which women first become pregnant or on how many pregnancies they experience. Socioeconomic status, education, availability and access to contraceptive methods, and the legal right to abortion represent the most routinely researched factors.

A CSS view (within which Krieger's "ecosocial" perspective represents only one model/theory) would, instead, *reconceptualize* pregnancy. In this reframing process, pregnancy becomes more than merely a risk factor or an "exposure" for breast cancer. Krieger writes:

> An ecosocial approach . . . would raise questions beyond social determinants of age at first pregnancy to inquire how pregnancy *itself* is conceptualized in relation to risk of breast cancer. Constructs of "embodiment," "pathways of embodiment," and the "dynamic and cumulative interplay between exposure, susceptibility and resistance" would require analyzing pregnancy in relation to developmental biology of the breast (especially maturation of lobules and ducts and also altered rates of apoptosis) as well as its effects on the endocrine system (synthesis of hormones within the breast plus alteration in magnitude and frequency of hormonal fluctuations) and cardiovascular system (increased vascularization of the breast). A concern with "accountability and agency," as well as scale and level, would additionally challenge gender-based views positing reproductive hormones as primary determinants of women's health. The net result would be to *re-conceptualize* pregnancy not simply as an "exposure" but also as a biological process capable of altering susceptibility to exogenous carcinogens.[31pp672-673(emphasis in original)]

A CSS view, however, not only questions long-held assumptions; it also proposes new constructs and a new language to define, frame, and name the phenomenon of interest. In the pregnancy example, new concepts/constructs Krieger suggests include *embodiment; pathways of embodiment; cumulative interplay between exposure, susceptibility and resistance*; and *accountability and agency*.[31p672] Equipped with new ways of "seeing," based on these and similar constructs, researchers understand better how pregnancy and breast cancer interact; this understanding, in turn, can highlight important leverage points for prevention and care.

Wittenborn, Rahmandad, and Hosseinichimeh[32] provide another example of how CSS approaches can question, challenge, and redraw the theoretical boundaries or assumptions underlying how scientists understand major depressive disorder (MDD). In 2016, the authors presented "the first broad boundary causal loop diagram of depression dynamics."[32p551] Before building the model, however, a literature review confirmed how prevalent a linear approach to studying MDD really is: Among the 12,060 studies identified, almost 93% assessed a *single* causal factor; only 7% examined two or more causes.[32]

Equipped with a CSS "lens," the investigators theoretically modeled MDD as emerging from the interactions among 13 reinforcing feedback loops "activated by exogenous factors."[32p559] The reinforcing loops either keep a person within depression's "vicious cycle" or, if intervened upon, can lead to healing, "even in the presence of original exogenous shocks."[32p559] The loops also can explain why different people, under similar conditions, experience dissimilar outcomes, based on the principle of sensitivity to initial conditions, as the "strength and relevance of different loops depend heavily on the stock variables on each loop and their speeds of change."[32p559]

Culling from available evidence, the model proposes feedback loops within the cognitive, social–environmental, and biological dimensions separately ("to simplify discussion"), but the authors note that several feedback loops reach across multiple dimensions. One example is the reinforcing loop connecting negative cognitive representations and social isolation: Depressed patients often engage in problem behaviors that push others away and weaken social networks; weak social networks and poor interpersonal ties "contribute to negative affect and processes and can lead to problematic responses (e.g., aggression) which, in turn, deplete interpersonal relationship quality. As depressed patients become further plagued by challenging relationships or isolation, their negative cognitive representations are reinforced" and may lead to dysfunctional behaviors, repeating the cycle.[32p556]

Reframing MDD as a dynamic system of interacting drivers and feedback loops can lead not only to better understanding this pernicious public health problem but also to developing better personalized treatment. Insisting in viewing MDD as resulting from one or two "common-cause factors"—as does much of the current research—can be, at best, ineffective and, at worst, iatrogenic or harmful[33]: Treating a patient whose depression is driven by a social isolation feedback loop with medication exclusively may, given the drugs' problematic side effects, help strengthen isolation; treating a patient whose depression is caused by an elevated (or chronic) cortisol response feedback loop with talk therapy or social support alone may also lead to adverse outcomes. MDD's epidemic proportions among US populations suggest our best efforts in managing the condition have not been very successful. Wittenborn, Rahmandad and Hosseinichimeh conclude, then, "Major public health problems often persist, despite best efforts to intervene, when they are more complex than the narrow frameworks used to understand them."[32p551]

6.6. IMPLICATIONS FOR PRACTICE, POLICY, AND TRAINING

It is probably safe to conclude that revolutionizing population health theory—questioning the boundaries of current theories and reframing the problems—will have indelible implications not only for population health's scientific enterprise but also for its practice, for policy development, and for training the future workforce.[34]

Abolishing the artificial separation between theory and practice, for instance, may be one valuable gain from this theory revolution. After all, the theorizing about population health, within a CSS perspective, demands input from stakeholders, especially from those embedded in systems that design, implement, and enforce health policies and services.

But a theory revolution will also affect other dimensions of population health practice. Gates summarizes the issue, claiming "STCS [systems thinking and complexity science] raises some new ways of thinking about and carrying out"[35p62] the main activities related to the planning, implementing and evaluating social/health interventions. Some scholars suggest that not only *how* we promote population health will change, even the term *health*, itself, might become a casualty.

Re-framing and redefining *health* will be required, because "doctors, patients, consumers, activists, pacifists, protesters, or policymakers," when holding conversations about health, "are not all talking about the same thing"[36p9]—and consensus is sine qua non for communication and improvement.

Alongside the impact on practice and on the concept of health, another dimension needing reassessment is the training and mentoring of future population health scientists and practitioners in these "new ways of thinking about and carrying out" public health interventions.[35p62] At a minimum, curricula in undergraduate and graduate training programs will require significant shifts. In a 2006 editorial, McLeroy[37] elaborated on this need when presenting work developed by the Systems Thinking Workgroup within the Association of Schools of Public Health. He outlined a few "critical themes" the group identified as essential to developing CSS competencies:

- Interconnectedness (a relational perspective);
- A non-reductionist approach;
- Integrating systems thinking into practice, including comparing and contrasting various systems models;
- A focus on context, particularly the idea of embedded systems;
- The nature of causality, particularly nonlinear relationships and the importance of feedback loops, stocks, and flows;
- The importance of progressive approximation for testing of models;
- The dynamic nature of systems across time;
- The importance of boundaries, including the subjective nature of the relationships between the observer and the observed;
- The importance of a multidisciplinary approach in systems thinking;
- Emergent properties, including the concepts of chaos and complexity;
- Autopoesis, or the self-organizing nature of some systems.[37p402]

Albeit slowly, efforts to incorporate CSS into training programs are emerging.[38] The Public Health Foundation, for example, lists "Leadership and Systems Thinking" as one among eight domains forming the core competencies for public health professionals.[39] Moreover, in 2016, the Interdisciplinary Association for Population Health Science made its debut as a professional organization,[40] claiming it arrives at a time in which "there is a *critical need for new approaches* to improving health and reducing health care costs."[41(emphasis added)]

These efforts may appear modest "appetizers" of potential transformations. Yet the future of population health holds tremendous promise for effective innovation and meaningful reform, through the lens of CSS. Yes, indeed, CSS *can* revolutionize population health theory and practice, and I sincerely hope readers who have had the patience to navigate this chapter will envision the possibilities and choose to join the revolution. Enlisting requires taking only three steps:

Step 1: *Accept nothing* at face-value, regarding theory, research, and practice in population health.

Step 2: *Theorize: Question the assumptions* grounding current narratives about population health, especially those whose uselessness has been outlived (cf. chapter's opening quote by McLuhan). Push, transcend, and transgress these narratives' boundaries.

Step 3: *Revolutionize* population health theory—and then practice!

REFERENCES

1. Revolutionize. English Oxford Living Dictionaries Web site. https:// en.oxforddictionaries.com/definition/revolutionize. Updated 2018. Accessed July 10, 2018.

2. Bacharach SB. Organizational theories: Some criteria for evaluation. *Acad Manage Rev.* 1989;14(4):496–515.

3. Goodson P. *Theory in health promotion research and practice: Thinking outside the box.* Sudbury, MA: Jones & Bartlett; 2010.

4. Miller JH, Page SE. *Complex adaptive systems: An introduction to computational models of social life.* Princeton, New Jersey: Princeton University Press; 2007.

5. Glanz K, Rimer BK, Viswanath K. *Health behavior and health education: Theory, research, and practice.* 4th ed. San Francisco: Jossey-Bass; 2008.

6. Roux AVD. Conceptual approaches to the study of health disparities. *Annu Rev Public Health.* 2012;33:41–58.

7. Halfon N, Hochstein M. Life course health development: An integrated framework for developing health, policy, and research. *Milbank Q.* 2002;80(3):433–479.

8. Thompson, DS, Fazio, X, Kustra, E, Patrick, L, Stanley, D. Scoping review of complexity theory in health services research. *BMC Health Services Research.* 2016;16:87.

9. Green LW, Kreuter, MW. *Health Program Planning: An Educational and Ecological Approach.* 4th ed. New York, NY: McGraw Hill, 2005.

10. Beckfield J, Krieger N. Epi + demos + cracy: Linking political systems and priorities to the magnitude of health inequities—evidence, gaps, and a research agenda. *Epidemiol Rev.* 2009;31:152–177.

11. Fang FC, Casadevall A. Reductionistic and holistic science (editorial). *Infect Immun.* 2011;79(4):1401–1404.

12. Crosby RA, Salazar LF, DiClemente RJ. Value-expectancy theories. In: DiClemente RJ, Salazar LF, Crosby RA, eds. *Health behavior theory for Public Health: Principles, foundations, and applications.* 2nd ed. Burlington, MA: Jones & Bartlett Learning; 2019:59–72.

13. Jayasinghe S. Conceptualising Population Health: From mechanistic thinking to complexity science. *Emerg Themes Epidemiol.* 2011;8(2):1–7.

14. Andersson C, Tornborg A, Tornberg P. Societal systems—complex or worse? *Futures.* 2014;63(July 15):145–157.

15. Goodson P. Researching genes, behavior, and society to improve Population Health: A primer in complex adaptive systems as an integrative approach. *Adv Med Sociol.* 2015;16:127–156.

16. Wagner CS, Roessner JD, Kamau B, et al. Approaches to understanding and measuring interdisciplinary scientific research (IDR): A review of the literature. *J Inform.* 2011;165:14–26.

17. DiClemente RJ, Crosby RA, Salazar LF. Stage models for health promotion. In: DiClemente RJ, Salazar LF, Crosby RA, eds. *Health Behavior Theory for Public Health: Principles, Foundations, and Applications.* 2nd ed. Burlington, MA: Jones & Bartlett Learning; 2019:94–115.

18. Abbott A. Transcending general linear reality. *Soc Theory.* 1988;6(2):169–186.

19. Valente TW. *Social Networks and Health: Models, METHODS, and applications.* New York, NY: Oxford University Press; 2010.

20. Christakis NA, Fowler JH. The spread of obesity in a large social network over 32 years. *N Engl J Med.* 2007;357:370–379.

21. Jacobs W, Goodson P, Barry AE, McLeroy KR. The role of gender in adolescents' social networks and alcohol, tobacco, and drug use: A systematic review. *J School Health.* 2016;86:322–333.

22. Jeon KC, Goodson P. Alcohol and sex: The influence of friendship networks on co-occurring risky health behaviors of US adolescents. *Int J Adolesc Youth.* 2016;21:499–512.

23. Klovdahl AS, Graviss EA, Musser JM. Infectious disease control: Combining molecular biological and network methods. *Soc Networks Health.* 2002;8:73–99.

24. Valente TW. Network interventions. *Science.* 2012;337:49–53.

25. Green LW. Public Health asks of systems science: To advance our evidence-based practice, can you help us get more practice-based evidence? *Am J Public Health.* 2006;96:406–409.

26. West G. Big data needs a big theory to go with it. *Sci Am.* https://www.scientificamerican.com/article/big-data-needs-big-theory/?print=true. Published May 1, 2013.

27. Carey G, Malbon E, Carey N, Joyce A, Crammond B, Carey A. Systems science and systems thinking for Public Health: A systematic review of the field. *BMJ Open.* 2015;5:e009002.

28. Flood RL, Carson ER. System science—making sense of the philosophical issues. In: *Dealing with Complexity: An Introduction to the Theory and Application of Systems Science.* 2nd ed. New York, NY: Springer Science+Business Media; 1993:245–256.

29. Ramalingam B, Jones H, Reba T, Young J. Exploring the science of complexity: Ideas and implications for development and humanitarian efforts. 2008; Working Paper 285.

30. Alvesson M, Sandberg J. *Constructing Research Questions: Doing Interesting Research.* London, UK: SAGE; 2013.

31. Krieger N. Theories for social epidemiology in the 21st century: An ecosocial perspective. *Int J Epidemiol.* 2001;30:668–677.

32. Wittenborn AK, Rahmandad H, Hosseinichimeh N. Depression as a systemic syndrome: Mapping the feedback loops of major depressive disorder. *Psychol Med.* 2016;46:551–562.

33. Mariotti H. Complexity is not systems thinking. https://www.linkedin.com/pulse/20140724182739-73571575-complexity-is-not-systems-thinking. Updated 2014.

34. National Academies of Sciences, Engineering, and Medicine. *Advancing the Science to Improve Population Health: Proceedings of a Workshop.* Washington, DC: The National Academies Press; 2017.

35. Gates EF. Making sense of the emerging conversation in evaluation about systems thinking and complexity science. *Eval Program Plann.* 2016;59:62–73.

36. Metzl JM. Introduction: Why Against Health? In: Metzl JM, Kirkland A, eds., *Against Health: How Health Became the New Morality*. New York, NY: New York University Press; 2010:1–6.

37. McLeroy K. Thinking of systems. *Am J Public Health*. 2006;96(3):402.

38. The National Academies Keck Futures Initiatives. *The National Academies Keck Futures Initiative: Complex systems: Task Group Summaries*. Washington, DC: National Academies Press; 2008. doi:10.17226/12622.

39. The Council on Linkages Between Academia and Public Health Practice. *Core Competencies for Public Health Professionals*. CDC/Public Health Foundation. http://phf.org/corecompetencies. Published 2014.

40. Bacharach CA, Daley DM. Shaping a new field: Three key challenges for Population Health science. *Am J Public Health*. 2017;107(2):251–252.

41. Interdisciplinary Association for Population Health Science. About IAPHS. https://iaphs.org/about-iaphs/. Updated 2018.

TAKE-HOME MESSAGES

Complex systems theory is defined by foundational concepts and properties that provide new ways of understanding and acting upon population heath challenges. Although complex systems science theories remain on the fringe of mainstream population health science, the applied examples in this section show a growing list of applications that suggest the tremendous potential of these new perspectives in generating future breakthroughs. Viewing population health as the product of complex adaptive systems of systems can overhaul our understanding of the determinants of population health and offers a path toward more meaningfully identifying targets for change that align with system structure—meaning they are more likely to work. Because we often strive for highly impactful actions, wonder why interventions have mixed feelings in different contexts, or wrestle with how and when to adapt components of interventions, a complex systems perspective is exactly what is needed to illuminate the way. Network approaches to population health provide a structured approach to seeing interconnections between system elements—people, organizations, or other entities—and analyzing the overall structure of complex systems. Networks are an integral component of complex adaptive systems of systems. Applying indicators of critical transitions, tipping points, and resilience can provide new insights into what it will take to create (or protect against, depending on the goal) change within population health systems.

It is for these reasons, along with many more identified throughout this volume, that complex systems science can advance population health theory. However, such a revolution would be accompanied by numerous consequences, many of which were explicated in Chapter 6. An additional consequence pertains to the fact that generating new theory grounded in complex systems perspectives is not without its difficulties. One key challenge is that complex systems theories—as is true of any theories in general—must be built and tested. The process of building and testing complex systems theories necessitate research designs and analytical methods not typically employed in population health science. Parts III and IV of this volume will explore these two dimensions of complex systems science in population health.

RESOURCES FOR FURTHER READING

Borsboom D, Cramer AOJ. Network analysis: An integrative approach to the structure of psychopathology. *Annu Rev Clin Psychol.* 2013;9:91–121.

Byrne D, Callaghan G. *Complexity Theory and the Social Sciences: The State of the Art.* New York, NY: Routledge; 2013.

Deffuant G, Gilbert N. *Viability and Resilience of Complex Systems: Concepts, Methods and Case Studies from Ecology and Society.* New York, NY: Springer; 2011.

El-Sayed AM, Galea S. *Systems Science and Population Health.* Oxford, UK: Oxford University Press; 2017.

Fang FC, Casadevall A. Reductionistic and holistic science. *Infect Immun.* 2011;79(4):1401–1404.

Gell-Mann M. Complex adaptive systems. In: Cowan G, Pines D, Meltzer D, eds. *Santa Fe Institute Studies in the Sciences of Complexity.* Santa Fe, NM: Santa Fe Institute; 1994:17–45.

Gell-Mann M. What is complexity? In: *Complexity.* New York, NY: Springer; 1995:16–19.

Goldenfeld N, Kadanoff LP. Simple lessons from complexity. *Science.* 1999;284 (5411):87–89.

Goodson P. Researching genes, behavior, and society to improve population health: a primer in complex adaptive systems as an integrative approach. In: Perry BL, ed. *Genetics, Health and Society.* Bingley, UK: Emerald; 2015:127–156.

Hammond RA. Complex systems modeling for obesity research. *Prev Chronic Dis.* 2009;6(3):1–10.

Holland JH. *Complexity: A Very Short Introduction.* New York, NY: Oxford University Press; 2014.

Louth J. From Newton to Newtonianism: Reductionism and the development of the social sciences. *Emergence: Complex Org.* 2011;13(4):63–83.

McKelvey B. Complexity science as order-creation science: New theory, new method. *Emergence: Complex Org.* 2004;6(4):2–27.

Miller JH, Page SE. *Complex Adaptive Systems: An Introduction to Computational Models of Social Life.* Princeton, NJ: Princeton University Press; 2009.

Mitchell M. *Complexity: A Guided Tour.* New York, NY: Oxford University Press; 2009.

Olde Rikkert MGM, Dakos V, Buchman TG, et al. Slowing down of recovery as generic risk marker for acute severity transitions in chronic diseases. *Crit Care Med.* 2016;44(3):601–606.

Prigogine I, Sengers I. *Order Out of Chaos.* New York, NY: Verso; 2017.

Resnicow K, Page SE. Embracing chaos and complexity: A quantum change for public health. *Am J Public Health.* 2008;98(8):1382–1389.

Scheffer M. *Critical Transitions in Nature and Society.* Princeton, NJ: Princeton University Press; 2009.

Scheffer M, Carpenter SR, Lenton TM, et al. Anticipating critical transitions. *Science.* 2012;338(6105):344–348.

Trefois C, Antony PMA, Goncalves J, Skupin A, Balling R. Critical transitions in chronic disease: Transferring concepts from ecology to systems medicine. *Curr Opin Biotechnol.* 2015;34:48–55.

Weaver W. Science and complexity. *Am Sci.* 1948;36:536–544.

Complex Systems and Methodology in Population Health Science

Introductory Material: Preview and Objectives

PREVIEW

Parts I and II of this volume describe fundamental concepts of complexity and argue for the importance of recognizing and accommodating complexity in theory, research, and population health practice. But how do we do this, and what are the ramifications of complexity for population health research and practice? This is the focus of Part III, which describes the unique ways that empirical and stakeholder-engaged research in population health, grounded in complex systems science, can be designed and conducted. Complex systems science-based methods are contextualized, with applications to pressing population health problems.

Chapter 7 discusses the process of designing population health research grounded in complex systems. Acknowledging increasing calls to use complex systems research approaches to address pressing population health problems, the authors suggest a step-by-step approach for designing research that generally follows traditional approaches but considers key elements of complex systems. Beginning with the initial stages of defining and narrowing the research objectives, these steps shape the subsequent research design, where systems mapping, computational modeling, and simulation methods are often needed. The chapter concludes with a discussion about the complementary and synergistic nature of complex systems and traditional research approaches.

Grounded in the premise that our mental models—how we understand phenomena in the real world—are inherently flawed in the presence of dynamic complexity, Chapter 8 describes how the systematic development of explicit models, through the act of modeling, provides means to mitigate these inherent shortcomings and can stimulate new ways of understanding and acting in population health that are grounded in "model thinking." For the study of complex systems, including many current examples in population health, a distinct class of modeling approaches grounded in mathematical and computational (simulation) modeling has emerged. Engagement in modeling can help overcome difficulties in learning imposed by the daunting complexity of the world, leading to transformed mental models and the proliferation of model thinking in population health research and action.

Chapter 9 illuminates the importance of community and stakeholder involvement in designing and conducting population health research. Complex systems science methods, designed to study "wholes" and to support decision-making in the context of complexity, can be transformative when used collaboratively with stakeholders that are impacted and capable of impacting key population health challenges. In this chapter, current best practices for engaging stakeholders in complex systems science methods—both mapping (qualitative model structuring) and modeling—are presented. A prominent focus of this chapter given the richness of extant methodological guidance, group modeling in the context of system dynamics modeling is described—an analytical method that will be further explored in Part IV. This group model building layer around simulation-informed learning has already begun to be extended and adapted for use with other approaches to complex systems science.

Chapter 10 encourages readers to consider why the overreliance on the Gaussian (i.e., normal) distribution in population health can lead to missing important insights about the structure of the complex systems determining population health. The normal distribution has been a dominant method for displaying and making inferences in population health for decades. As this chapter describes, while the normal distribution has been useful to the field, not all outcomes in population health are normally distributed. It points out several situations in which assuming outcomes are normally distributed and carrying on with analysis will lead to overly generalized (at best) or incorrect (at worst) conclusions within population health research.

OBJECTIVES

The objectives of this section are as follows:

1. Aligned with common population health approaches, to describe the steps in a research design process that accommodates complexity and complex systems science.
2. Describe the value of models and modeling in learning and transforming mental models.
3. Explain the power of model thinking, computational modeling and simulation, and the many-model approach in population health research and action.
4. Explicate current best practices in stakeholder engagement designed to elicit, challenge, integrate, and use their mental models to inspire action.
5. Highlight the importance of recognizing non-normally distributed phenomena in population health and appreciating the value of studying them differently to learn about important complex system structure, which can underpin more impactful action.
6. Describe power laws and fat-tailed distributions in population health science and the phenomena that generate them.

7

Designing Population Health Research Grounded in Complex Systems Science

LEAH FRERICHS AND NATALIE R. SMITH

7.1. INTRODUCTION

In recent decades, there has been increasing acknowledgement that research has fallen short of helping to address many pressing population health problems such as obesity, antibiotic resistance, and violence. Many of the advances made in population health over the past century have resulted from research using traditional deductive approaches. For example, these approaches have been used to identify proximal causes of major infections (polio, measles, human papillomavirus) and helped drive the creation of vaccines. Yet, these same approaches fall short of advancing research surrounding more complex population health problems that do not have a single proximal cause, such as the recent antivaccine movement. To help advance scientific knowledge about complex problems, there has been an increased interest in using scientific approaches grounded in systems thinking and complexity science.[1,2] To promote the adoption of complex systems approaches, we must change how we design research. In contrast to deductive research designs that attempt to isolate a single relationship of interest, research grounded in complex systems requires us to embrace a holistic understanding of the interdependent and dynamic influences on population health problems.

Population health research design typically follows these basic steps: (1) Find your focus (identify the research problem, objectives and questions); (2) narrow your focus (decide on study type, design, sample, and measures); (3) define data collection and management procedures (decide on mechanics

Leah Frerichs and Natalie R. Smith, *Designing Population Health Research Grounded in Complex Systems Science* In: *Complex Systems and Population Health*. Edited by: Yorghos Apostolopoulos, Kristen Hassmiller Lich, and Michael Kenneth Lemke, Oxford University Press (2020). © Oxford University Press. DOI: 10.1093/oso/9780190880743.003.0007 of data collection and develop data management plans); (4) consider external logistics (consider research scope, context); and (5) document the research plan (develop protocols and dissemination plans).[3] Designing research with a complex systems approach can be aligned with these same basic steps but will require new thinking and new tools within each step. This is especially true in the initial stages of finding and narrowing one's focus. Across all steps, research design must account for elements of dynamic complexity that are discussed in Chapters 1, 2, and 20 of this text. These elements include key characteristics of complex systems such as nonlinearities, interdependencies, sensitivity to initial conditions/path dependence, resilience, and critical transitions/tipping points.

This chapter provides an overview of designing research grounded in complex systems. It details steps in a research design process using a complex systems approach in alignment with the same steps generally followed in population health. All steps are described, emphasizing the initial stages of defining and narrowing the research focus.

7.2. FINDING YOUR FOCUS WITH A COMPLEX SYSTEMS APPROACH

Similar to traditional research, a research approach grounded in complex systems is typically driven by a broad theoretical or real-world problem. In traditional deductive research designs, research objectives and questions are developed to reduce phenomena into constituent parts and study specific cause-effect relationships among these individual parts.[2,4] This approach leads to important questions about specific components of an issue and is valuable when trying to understand issues that can be disentangled from the contexts in which they are embedded and that are otherwise amenable to reduction. However, as described in Chapter 2, population health challenges with complex system characteristics are not amenable to reduction and require researchers to instead consider the structure of problems. Complex systems characteristics and properties compel researchers to define objectives and ask questions about how factors such as interconnections, delays between cause and effect, and nonlinear relationships influence outcomes of interest. The following provides a description of how research objectives and questions might be defined from a complex systems research approach using relevant population health examples.

7.2.1. Research Objectives

Research objectives are an important first step to define what a research study intends to accomplish. The objectives (also sometimes called aims) typically begin with "to," followed by a verb such as identify, explore, describe, explain, compare, assess, or test. In general, the word choice for research objectives will suggest a general research approach. Traditionally, the word choice suggests whether the research design is exploratory or descriptive versus a more structured assessment of associations, relationships, or causes. For example, consider the two research objectives articulated in traditional research thinking and language:

- To identify patient- and provider-level factors influencing colorectal cancer screening rates in community X.
- To assess the effect of intervention A on colorectal cancer screening in clinics X and Y.

When using a complex systems approach, the research objectives may also suggest either exploratory, descriptive, or more structured assessments. However, the research objective should make it clear that the study will involve characteristics of complex systems. For example, the two traditional research objectives above could be reframed to illuminate complex system structure:

- To identify *feedback loops between* patient- and provider-level factors that could influence colorectal cancer screening rates in community X.
- To assess the *potential impact* of intervention A on colorectal cancer screening in clinics X and Y *considering heterogeneous effects based on patient demographics and clinic context.*

Complex-systems–grounded research may also require development of objectives that are not merely adaptations of more traditional objectives. This is especially relevant when the issue of interest is influenced by individuals whose decisions are all interdependent, resulting in continual adaptation and emergence of new behaviors over time. For example, traditional research on colorectal cancer screening has often focused on one facet of the screening process (e.g., patient-targeted interventions, provider- or clinic-level interventions). However, colorectal cancer screening involves the interconnected decisions of multiple stakeholders—patients, providers, insurers, and clinic personnel. Thus, research objectives also need to focus on how interdependencies, gaps, or misaligned incentives across these stakeholders could influence the colorectal cancer screening process and outcomes. Some example research questions could be:

- To explore how changes in patient demand for fecal occult blood testing impact clinic workflow.
- To construct a diagram of colorectal cancer screening processes and identify potential intervention leverage points.
- To quantify how geographic distribution of colonoscopy capacity may influence screening outcomes.
- To analyze how differential demand across heterogeneous sociodemographic groups may influence screening outcomes.

7.2.2. Research Questions

The next step in designing a study is to translate research objectives into research questions and hypotheses. The traditional research approach is oriented toward questions that seek to identify risk and protective factors and evaluate interventions that address these factors independently (or a few at a time). However, population health challenges with complex systems characteristics are unlikely to respond well or expediently to this approach. Complex systems approaches should focus on understanding how a system's parts interrelate to influence the whole and require thinking beyond two (or a few) factors or pinpointing proximal effects. The approach compels research questions that focus on understanding how the interconnections among components (including actors) and micro rules/behaviors give rise to population-level outcomes or behaviors of systems as a whole. This means that research questions grounded in complex systems approaches nearly always involve a relational component and are rarely focused on assessing causal relationships (at least not by traditional epidemiological definitions of *cause* such as the Bradford Hill guidance[5]).

Thus, the traditional population health research question categories: (1) descriptive or exploratory (understanding a problem when little is known), (2) relational (understanding relationships between concepts or measures), or (3) causal (testing whether one variable causes changes in another outcome variable of interest)[3] are not ideal for a complex systems approach. In contrast, three general categories of research questions more aligned with a complex systems approach are (1) descriptive or exploratory, (2) mechanistic, or (3) forecasting. The PICOTS (patient/population, intervention, comparison, outcome, time, setting)[6] is also a useful framework that has been commonly used to highlight how to formulate research studies in population health research. However, when PICOTS component definitions are used to help guide complex systems science research, they require slightly different definitions (as highlighted in Table 7.1).

As an applied example, consider how researchers have uncovered geographic patterns of different types of food outlets in association with diet-related health disparities. Specifically, evidence supports a higher prevalence of diet-related health disparities among low-income and minority communities in association with limited access to healthy foods and to a higher density of fast-food outlets and convenience stores in those areas.[7,8] Yet, fast-food zoning ordinances to reduce the consumption of fast food have had disappointing, sometimes null outcomes.[9] As discussed in a commentary by Brown and Brewster (2015), our traditional research approaches can lead us to focus on narrowly defined and potentially ineffective targets.[10] From a complex systems approach, researchers interested in the noted diet-related health disparities would ask questions about how observed patterns of dietary behaviors emerge from a set of rules shaped by social norms, food access, market forces, food manufacturing, and distribution systems.

Table 7.1. COMPARISON OF THE TRADITIONAL PICOT DEFINITIONS TO
A COMPLEXITY SCIENCE APPROACH

PICOT component	Traditional Definition[a]	Complex Systems Science Definition
(P) Patient/ population	Population refers to the sample of subjects you wish to recruit for your study.	Population refers to the cohort(s) of individuals and their characteristics that are relevant to the issue of interest. There will likely be a balance between defining the most detailed population of interest and one for which data will be available or obtainable.
(I) Intervention	Intervention refers to the treatment that will be provided to subjects enrolled in your study.	Intervention (if applicable) refers to the counterfactuals or "what if" scenarios, where the effects of changing various parameters of a model (analogous to different experimental conditions) can be simulated.
(C) Comparison	Comparison identifies what you plan on using as a reference group to compare with your treatment intervention. Many study designs refer to this as the control group.	Comparison identifies a baseline or 'status quo' scenario (i.e., what will happen if no changes occur) that can be used as the main comparator for the counterfactual scenarios within simulation modeling approaches.
(O) Outcome	Outcome represents what result you plan on measuring to examine the effectiveness of your intervention.	Outcome represents the result (or results) that are key factors in decision-making processes for intervention and policy. There is likely a need to consider multiple outcomes such as health and economic outcomes and across different heterogeneous subgroups of interest.
(T) Time	Time describes the duration for your data collection	Time describes the scale and speed that is appropriate to observe changes in model behavior and outcomes. Decisions regarding time should reflect the known natural history of the issue of interest (e.g., the speed and scale to observe an infectious disease may considered in time units of hours over the course of several months whereas a chronic disease may require one-year units over decades). Decisions can be made to run scenarios at different time scales.
(S) Setting	Setting describes the place(s) where the study is taking place and/or the intervention is reaching the patient/population	Setting identifies the environment(s) that provide the context for the population. The setting can represent multiple types of environments that are relevant to the research question. In some cases, the settings can have their own properties, which can change over time.

[a]Sources: Guyatt G, Drummond R, Meade M, Cook D. *The Evidence Based-Medicine Working Group Users' Guides to the Medical Literature.* 2nd ed. Chicago: McGraw Hill; 2008; Riva JJ, Malik KM, Burnie, SJ, Endicott AR, Busse JW. (2012). What is your research question? An introduction to the PICOT format for clinicians. *Journal of the Canadian Chiropractic Association,* 56(3), 167–171.

More specifically, exploratory and descriptive research questions from a traditional perspective often seek to answer questions such as:

- What are the risk and protective factors for healthy diets?
- Who are the stakeholders related to healthy diets?

In contrast, research questions from a complex systems approach can be similarly exploratory but should also be relational. For example, the previous questions become:

- How do risk and protective factors *interconnect to influence* healthy diets?
- How do stakeholders related to healthy diets *influence each other's actions and decisions?*

Further, from a complex systems approach, mechanistic questions should focus on assessing the specific interconnected pathways of influence within a system and the extent to which they explain behavior. These types of questions have not typically been present in traditional research. A mechanistic question developed using a complex systems approach might ask:

- To what extent can reinforcing feedback loops among social norms, healthy food demand, and food supply explain changes in dietary behaviors?

Complex systems approaches are also not generally used to pinpoint proximal cause and effect relationships that are common in traditional research. In contrast, the approach is more concerned with understanding and/or forecasting how interconnected causal pathways potentially affect outcomes over time. This can, however, involve consideration of how small changes in specific factors may lead to large outcomes within a system of interest (i.e., tipping points) or understanding how to optimize interventions. For example, forecasting research questions would be:

- What is the potential impact of combining a social marketing campaign with an increase in grocery store density on healthy diets, compared to implementing each independently?
- What is the potential impact of increasing the density of grocery stores on healthy diets, given interconnections of social norms, healthy food demand, and food supply?
- How does neighborhood context influence the effectiveness of increasing grocery store density and social marketing campaigns?

Finally, it must be noted that traditional research questions also translate relational and causal research questions into hypotheses. Hypotheses are *sometimes* applicable to complex systems mechanistic and forecasting research questions. However, the same types of statistical testing traditionally used in population health research that are geared toward falsifying a null hypothesis are often not appropriate. Although it is possible to use hypothesis tests and confidence intervals (or, more accurately, uncertainty intervals) to objectively compare counterfactual scenarios from complex systems analysis tools, statistical assumptions such as independence of observations are often not satisfied. Thus, along with the shift in research questions, we must shift away from traditional statistical methods that focus on falsifying null hypotheses.

7.3. NARROWING YOUR FOCUS

7.3.1. Specifying Research Methods

After the research focus is defined, the next step is to determine the best research methods and specific data required to answer the research questions. Traditional population health study designs (e.g., case-control studies, cohort studies, randomized trials, quasi-experimental studies) may play a role in complex systems approaches; however, they will not typically be the primary design. For example, a cohort study may be useful to obtain data on variables relevant to your questions of interest, but complex systems research questions more often will involve either *qualitative systems mapping* or *computational modeling and simulation*, among other tools appropriate for complex systems. Exploratory and descriptive research questions are likely to involve qualitative or mixed-methods designs and should draw upon systems mapping methodologies (see Chapter 9 of this volume). In brief, these are digital or pen-and-paper tools that help researchers visually describe system components and their relationships. The tools are particularly useful to improve understanding of and communicate a system by making both abstract (e.g., policies, values) and concrete (e.g., people, spatial locations) components of a system and their relationships explicit in ways that written and oral narratives do not readily convey. Mechanistic and forecasting research questions in complex systems approaches will often involve *computational modeling and simulation* analytical methods (although these tools can also be applied to exploratory and descriptive research questions).

Computational modeling and simulation analytical methods allow us to create and use digital representations of real-world, complex phenomena to understand influences on population health problems and evaluate how different intervention and policy choices could influence outcomes.[11] Computational modeling and simulation has been made possible with advancements in computing technology that have led to some of the most innovative methodologies currently available to population health scientists for researching complex systems challenges.[1,12] These methodologies have been described as a "third way" of engaging in research (the other two being induction and deduction), where a model that represents a dynamically complex system is run over a period of time to generate data.[11,13] Simulation models represent "virtual worlds"[14]—in silico laboratories for rigorously exploring any number of dynamic theories and hypotheses. The approaches can capture vexing nonlinearities by including hypothesized causal factors across multiple levels and spatiotemporal scales, account for interrelationships, feedbacks, and interactions among these factors and also provide insights into the emerging aggregate patterns produced by these complex systems.[15]

Computational modeling and simulation methodologies can be used for many different purposes and are of value across many stages of scientific inquiry in population health science, spanning from hypothesis generation, to knowledge synthesis and the identification of research gaps, to virtual experimentation.[13,16] Very simple and conceptual simulation models that do not rely on concise testing, and validation can be developed and used by researchers as proof-of-principle exercises and are especially valuable for engaging in thought experiments and generating new research questions and hypotheses.[13,14] Simple models can also be used to test initial research questions about complex system mechanisms, and as these tentative ideas are refined over time, the simple models can be modified to be more complex and include more scientific knowledge.[14,17] Building up complexity in models allows researchers to synthesize the best available data from multiple sources. Through this process researchers might also identify gaps in current knowledge or data availability that could lead to new research questions.

Models can also be used for virtual experimentation. These models can help answer questions that seek to provide more accurate quantitative answers to mechanistic and forecasting research questions. Though, it is important to note that the quantities of focus are more often the patterns and trends versus specific effect sizes of outcomes. Models built for virtual experimentation are especially powerful for testing counterfactuals, or "what if" scenarios, where the effects of changing various parameters of the model (analogous to different experimental conditions) can be simulated.[17] Counterfactuals can be simulated in the context of identifying causal relationships within the dynamically complex system or evaluating intervention or policy change strategies.[11] Simulation modeling confers numerous advantages to researchers over the in vivo (real-world) experimental and quasi-experimental study designs. In particular, simulation modeling provides researchers with an unprecedented degree of experimental control and allows for the systematic exploration of limitless counterfactuals—including those that need to be evaluated across very long time periods[17]—that would not be possible using in vivo methodologies due to a number of logistical and ethical challenges. However, it must be noted that the limitless counterfactuals that simulation modeling provides also typically requires the researcher to make numerous assumptions and carefully consider uncertainty. Rigorous testing of simulation models built for virtual experimentation is critical. Importantly, there are many simulation modeling approaches, and the research question should help define the type of modeling approach. Detailed guidance on how to determine the best type of simulation model is provided in Chapter 12 of this volume.

7.3.2. Clarifying Data Needs and Analysis Plans

Another important step is to define measures and the types of data that are needed. The measures should align with the factors and relationships defined by the complex system of interest and define, more precisely, how they will be measured. This process should help determine the data or literature needed to obtain measures. Depending on the research question and scope of the complex issue, literature reviews may be required across multiple components of an issue, which are often more extensive than those required for deductive research approaches. During this step, knowledge or data gaps could be identified that require researchers to make pragmatic decisions about their modeling approach. For example, if it is determined that a model parameter is unknown and unavailable from the current literature or data sources, a researcher may decide to use expert opinion for an estimate and designate the parameter for extensive sensitivity analyses. In other cases, new secondary data analyses or primary data collection might be needed.

Also, the iterative nature of the research process may influence this step. Specifically, it is common to identify new measures and data needs in the process of developing a complex systems model. Sometimes the identified measures are difficult to obtain or unmeasurable. In these cases, the researcher may need to use model calibration (i.e., optimizing the model fit to other observable data by fine-tuning the unmeasurable parameter). Other times the identified measures require primary data collection or new analyses of existing data. Thus, this stage often requires more time and support than that of traditional research.

7.3.3. Validity and Credibility

The accuracy and trustworthiness of study findings are an important consideration in population health research. With the switch in research designs and tools, the commonly encountered threats to validity in public health research (e.g., selection bias, regression to the mean, etc.)[3] are relevant when assessing the data used as inputs to simulation models, but less relevant for assessing modeling outputs. In contrast, more attention is needed to methodology that builds credibility in the model by comparing the simulation model outputs to real-world data, conducting analysis that examine uncertainty in model parameters, and constructing clear visualizations (e.g., histograms, box plots, scatter plots) comparing counterfactual results. Strengthening credibility in a complex systems models can involve:

- Data credibility—Are the data used to build and perform experiments appropriate, accurate, and sufficient? Have all data transformations, (dis) aggregations, and functions been defined correctly?
- Conceptual/structural credibility—Are the theories, relationships, assumptions underlying the model structure correct? Does the model "reasonably" represent the problem entity for the intended purpose of the model?
- Behavioral/operational credibility—How accurately does the model reproduce major behavioral/outcome patterns observed in the real world?

More details about building credibility and verifying simulation models and the specific techniques can be found in Part IV of the book.

7.4. DATA MANAGEMENT AND EXTERNAL LOGISTICS

Similar to traditional research, data management remains a critical part of research approaches grounded in complex systems. Questions about how to securely store, link, and transfer data must be addressed. In some cases, complex-systems approaches involve computationally expensive tools that require special consideration. For such projects, resources for high-performance computing and storage may be required beyond what is typically available from general-purpose computers. Studies may also consider platforms that enable data- and code-sharing (e.g., GitHub) as well as those that enable stakeholders to interact with simulation models.

7.5. DOCUMENTING RESEARCH PROTOCOLS

As with any research study, formal documentation of procedures is critical. Proper and rigorous documentation helps tighten research procedures and is an important communication tool for the research team. Further, replication is an essential step in complex systems methodologies.[13] Simulation model replication has been hindered by numerous factors, especially those related to a lack of consensus in simulation model development and testing and relatively small community of researchers who engage in computational modeling and simulation.[4,13] At the same time, the computer-based nature of simulation modeling enables for rapid dissemination, such as by sharing applets, source codes, or downloadable model files amongst researchers, which suggests that replication can be much easier using these methodologies than it is in experimental or quasi-experimental designs. Model replication is important for several reasons, such as for checking for errors; evaluating the inferences drawn from models; and identifying strengths, limitations, and redundancies among similar models.[13] Recommendations and guidelines have been published regarding best practices for providing documentation of simulation models.[18-20]

7.6. CONCLUSIONS

Complex systems science should not be considered a replacement to or antagonistic with traditional approaches; instead, they should be viewed as approaches that are *synergistically iterative*. Either approach may be more or less valid for investigating any given research question; therefore, the value of either approach is context-dependent, and no one approach is inherently better than the other.[21] Similarly, both approaches have their own distinct limitations that must be acknowledged by researchers when considering a given problem.[21] We summarize some of the most important similarities and differences in Table 7.2.

Table 7.2. COMPARISON TRADITIONAL AND COMPLEX SYSTEM RESEARCH APPROACHES

Step	Similarities	Differences
Finding your focus		
Research objective	Typically begin with "to," followed by a verb such as: identify, explore, describe, explain, compare, assess, test	In a complex systems approach, the objective should suggest that the study will involve characteristics of complex systems such as feedback loops, nonlinearity, delays, and interconnections.
Research question	Both approaches can define descriptive / exploratory research questions. Questions should align with research objectives	General categories of traditional questions: (1) exploratory/descriptive, (2) relational, (3) causal General categories of complex systems questions: (1) exploratory/descriptive, (2) mechanistic, and (3) forecasting, all of which should contain a relational component
Narrowing your focus		
Specifying research method	Methods should follow the research question	Complex systems approaches will typically use systems mapping or simulation modeling approaches versus traditional research designs such as randomized controlled trials, case-control, and observational cohort designs.
Data needs and analysis plan	Data requirements should flow directly from the research question and hypothesis	Complex systems approaches may require additional literature review, secondary data analyses, or primary data analyses to structure a qualitative or computational systems model
Validity and credibility	Both approaches should be validated	Complex systems approaches should focus on validating model structure and data inputs
Data management and logistics	Both approaches need to consider data security, linkage, and transfer	Simulation models may require additional computing resources
Documenting research protocols	Formal documentation of procedures is critical, and all designs should be replicable	The nature of documentation is different for simulation modeling and research designs should make use of published guidance

In addition to their individual contributions to population health, combining complex systems and traditional approaches has profound implications for data collection and measurement. Simulation models rely on traditional data collection methodologies and cause–effect analyses for model parameterization, testing, and validation. As a result, simulation models provide ways to synthesize existing data and research findings from disparate sources in integrative frameworks, as well as uncover important gaps in data and understanding that can be explored using subsequent deductive approaches.[14,15,22] On the other hand, simulation modeling generates novel synthetic data, which can be analyzed using deductive analytical techniques such as linear statistical modeling.[13] These data are typically "cleaner" than those that are derived from in vivo studies because they are not subject to the same difficulties as in vivo studies such as missing data, confounding variables, or unreliable measurement.[13] Further, the process of aligning reductionist- and complex-systems–grounded models, often called *docking models*, can be employed to refine theory by combining and comparing models from across these paradigms to examine the robustness of causal inference, explore underlying mechanisms, and test and refine dynamic hypotheses or theories.[17]

Ultimately, complex systems approaches should be viewed as complementary to the traditional approaches that currently dominate population health research, rather than a panacea that will allow researchers to solve all of the most pressing challenges in these fields.[14,15] The greatest potential of infusing complex systems approaches into these domains is likely from the potential synergy between these novel and current approaches.[21] As readers will learn in other chapters in this volume, traditional approaches are essential to the development of computational simulation models, which in turn reveal new research questions that may be investigated using traditional approaches—representing an iterative relationship[14,15] and synergy.

REFERENCES

1. Andersson C, Törnberg A, Törnberg P. Societal systems: Complex or worse? *Futures*. 2014;63:145–157.
2. Louth J. From Newton to Newtonianism: Reductionism and the development of the social sciences. *Emergence: Complexity and Organization*. 2011;13(4):63–83.
3. Reynolds H, Guest G. Designing research. In: Guest G, Namey E, eds. *Public Health Research Methods*. London: SAGE; 2015:33–68.
4. Marshall B, Galea S. Formalizing the role of agent-based modeling in causal inference and epidemiology. *American Journal of Epidemiology*. 2015;181(2):92–99.
5. Bradford Hill A. The environment and disease: association or causation? *Proceedings of the Royal Society of Medicine*. 1965;58:295–300.
6. Guyatt G, Drummond R, Meade M, Cook D. *The Evidence Based-Medicine Working group Users' Guides to the Medical Literature*. 2nd ed. Chicago, IL: McGraw Hill; 2008.
7. An R, Sturm R. School and residential neighborhood food environment and diet among California youth. *American Journal of Preventive Medicine*. 2012;42(2):129–135.

8. Hattori A, An R, Sturm R. Neighborhood food outlets, diet, and obesity among California adults, 2007 and 2009. *Preventing Chronic Disease.* 2013;10(E35):1–11.

9. Sturm R, Hattori A. Diet and obesity in Los Angeles County 2007–2012: Is there a measurable effect of the 2008 "Fast-Food Ban"? *Social Science & Medicine.* 2015;133:205–211.

10. Brown DR, Brewster LG. The food environment is a complex social network. *Social Science & Medicine.* 2015;133:202–204.

11. Cioffi-Revilla C. Computational social science. *Wiley Interdisciplinary Reviews: Computational Statistics.* 2010;2(3):259–271.

12. Castellani B. Focus: Complexity and the Failure of Quantitative Social Science. 2014; http://discoversociety.org/2014/11/04/focus-complexity-and-the-failure-of-quantitative-social-science/. Accessed April 1, 2016.

13. Axelrod R. Advancing the art of simulation in the social sciences. In: Rennard J-P, ed. *Handbook on research on nature inspired computing for economy and management.* Hershey, PA: Idea Group; 2005.

14. Diez-Roux AV. Complex systems thinking and current impasses in health disparities research. *American Journal of Public Health.* 2011;101(9):1627–1634.

15. Galea S, Riddle M, Kaplan GA. Causal thinking and complex system approaches in epidemiology. *International Journal of Epidemiology.* 2010;39(1):97–106.

16. Balestrini-Robinson S, Zentner JM, Ender TR. On modeling and simulation methods for capturing emergent behaviors for systems of systems. 12th Annual Systems Engineering Conference; 2009; San Diego, CA.

17. Auchincloss AH, Diez Roux AVD. A new tool for epidemiology: The usefulness of dynamic-agent models in understanding place effects on health. *American Journal of Epidemiology.* 2008;168(1):1–8.

18. Eddy DM, Hollingworth W, Caro JJ, Tsevat J, McDonald KM, Wong JB. Model transparency and validation: a report of the ISPOR-SMDM Modeling Good Research Practices Task Force-7. *Medical Decision Making.* 2012;32(5):733–743.

19. Grimm V, Berger U, DeAngelis DL, Polhill JG, Giske J, Railsback SF. The ODD protocol: a review and first update. *Ecological Modelling.* 2010;221(23):2760–2768.

20. Muller B, Bohn F, Derebler G, et al. Describing human decisions in agent-based models-ODD+ D, an extension of the ODD protocol. *Environmental Modelling & Software.* 2013;48:37–48.

21. Fang FC, Casadevall A. Reductionistic and holistic science. *Infection and Immunity.* 2011;79(4):1401–1404.

22. Agar M. Complexity theory: An exploration and overview based on John Holland's work. *Field Methods.* 1999;11(2):99–120.

8

Model Thinking and Formal Modeling to Improve Our Mental Models in Population Health Research

MICHAEL K. LEMKE

8.1. INTRODUCTION

We inhabit a world that is inherently complex, and we are surrounded by innumerable complex systems in our daily lives. When encountering this ubiquitous complexity, the human mind (typically by default) applies various heuristics to provide order and simplify this flood of information and make sense of it all. From these heuristics, our *mental models*—how we understand phenomena in the real world—emerge, which shape our decisions. Unfortunately, the same limitations that confound our judgment and decision-making heuristics similarly cloud our mental models and result in fundamental misunderstandings about those complex systems that make up our world and lead to flawed decisions about how to act upon them.

The development of *models*, through the act of *modeling*, provide means to mitigate inherent shortcomings in our cognitive abilities and mental models and can stimulate new ways of understanding and acting in population health, grounded in *model thinking*.[1] For the study of complex systems in particular, including those that define many of the key domains of population health research and action, a distinct class of modeling approaches grounded in *computational simulation modeling* have emerged in recent decades to enable novel scientific inquiry and facilitate decision-making. Engagement in modeling can also overcome the difficulties in learning imposed by the daunting complexity of the world, leading

Michael K. Lemke, *Model Thinking and Formal Modeling to Improve Our Mental Models in Population Health Research* In: *Complex Systems and Population Health.* Edited by: Yorghos Apostolopoulos, Kristen Hassmiller Lich, and Michael Kenneth Lemke, Oxford University Press (2020). © Oxford University Press.
DOI: 10.1093/oso/9780190880743.003.0008

to transformed mental models and the proliferation of model thinking in population health research and action.

8.2. HOW WE INADEQUATELY MAKE SENSE OF THE WORLD AND WHY IT IS PROBLEMATIC

The dynamic complexity of those systems that impact us, and the bewildering amount of information and phenomena they produce, overwhelm the ability of our information processing and cognitive systems to understand them and render simplification necessary.[2,3] We selectively attend to only a portion of this flood of information, filtering out most and ultimately processing only a small amount of what our senses actually encounter.[3] Based on what we learn from the information we cognitively process over time, we form innumerable mental models—our internal, simplified representations of the real world. Mental models are generally enduring and resilient, and they represent our understanding of the world (e.g., cause–effect relationships) and shape our behaviors (i.e., how we act upon the world).[3-5] A positive (reinforcing) feedback loop exists between mental models and perceptual filtering: Our mental models tell us which information is important, such as those data that conform with what we "know" about the world.[3] Other information is subsequently deemed to be unimportant and filtered out,[3] confirming our prior models.

Although necessary, these cognitive strategies are wholly inadequate for understanding our inherently complex world. These failings are especially apparent when considering mental models, which are hampered by our own misperceptions and biases and are commonly inconsistent, unreliable, and too narrow.[6-8] Even worse, our mental models have been shown to be wrought with numerous shortcomings that cause them to break down when encountering complex phenomena.[9] Consistently, our mental models have been shown to fall short in capturing key characteristics of complex systems, including interconnections and interactions,[4,10] nonlinear relationships,[7,10-12] feedback structures,[3,7,8,10-13] time delays,[7,10-13] and accumulations,[3,7,12,13] to name a few. We also consistently take an exogenous, rather than an endogenous, viewpoint—attributing key outcomes as arising from factors beyond our control (external forces), rather than our own actions[13]—and we underestimate the importance of the system structure in how people behave (i.e., the fundamental attribution error).[3] Due to these (and other) fallacies, cause and effect judgments in our mental models are often erroneous, as we assume single causes for outcomes, focus on spatially and temporally proximal cause–effect relationships, and settle the first satisfactory explanation we find.[7,10] In instances of complexity—with distal temporal and spatial cause and effect— these judgments become even more spurious.[7]

Shortcomings in our mental models when confronted with dynamic complexity have been repeatedly demonstrated. One such example is in the "Beer Game," which is a simulation game that mimics a beer production and distribution system that features a delay between when an order is placed and when it is filled.[14] In the Beer Game, players fill one of four positions: factory, distributor, wholesaler, and retailer.[14] Players have one goal, which is to minimize costs, and have one decision to make—how much beer to order—and are instructed not to communicate with one another outside of the product ordering process.[14] Customer demand is consistent through the beginning of the game, but later increases and stays at that level throughout the remainder of the game.[14] This relatively small and one-time change in customer demand in the game disrupts equilibrium and results in ordering decisions that generate widespread oscillation and instability.[14] When players are asked about the instability that followed the increase in customer demand, they typically blame an outside factor out of their control, when, in reality, the instability largely results from flawed decision-making among the players, reflective of the shortcomings of the mental models they bring to bear while playing the game. In particular, the players focus on their own decisions in isolation, rather than looking at the larger system (i.e., all the players in the game), and their solutions address symptomatic (i.e., making an ordering decision based on their immediate supply), rather than root (i.e., the delays inherent to the ordering process in the game) causes of the problem initiated by the change in customer demand, which end up being exacerbatory.[14]

Other shortcomings in our mental models have been uncovered by social scientists when considering the phenomenon of emergence. Two everyday examples of emergence are bird flocks and traffic jams. With respect to the former, when individuals are asked how migratory birds form V formations, they typically attribute these patterns to following a pecking order, such as the other birds following a lead bird; essentially, they identify one centralized cause, and they view V formations as deterministic.[15] However, in reality, V formations have been proven as *emergent* from individual birds who are following a very simple set of rules, without the presence of a centralized controller.[15] Similarly, when individuals are asked to identify the origin of traffic jams, they typically identify one centralized cause, such as a roadway accident.[15] However, these individuals rarely identify factors that do not represent a centralized cause, such as randomness from cars merging onto the roadway.[15] Together, these fallacies in thinking are attributed to a cognitive pattern that has been labeled as the "deterministic-centralized mindset," which leads individuals to view randomness as destructive of patterns, rather than the source of creating these patterns (the "deterministic" part), and to describe patterns as being caused from a centralized controller or cause (the "centralized" part).[15,16]

These same shortcomings in our mental models that undermine our understanding of real-world phenomena also reduce our ability to act on the world in the way that we intend, as most of our decisions are grounded in the understanding of the world that we derive from our mental models.[4] The term *policy resistance* describes the scenario where our inadequate understanding of a complex system we are trying to act on leads to solutions that are either ineffective or make things worse, creating what we see as "side effects" and leading to frustration and helplessness.[7,10] In other words, when trying to act on complex systems, the mental models we bring to bear are not up to the task, and then we are surprised when unexpected outcomes—that are given the misnomer side effects—occur.[3,4,10] The complex systems that we try to change are interrelated and interconnected,[3] non-linear,[10] inundated with feedbacks,[3,7,10] exhibit time delays,[3,7,10] and endogenous[3]—and, as a result of all of these characteristics (and many more), they are policy resistant.[10]

Scientists are not excluded from the limitations of our mental models and our frequent inability to effectively act on our world.[3] The Newtonian paradigm, grounded in reductionism, makes sense to many of us in the context of the characteristics of our mental models.[17] Intuitively, the type of mechanistic thinking it purports aligns with how many of us tend to view the world,[17] and indeed it has been, and continues to be, the dominant paradigm in population health.[17] The mental models of population health researchers critically influence research and action by shaping, for example, what research questions we ask to address population health issues, which usually assume cause and effect relationships that are spatially and temporally proximal and focus on risk-factor epidemiology; how we go about answering those research questions, which typically focuses on variable isolation; what actions we take to fix population health problems, which are most commonly oriented toward symptoms rather than root causes; and what we teach students in population health curricula. The deep-seated influences of mental models in population health are demonstrated by the body of knowledge accumulated in the field, as well as the persistent gaps in knowledge; those problems that have been effectively addressed and those that seem stubborn, worsening, or intractable; and the explicit educational backgrounds and training—and gaps in learning, understanding, and expertise—among population health researchers.

It is clear that our mental models are unable to cope with the dynamic complexity inherent to the world around us.[10,12] Thus, to better understand the complex world that we live in, and to meaningfully be able to act upon it, requires both amending our own incorrect mental models and, as described in Chapter 9 of this volume, transformatively integrating the incomplete mental models held by many, to better correspond with how things really are. The solution is to engage in new ways of thinking—to become *model thinkers*[1]—to overcome the failings of our mental models, to better understand those complex systems that constitute our world, and to effectively act upon them.[3,7,10] However, to become model thinkers, we need help—we need frameworks and tools that can help to bridge the gap between the shortcomings of our cognitive capabilities and resulting mental models and the dynamic complexity of the world.[10] Therefore, we turn to models, and formal models in particular, as critical enablers of understanding that "make us smarter"[1] and therefore better prepared to make decisions to change the world. The growing prevalence of models across professional fields, including academia,[1] provides evidence of the growing appreciation of their diverse value and, indeed, necessity in understanding and acting in the modern world. In the case of complex systems, a specific set of modeling methodologies and tools have been developed that rely on computational simulation modeling, that allows for experimentation using simulation based on virtual worlds.[3,7,18]

8.3. MODEL THINKING AND FORMAL MODELING
TO UNDERSTAND POPULATION HEALTH CHALLENGES

The term *model* refers to a simplified version of something in the real world.[19] The concept of simplification is key: Because our cognitive abilities are overwhelmed by the complexity of the real world, we instead study models that pare down reality by taking that aspect of the real world it represents and making it smaller, or with fewer details, or with less complexity[20] because it allows for comprehension.[21] Thus, models have purpose—they are "purposeful representations" of reality[18] that allow us to understand the world around us.[21] However, the application of models has been vast in scope, and the uses of models include (but is not limited to) the following: reasoning, explaining, designing, communicating, acting, predicting, exploring, guiding data collection, discovering new research questions, training, and education.[1,5,22]

Models can take many forms, depending on their purpose, as we are surrounded by models throughout our daily lives. One way that models can be distinguished is by whether they are *implicit* or *explicit*. Implicit models are distinctly nonscientific, as their relation to data is unknown, and they are marked by unclear underlying assumptions, untested internal consistency, and other potential flaws.[22] Mental models are examples of implicit models that are internal (psychological) models: They are our internal, simplified representations of phenomena in the real world. In contrast, explicit models are out in the world and laid out in such a way that they can be evaluated by others.[22] Video games are examples of explicit computer-based (in-silico) models: For example, the Civilization series allows players to control the rise and fall of civilizations across millennia in a matter of hours from their laptop by paring down reality in countless ways. There are also explicit physical models: Hobbyists can purchase kits to construct scale models that allow them to have an appealing (but greatly simplified and reduced) version of an object of interest—such as Wrigley Field—on display in their homes. However, for becoming model thinkers, especially in the context of population health, we are most interested in developing *formal models*—models that precisely and systematically represent some aspect of the real world, typically in a scientific or modeling language (e.g., mathematics, diagrams, computer algorithms), that provides transparency in its assumptions and allows for testing and analysis.[1,18]

8.4. FORMAL MODELING IN POPULATION HEALTH RESEARCH

A distinct set of formal modeling approaches, collectively known as computational simulation modeling, have been developed as the primary means to study complex systems.[8,23] These approaches enable development of formal models that represent attributes of complex systems (as discussed in Chapter 2 of this volume), including those attributes—interconnections and interactions, nonlinear relationships, feedback structures, distal cause and effect relationships, and emergence—that confound only our cognitive abilities and mental models.[24] Further, these methods can be used to represent the structures of those complex adaptive systems and complex adaptive systems-of-systems (as discussed in Chapter 3 of this volume) that shape key domains of inquiry in population health.[23,24]

Referred to as a "third way of doing science" (with induction [statistics] and deduction [mathematics] being the other two),[5] the hallmark of computational simulation modeling is simulation, which is a particular type of modeling that allows us to conduct in-silico experiments on computer-based virtual worlds.[5,9,20] As a virtual laboratory, simulation modeling has been applied to allow researchers to conduct experiments and gather evidence in instances when that would normally be impossible, such as when in vivo experimentation would be infeasible, unethical, too expensive, or too time consuming.[3,10,20] Even when in vivo experimentation is possible, simulation models will still usually be needed to study complex systems, as the types of hypotheses that are investigated in these systems are best explored by taking advantage of the tremendous power of these techniques—especially when our key research questions assume nonlinear relationships, interdependencies, and other such fundamental attributes of complex systems.[3,20,23] Another key domain of applications for simulation models has been for decision-making, as the implications of various arrays of policies and other actions can be simulated across potentially long time horizons, and their consequences examined.[4] Additional applications of simulation modeling include (but are not limited to) theory development, prediction, data collection guidance, communication, training, and even entertainment.[4,20]

8.5. TRANSFORMING OUR MENTAL MODELS USING COMPUTATIONAL SIMULATION MODELING

Although our mental models fall short when understanding complex systems, we can engage in modeling and use formal models—and computational simulation models in particular—to learn and transform these deeply held internal understandings of the world. Models are valuable for all the reasons stated in this chapter (and many more), but perhaps none more than to overcome barriers to learning that the complexity of the world presents. Not only does complexity reduce the amount of evidence that is generated and available to us, it also reduces our ability to learn from the evidence that is present.[3] Those "usual suspects" that confound our mental models in the presence of complexity—such as time delays, feedbacks, accumulations—additionally hinder our ability to learn.[3] In particular, our misperceptions of feedback—which is an essential process in learning—confound our ability to learn about complex systems and lead to distorted mental models. To transform our mental models, a new type of learning must take place: we need to shift from *single-loop learning*, where we learn how to pursue our goals grounded in the context of our initial mental models and modify our actions based on what happens along the way, to *double-loop learning*, where those initial mental models actually change along the way as well—leading to new understanding of the world and new ways of acting upon it.[3]

Computational simulation modeling provides the tools capable of making this shift and overcoming those barriers to learning in the presence of complexity.[8,9,12] These approaches provide numerous advantages for learning about complex systems that have been shown to transform the mental models of both modelers and model consumers (e.g., community stakeholders).[4,12,25-28] However, the use of simulation models in particular can provide that "second loop" for double-loop learning, as these virtual worlds provide learning platforms that circumvent the barriers to learning that are present in the real world.[3] Here, individuals can see the immediate consequences of any number of potential actions; they can take actions that they could, or would not, do in the real world and learn from the consequences of those actions; they can be asked to repeat their actions in different conditions and contexts to see how the consequences may change; and they receive clear and near-instantaneous feedback from their actions— leading to learning that can transform mental models.[3,7] Unlike the real world, which is hopelessly complex, simulation models are just that—*models, simplified representations of reality*. More specifically, they are formal models; therefore, unlike the "black box" cause–effect relationships that permeate reality, simulation models are transparent "under the hood" (e.g., the assumptions of the model) to both modelers and model users, which provides additional opportunity for learning and for improving the simulation model itself.[3,4,7]

There are several types of computational simulation modeling approaches that can be used to facilitate learning and transform mental models. Chapter 12 of this volume provides a thorough discussion of their assumptions, strengths, and weaknesses, and subsequent chapters in this volume provide nuanced descriptions of their application in key domains of population health. However, two of these techniques—system dynamics modeling (SDM) and agent-based modeling (ABM)—are highlighted in the following discussion to demonstrate their value as learning tools to improve our understanding of complex systems in population health and transform our mental models.

8.5.1. The Beer Game: System Dynamics Modeling in Chronic Disease Prevention

SDM is a typically (but not exclusively) top–down, aggregate-oriented computational modeling approach that emphasizes uncovering the structure of the dynamically complex systems and determining how to leverage this structure to create desirable change in outcomes.[29,30] Chapter 13 of this volume provides an in-depth description of another application of SDM in these domains. As discussed previously, participants in the Beer Game demonstrate overly narrow thinking that leads them to focus on their own decisions in isolation, rather than looking at the larger system; further, their solutions focus on addressing symptomatic, rather than root, causes of the problem. The Beer Game is analogous to the mental models that are typically brought to bear in population health, and the same limitations that are observed in the game are also observed in population health research, where causal inference is primarily focused on methodological variable isolation, rather than on viewing population health systems holistically and on exploring proximal (e.g., behavioral) rather than distal (e.g., public policy) factors. Similarly, many public health interventions are often compartmentalized and address only a small number of proximal factors, rather than considering the system that generates the problems they seek to address as a whole, and they typically address symptomatic rather than root (i.e., structural) causes.[31]

In recognition of this, Jack Homer and Gary Hirsch engaged in an SDM effort to evaluate broad categories of chronic disease interventions.[31] They built a relatively simple system dynamics model that simulated two types of chronic disease prevention: Upstream prevention of disease onset (root causes) and downstream prevention of disease complication (symptomatic causes).[31] The model was simulated across 50 years for three different policy scenarios: Status Quo (no intervention), More Complications Prevention (intervention that addresses symptomatic causes), and More Onset Prevention (intervention that addresses root causes).[31] The results of their SDM effort revealed the power of understanding system structure and time delays in chronic disease prevention efforts. While the More Complications Prevention intervention scenario initially leads to reduced deaths from chronic disease complications, in the long term it leads to more people in the population with chronic disease and greater need for prevention for these complications, which creates a reinforcing loop that creates a "vicious cycle" leads to greater deaths from chronic disease complications in the long term.[31] In contrast, the More Onset Prevention intervention scenario formed a reinforcing loop that created a "virtuous cycle" that led to declines in chronic disease prevalence and deaths from chronic disease prevalence over time.[31] Because of the inherent shortcomings in our mental models and in Newtonian approaches regarding system structure, feedback loops, and time delays, it is unlikely that these valuable insights for understanding and interventions could have been learned otherwise.

8.5.2. Bird Flocks and Traffic Jams: Agent-Based Modeling in Alcohol Prevention

In contrast to SDM, ABM is a typically (but not strictly) bottom–up computational modeling approach that seeks to model macro-level outcomes from the interaction of micro-level elements.[30] Chapter 14 of this volume provides an in-depth description of another application of ABM in population health.

To reiterate from earlier in the chapter, misattribution of observed patterns in bird V-flocks and traffic jams is due to the deterministic-centralized mindset, where the roles of randomness and centralized control in creating such patterns are often misconstrued. As demonstrated by this mindset, emergent properties are difficult for our mental models to embody; analogous to this, most population health research is oriented toward risk-factor epidemiology, rather than those individual-level actions and decisions driven by human agency[32] that are inherent in many of the complex systems. The deterministic-centralized mindset is also found in substance prevention research, where emergence and other related properties, such as stochasticity, self-organization, co-evolution, and adaptation, are often overlooked.[33] Hence, the explicit purpose of ABM in understanding emergent properties in dynamically complex systems has particular value in transforming mental models in substance prevention research and action, where population-level patterns in use and abuse are emergent from the interactions of individual users and their environments that are often random and are not centrally controlled.[33,34]

Given the potential value of ABM in substance use prevention, researchers constructed an agent-based model of drinking behavior that examined how the patterns of interactions change upon the introduction of an alcohol outlet into the environment among three types of agents: Susceptible nondrinkers, current drinkers, and former drinkers.[34] The ABM showed several counterintuitive patterns: Introducing even one current drinker into a population of susceptible drinkers could cause the entire population to become current drinkers over time, and introducing an alcohol outlet into the environment actually reduced the ability of current drinkers to convert susceptible drinkers because it led the current drinkers to cluster away from them.[34] These patterns, which have potentially critical implications for alcohol prevention initiatives, would be difficult, if not impossible, to anticipate using only mental models, and it is unlikely that Newtonian approaches would have been able to expose them.

8.6. CONCLUSIONS

To effectively understand, act, and learn in our inherently complex world—to become model thinkers—we need formal models, and computational simulation models in particular. However, formal models are not a panacea. First, before developing formal models in the first place—and especially computational simulation models, which are typically more taxing—the value of that model beyond, say, our mental models needs to be weighed.[35] Sometimes the simpler solution, or an existing model already available to us, will suffice. Models must have suitable assumptions and, especially in the realm of population health, be based on solid theory and data.[23] Models are the products of human judgment: They require practice, are prone to mistakes, and rely on our existing knowledge of the real-world object they intend to represent.[1,5] Models, and simulation models in particular, are not necessarily a substitute for the way we currently engage in science—in silico experimentation is fundamentally different than in vivo experimentation: With the latter, we are experimenting with the actual object we wish to investigate, while with the former we are only experimenting with the *model* of that object.[20]

Additionally, relying on one model to understand any (inherently complex) aspect of reality will more than likely be insufficient.[1] Thus, along with being model thinkers, we also need to be "many-model thinkers": applying multiple models to understand parts of our world.[1] This is especially true for complex systems, which are especially difficult to learn about, understand, and effectively act upon.

Engaging in many-model thinking and applying multiple models to complex systems allows us to take advantage of the strengths of each model, while covering up the flaws inherent in each individual model.[1] For computational simulation modeling, each approach has its own strengths and weaknesses (as discussed in Chapter 12 of this volume); by combining approaches, such as by engaging in complementary hybrid approaches (as discussed in Chapter 15 of this volume), our modeling endeavors can attain synergies that we could not achieve otherwise.[4]

Despite the caveats of modeling, we need formal models, and especially computational simulation models, to become model thinkers as we engage in population health research and action. Our cognitive abilities are not up to the task of the flood of information we receive from the world. Our heuristics and mental models suffer from a host of shortcomings and failings that leave us woefully unable to learn, understand, and act upon the world, and this is exacerbated tenfold in the presence of complexity. John Sterman once said, "All decisions are based on models, and all models are wrong . . . yet accepting them is central to effective systems thinking."[12p525] Thus, computational simulation models are powerful tools for thinking in new ways in population health—for engaging in double-loop learning, and transforming our mental models as we try to understand and change the world around us.

REFERENCES

1. Page SE. *The model thinker.* New York, NY: Basic Books; 2018.
2. Louth J. From Newton to Newtonianism: Reductionism and the development of the social sciences. *Emergence Complex Org.* 2011;13(4):63–83.
3. Sterman JD. Learning from evidence in a complex world. *Am J Public Health.* 2006;96(3):505–514.
4. Osgood N. What tools does complex systems modeling provide for understanding population health and health disparities? Conference on Complex Systems, Health Disparities and Population Health: Building Bridges; February 24–25, 2014; Washington, DC.
5. Madey G, Kaisler SH. Computational modeling of social and organizational systems. http://www3.nd.edu/~gmadey/Activities/CMSOS-Tutorial.pdf. Published 2008. Accessed October 25, 2015.
6. Milstein B, Homer J. System dynamics simulation in support of obesity prevention decision-making. Institute of Medicine Committee on an Evidence Framework for Obesity Prevention Decision-Making; March 16, 2009; Irvine, CA.
7. Sterman JD. Systems dynamics modeling: Tools for learning in a complex world. *Calif Manage Rev.* 2001;43(4):8–25.
8. Vennix JAM. Group model-building: Tackling messy problems. *Syst Dynam Rev.* 1999;15:379–401.
9. Andersson C, Törnberg A, Törnberg P. Societal systems: Complex or worse? *Futures.* 2014;63:145–157.
10. Sterman JD. Sustaining sustainability: Creating a systems science in a fragmented academy and polarized world. In: Weinstein MP, Turner RE, eds. *Sustainability*

science: The emerging paradigm and the urban environment. New York, NY: Springer; 2012:21–58.

11. Minami N, Madnick S. *Using system analysis to improve traffic safety.* Cambridge, MA: Massachusetts Institute of Technology; 2010.

12. Sterman JD. All models are wrong: Reflections on becoming a systems scientist. *Sys Dynam Rev.* 2002;18(4):501–531.

13. Sterman JD. Modeling managerial behavior: Misperceptions of feedback in a dynamic decision making experiment. *Manag Sci.* 1989;35(3):321–339.

14. Goodwin JS, Franklin SG. The Beer Distribution game: Using simulation to teach systems thinking. *J Manag Dev.* 1994;13(8):7–15.

15. Wilensky U, Rand W. *An introduction to agent-based modeling: Modeling natural, social, and engineered complex systems with NetLogo.* Cambridge, MA: MIT Press; 2015.

16. Wilensky U, Resnick M. Thinking in levels: A dynamic systems approach to making sense of the world. *J Sci Ed Tech.* 1999;8(1):3–19.

17. Dekker S, Cilliers P, Hofmeyr J-H. The complexity of failure: Implications of complexity theory for safety investigations. *Safety Sci.* 2011;49(6):939–945.

18. Railsback SF, Grimm V. *Agent-based and individual-based modeling: A practical introduction.* Princeton, NJ: Princeton University Press; 2011.

19. Meadows DH, Wright D. *Thinking in systems: A primer.* White River Junction, VT: Chelsea Green; 2008.

20. Gilbert N, Troitzsch K. *Simulation for the social scientist.* Berkshire, UK: McGraw-Hill Education; 2005.

21. Puccia CJ, Levins R. *Qualitative modeling of complex systems: An introduction to loop analysis and time averaging.* Cambridge, MA: Harvard University Press; 1986.

22. Epstein JM. Why model? *J Artif Societ Soc Simul.* 2008;11(4):12–16.

23. Miller JH, Page SE. *Complex adaptive systems: An introduction to computational models of social life.* Princeton, NJ: Princeton University Press; 2009.

24. Kaplan GA, Simon CP, Diez Roux AV, Galea S. Introduction: Bridging complex systems, health disparities, and population health. In: Kaplan GA, Diez Roux AV, Simon CP, Galea S, eds. *Growing inequality: bridging complex systems, population health, and health disparities.* Washington, DC: Westphalia Press; 2017.

25. Marshall D, Burgos-Liz L, Ijzerman MJ, et al. Selecting a dynamic simulation modeling method for health care delivery research—Part 2: Report of the ISPOR Dynamic Simulation Modeling Emerging Good Practices Task Force. *Value Health.* 2015;18(2):147–160.

26. Royston G, Dost A, Townshend J, Turner H. Using system dynamics to help develop and implement policies and programmes in health care in England. *Syst Dynam Rev.* 1999;15(3):293–313.

27. Wolstenholme E. A patient flow perspective of UK health services: exploring the case for new" intermediate care" initiatives. *Syst Dynam Rev.* 1999;15(3):253–271.

28. Hovmand PS, Andersen DF, Rouwette E, Richardson GP, Rux K, Calhoun A. Group model-building "scripts" as a collaborative planning tool. *Syst Res Behav Sci.* 2012;29(2):179–193.

29. Figueredo GP, Siebers P-O, Aickelin U, Whitbrook A, Garibaldi JM. Juxtaposition of system dynamics and agent-based simulation for a case study in immunosenescence. *PLoS One.* 2015;10(3):e0118359.

30. Balestrini-Robinson S, Zentner JM, Ender TR. On modeling and simulation methods for capturing emergent behaviors for systems of systems. 12th Annual Systems Engineering Conference; 2009; San Diego, CA.

31. Homer JB, Hirsch GB. System dynamics modeling for public health: Background and opportunities. *Am J Public Health.* 2006;96(3):452–458.

32. Olaya C. Cows, agency, and the significance of operational thinking. *Syst Dynam Rev.* 2015;31:183–219.

33. Apostolopoulos Y, Lemke MK, Barry AE, Hassmiller Lich K. Moving alcohol prevention research forward—Part I: Introducing a complex systems paradigm. *Addiction.* 2018;113(2):353–362.

34. Gorman DM, Mezic J, Mezic I, Gruenewald PJ. Agent-based modeling of drinking behavior: A preliminary model and potential applications to theory and practice. *Am J Public Health.* 2006;96(11):2055–2060.

35. Homer JB. A system dynamics model of national cocaine prevalence. *Syst Dynam Rev.* 1993;9(1):49–78.

9

Engaging Stakeholders in Mapping and Modeling Complex Systems Structure to Inform Population Health Research and Action

KRISTEN HASSMILLER LICH AND JILL KUHLBERG

9.1. INTRODUCTION

It is critically important that population health researchers and leaders meaningfully collaborate with stakeholders in any health initiative to identify problems and priorities, to integrate and transfer evidence, to grow (shared) understanding, and to generate theory and test hypotheses. Such collaboration is also critical for eliciting feasible action ideas that are aligned with the motivating problem and make use of available assets. Failure to coordinate research and real-world practice, as has all too often been the case whether or not the focal problem is complex, results in only a minority of research evidence actually reaching—and that after a nearly two-decade average delay.[1] Bodies of work around knowledge translation, participatory action research, community-based participatory research, and dissemination and implementation (to name a few) have developed to improve bidirectional coordination between research and practice and to speed up the rate at which relevant research is translated into action. While this emerging work has had a profound impact on population health, it must expand to accommodate a complexity science perspective. In this chapter, we present current best practices and call the reader to join in efforts to use, evaluate, adapt, and innovate—building a science around stakeholder engagement in the presence of complexity.

Kristen Hassmiller Lich and Jill Kuhlberg, *Engaging Stakeholders in Mapping and Modeling Complex Systems Structure to Inform Population Health Research and Action* In: *Complex Systems and Population Health.* Edited by: Yorghos Apostolopoulos, Kristen Hassmiller Lich, and Michael Kenneth Lemke, Oxford University Press (2020). © Oxford University Press. DOI: 10.1093/oso/9780190880743.003.0009

9.2. WHY INVOLVE STAKEHOLDERS IN MODELING COMPLEX PROBLEMS?

In this chapter, we define stakeholders as " people or organisations with an interest in the (wicked) problem and its (re-)solution."[2p35] We encourage broad engagement, including all who affect the problem in some way or must contribute to the solution. A key component of fostering collaboration is aligning incentives and efforts among multiple stakeholders.[3] Stakeholders possess their own mental models of the origins and drivers of the problem at hand and what it would take to address it. And, as described in Chapter 8 of this volume, for stakeholders working to address complex problems or problems embedded in complex systems, this is especially challenging since human cognition is notoriously impaired in simulating the delays, feedback effects, and nonlinearities present in complex systems that impact their proposed strategies' ability to effect desired change.[4-6] This extends to challenges intuiting how complex micro-level rules can generate emergent system phenomenon.[7] Since formal models (i.e., system dynamics [SD] models, agent-based models, discrete event simulation models, etc.) support individuals in refining and improving their mental models and decision-making efficacy, the involvement of stakeholders in building those models has shown to be effective in supporting them in making better decisions and the implementation of planned action.[8] Hovmand[9] also argues that the call to involve stakeholders in the model-building process comes from a need to build support and advocacy for action and policy change to address complex societal issues from the bottom up, that is, from the constituents affected by policies and programs, aware of assets and constraints, and approaching decision-making informed by model-building activities.

9.3. GROUP MODEL BUILDING IN SYSTEM DYNAMICS

Group model building (GMB) is one of the oldest practices of involving stakeholders in the model-building process, developed simultaneously by two groups of system dynamicists in the late 1980s.[10] GMB was initially conceptualized to engage stakeholders in every step of the often iterative and nonlinear GMB process, which includes defining the problem, hypothesizing key system structure producing the problematic system behavior/outcomes, creating and formulating a quantitative model of the system structure, testing/building confidence in the model and analyzing it, and, using the resulting model to inspire/formulate and evaluate action ideas.[10,11] Several threads of GMB have evolved since; for example, participatory SD modeling allowed for more flexibility in when stakeholders are/are not engaged[12] and community-based SD (CBSD) designed to use and grow capacity for ongoing use of GMB within communities.[9] While it has been argued that different threads of GMB practice can be characterized by their conceptualization of participation as normative, substantive, instrumental, or transformative,[13] all GMB projects typically entail one or more of the following components: (1) involving the stakeholders in the often iterative process of model conceptualization (e.g., identification of relevant factors and how they are related), (2) generating policy options and scenarios for testing using the model with stakeholders, (3) facilitating discussion about model-based insights from the modeling process, and/or (4) model analysis.[14]

9.3.1. Goals and Dimensions of GMB Practice

Goals of GMB span multiple levels, from the individual to the group, to the larger organization or community.[15] At the individual level, the goal of the GMB process is to generate a positive reaction to the learning and mental model refinement supported by the process and, through that, engage commitment and trigger change in behavior(s). Targeted changes in behavior may involve a shift in policy, in the information/data used to inform decisions, or in the way that data are interpreted and acted upon. At the group level, the aim of participation in the modeling process is to foster greater alignment of mental models around a specific problem and a commitment to a coordinated response to address it. At the organization or community levels, the goal is to see changes in the system, evidence of system improvement, or problem alleviation. The development of CBSD has advanced another goal in line with its normative value of participation, which is the increased capacity of the stakeholders involved in the process to use modeling to address problems in the future.[9]

With these goals in mind, there are four dimensions over which GMB projects can vary.[11] The first dimension asks, *Who defines the problem?* Dynamic problems can be identified and defined by the stakeholder group(s) or by outsiders (i.e., researchers, governing boards, nongovernmental organizations, etc.). The second asks, *How structured the process will be?* The activities employed in the process of GMB range from completely open-ended and improvised to highly structured. Structured processes can involve "scripts," which describe team roles and steps organized toward a certain objective (i.e., creation of a causal loop diagram, list of potential policies to improve outcomes, elicitation of parameter values or functional forms within the simulation model).[14,16] Third, *what kind of model(s) will be developed or is(are) required to support the insights the stakeholders need to address the identified problem?* System dynamics is unique as a systems science method as it draws insights from both qualitative maps/diagrams and quantified computer simulation models.[17] The nature and objectives for certain problems warrant pursuing one or both types.[9] Lastly, modelers are asked to consider *if, in the modeling process, the GMB project will begin with a blank slate—letting participants define the initial model structure—or whether an existing model will be used (perhaps large or small; qualitative or simulating; accurate or intentionally wrong to spur discussion and iteration) as a starting point to build upon or refine in some way?*

The decisions made for each of these dimensions in the beginning of a project and as the modeling process unfolds are the result of the nature of the problem at hand, resources available (including time, participants, modeling and facilitation expertise, funding, etc.), values of those involved in the planning and steering of the project (often referred to as the core modeling team), and the sociocultural context where the modeling is taking place.[9] In addition to varying along the previously identified four dimensions, GMB practice can also vary in terms of when in the modeling process certain stakeholder groups or individuals are involved and how much they participate (i.e., providing information to modelers on the system or building/drawing model structure themselves, etc.). For examples of such variation on SD projects involving cross-sector collaborations in population health, see Cilenti et al.[18]

Since GMB's initial development nearly 30 years ago, its reported effectiveness in supporting individual and collective changes[8,19] has brought an exponential increase in its use in a range of contexts addressing complex problems related to population health. Cilenti et al.[18] found over 30 applications of GMB in collective learning and action planning for community health alone.

9.4. THE ICEBERG AS A COMPLEXITY SCIENCE METAPHOR

The iceberg as a metaphor for systems thinking is incredibly useful for reminding us—as researchers and practitioners in population health—of the importance of learning, for a given problem, the underlying determinants that are so often complex and hidden from ready view (Figure 9.1).[20] At the tip of the iceberg, above the waterline, is a problematic event—what we see that causes pain and a need to react. For example, an avoidable death, a poorly controlled disease outbreak, or a critical healthcare service provider becoming financially nonviable. It might also represent problematic symptoms of a more fundamental underlying problem— for example, a cluster of maternal deaths among African-American women in a community masking underlying structural racism or long wait times in an emergency department triggered by an underresourced community mental health system rendering the emergency department a last-resort safety net for care. More systems-aware methods for problem identification and prioritization exist. As one example, concept mapping is a systematic approach that can be used to document problematic events, organize them into meaningful clusters, and rank each in terms of relative importance and feasibility to change across key stakeholder groups. While it is fundamentally an approach to making sense of stakeholder responses, it can also be used as input to other approaches used to dive under the waterline.[21]

If the problematic event we seek to address is shaped by or embedded within a complex system, we are not likely to understand it well without using methods aligned with deeper levels of the iceberg. If we fail to appreciate the patterns of events (first level below the waterline), our sense of what the problem is might be off. For example, we might attribute an isolated event to a bigger trend or assume the characteristics of a recent event or outcome in one subgroup or community represent the context without testing that assumption. Ultimately, to improve outcomes, we need to understand the structure of the system producing problematic patterns

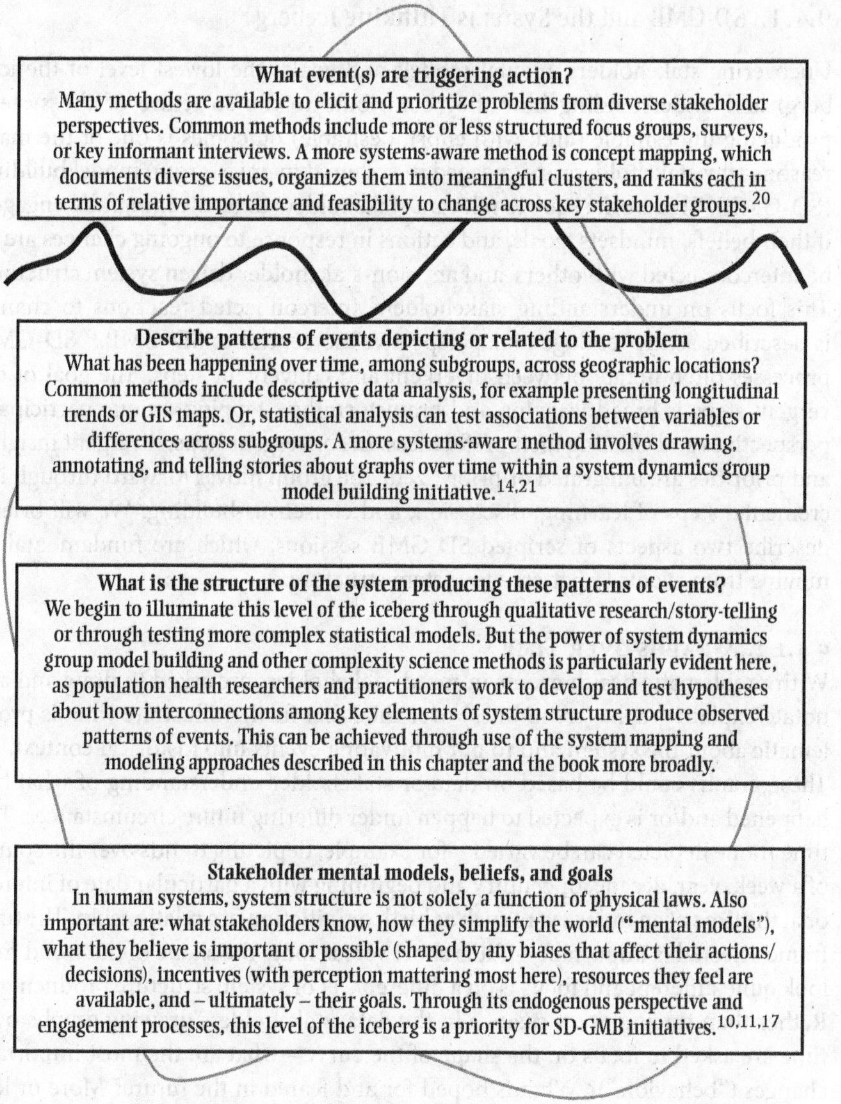

What event(s) are triggering action?
Many methods are available to elicit and prioritize problems from diverse stakeholder perspectives. Common methods include more or less structured focus groups, surveys, or key informant interviews. A more systems-aware method is concept mapping, which documents diverse issues, organizes them into meaningful clusters, and ranks each in terms of relative importance and feasibility to change across key stakeholder groups.[20]

Describe patterns of events depicting or related to the problem
What has been happening over time, among subgroups, across geographic locations? Common methods include descriptive data analysis, for example presenting longitudinal trends or GIS maps. Or, statistical analysis can test associations between variables or differences across subgroups. A more systems-aware method involves drawing, annotating, and telling stories about graphs over time within a system dynamics group model building initiative.[14,21]

What is the structure of the system producing these patterns of events?
We begin to illuminate this level of the iceberg through qualitative research/story-telling or through testing more complex statistical models. But the power of system dynamics group model building and other complexity science methods is particularly evident here, as population health researchers and practitioners work to develop and test hypotheses about how interconnections among key elements of system structure produce observed patterns of events. This can be achieved through use of the system mapping and modeling approaches described in this chapter and the book more broadly.

Stakeholder mental models, beliefs, and goals
In human systems, system structure is not solely a function of physical laws. Also important are: what stakeholders know, how they simplify the world ("mental models"), what they believe is important or possible (shaped by any biases that affect their actions/decisions), incentives (with perception mattering most here), resources they feel are available, and – ultimately – their goals. Through its endogenous perspective and engagement processes, this level of the iceberg is a priority for SD-GMB initiatives.[10,11,17]

Figure 9.1 The iceberg as a systems thinking metaphor.

of events—including the effects of diverse stakeholders' mental models and goals (the second and third levels of the iceberg, below the waterline). We need to design actions that are aligned with system structure—leveraging opportunities for change and/or correcting system failures. But doing so requires understanding what lies beneath the waterline. You may have heard a colleague say something like "Outcomes are terrible, the system is just broken." We argue that the system is functioning exactly as it is designed to do—we just need to understand why it is producing observed outcomes and what it would take to create change.

9.4.1. SD-GMB and the Systems Thinking Iceberg

Uncovering stakeholders' mental models and goals (the lowest level of the iceberg) and understanding how they contribute to the structure of the system producing undesirable (and, with effort, desirable) outcomes is one of the main reasons why stakeholders are engaged in system dynamics-group model building (SD-GMB). This work requires relevant stakeholders to be meaningfully engaged if their beliefs, mindsets, goals, and actions in response to ongoing changes are to be interconnected with others' and any non-stakeholder driven system structure. This focus on understanding stakeholders' interconnected reactions to change is described as the "endogenous perspective" so central to SD-GMB.[17] SD-GMB processes often iterate between divergent and convergent steps. The goal of divergent steps is broad learning and brainstorming—tapping unique participant perspectives and eliciting their preferences. In convergent steps, divergent insights and priorities are integrated or prioritized. The group moves forward through incremental steps of learning, discussion, and consensus-building. We will briefly describe two aspects of scripted SD-GMB sessions, which are fundamental to moving from events to patterns to system structure.

9.4.1.1. GRAPHS OVER TIME

With problematic health events in mind, stakeholders are asked to draw and annotate/explain graphs (trend lines) over time that further illustrate what is problematic about the system and to put motivating events into historical context.[14,22] These graphs could be based on data or stakeholder understanding of what has happened and/or is expected to happen under differing future circumstances. The time frame depicted can be varied—for example, depicting trends over the course of a week, year, decade, or century and beginning with a particular date of interest or at the time of an index event such as birth or initiation of a relationship. The time frame selected is important—if it is short versus long, the shape of the trend may look quite different and focus is on a different set of system structure producing it. Rather than tracing every nuance in the data, stakeholders drawing graphs over time are asked to focus on the shape of the curve—what are the most important changes ("behaviors")? What is hoped for and feared in the future? More or less time can be allocated to drawing, discussing, and prioritizing graphs representing the problem to be studied. But once the key graphs over time to be explained, or "reference modes," are identified, additional graphs over time are drawn to depict key changes contributing to the reference mode behavior. As an example, important changes that might affect a reference mode depicting disparities in maternal mortality trends by race over the past 30 years might include changes in the prevalence of key risk/protective factors, access to healthcare, or the likelihood problematic conditions are diagnosed by providers seeing mothers in the first year after giving birth. Drawing, annotating, and describing graphs over time encourages rich and dynamic storytelling about key aspects of system structure—including the dynamics (a change in X triggers a change in Y quickly/slowly/after some delay/once a tipping point is reached) and interconnections between variables that are often missed when relevant but disconnected variables are brainstormed.

9.4.1.2. QUALITATIVE MODEL CONCEPTUALIZATION

Other structured activities guide GMB participants in drawing an explicit representation of their understanding of key system structure capable of producing reference mode trends in the form of a qualitative diagram(s) depicting central stocks, flows, feedback loops, and delays.[5,14] These causal loop and stock and flow diagrams are described more fully in Chapter 13 of this book. As these "dynamic hypotheses" are developed and discussed, they may trigger refinement of the problem definition or lead to hypothesis testing and iteration after soliciting feedback from other stakeholders, reviewing the research literature, or considering/analyzing data.

9.4.2. Simulation Modeling and the Systems Thinking Iceberg

The later stages of SD-GMB focus on transforming system structure diagrams into quantified simulation models, which are then subjected to programming verification (does model code depict intended system structure?), face validity checks with additional stakeholders, and testing to assess consistency with available data. Model iteration continues until confidence is built that it appropriately represents system structure to support analysis objectives.[5] This simulation model is a more sophisticated way to represent system structure (the second level below the waterline in Figure 9.1). The model can be used with stakeholders to help them identify and agree on new goals and actions that are capable of producing desired patterns/outcomes in the simulated (and hopefully the real) world.

Although GMB and the literature focused on refining and improving its use has evolved within SD practice, more recently, modelers from other systems science approaches have worked to adapt GMB practices to support a broader set of simulation methods. Drawing on established activities from GMB,[14] but developing their own activities tailored to suit the unique needs and questions posed by the use of agent-based models,[23,24] researchers are increasingly pushing the boundaries of participatory practices to support model building and use to address complex population health (and other) challenges.

9.4.3. Other System Mapping Methods and the Systems Thinking Iceberg

SD is quite advanced in its approach to engaging stakeholders in building models to uncover the structural determinants of problematic real-world trends and using these models to inform improvement efforts. SD-GMB is particularly powerful when stakeholders' actions, for which they have agency, are a central part of the problem. SD is designed for *dynamically complex* problems, in which complexity stems from nonlinear and feedback dynamics, accumulations over time, and delays. As evidenced by the breadth of complexity science methods discussed in this book, it is not the only approach for studying complex systems problems, nor is dynamic complexity the only type of complexity that can threaten population health. In this section, we briefly highlight alternatives to SD casual loop and stock and flow diagramming that could be conducted with stakeholders using some of the scripted SD-GMB processes[14] and/or woven into SD-GMB initiatives to uncover aspects of the iceberg. We will describe four distinct collaborative system mapping approaches (far from all relevant approaches) that we have found useful in illuminating aspects of system structure relevant to complex population health outcomes.

9.4.3.1. THE FIVE RS

Recognizing the need for a simple approach to understanding system structure, the Five Rs[25] was developed to guide a stakeholder group in understanding system structure related to a problem they are working on in terms of its roles, results, resources, relationships, and rules. With extensive use of this framework with collaborations, we find it helpful to begin by brainstorming what success looks like (*results*), encouraging inclusion of both currently measured and nonmeasured but meaningful constructs. Clustering results and prioritizing a subset can help bound a project more reasonably before the remaining Rs are brainstormed (an example of divergent brainstorming followed by convergent consensus-building typical of the previously described GMB processes). This first step aligns with the tip of the iceberg (Figure 9.1) and can be extended to depict problematic trends (second level of the iceberg), potentially overlapping with problem identification and graph over time elicitation from the SD-GMB process. Next, the group should name stakeholders with a *role* in affecting change in these results (or who are affected by change in them). These are stakeholders who might be important to engage in a GMB process, and certainly further system mapping. *Resources* include assets that can be leveraged to create change—including, for example, personnel, grant or other funding, data, influence, etc. Next, the collaboration should describe key *relationships* that should be attended to support change—for example, improving hand-offs in care or data sharing between two organizations. Lastly, *rules*—both informal and formal—shape how things work within the system, or the other Rs (e.g., results that must be tracked, who has a role, what resources are available, the nature of relationships). Brainstormed Five Rs should be documented and iterated over time as new perspectives are incorporated or as the system itself changes—and used to inform understanding of complex systems and how to improve them. We have found the Five Rs to be an accessible way to map system structure (third level of the iceberg) and to support early GMB efforts by drawing out potentially important variables to include in system diagrams and models. Discussion of resources, rules, and relationships often begin to describe aspects of stakeholder mental models, biases, incentives, and goals (fourth level of the iceberg).

9.4.3.2. PROCESS FLOW DIAGRAMMING

Process flow diagrams, often used within more narrowly focused quality improvement initiatives,[26,27] can be useful for visualizing complex processes in terms of starting and stopping conditions, process steps or activities completed by various stakeholders, and branching points that might trigger different process pathways. Process steps can be organized into stakeholder specific "swim lanes" to illuminate who does which tasks and handoffs between stakeholders.[28-30] Process flow diagrams developed by a collaboration can be an invaluable tool for visualizing broad processes—either as they currently exist or in terms of a desired future state. We have found that sometimes, when a population health initiative is sufficiently complex, process flow diagramming is necessary to get stakeholders on the same page before other collaborative system mapping methods can begin (e.g., SD-GMB, which might focus on the dynamics, delays, and feedback forces that promote or limit the initiative's success or the Five Rs, which describes the system into which the complex intervention is/will be implemented). Process flow diagramming resides at the third level of the iceberg (system structure).

9.4.3.3. System Support Mapping

System Support Mapping[31,32] is a structured mapping exercise that can be completed by individuals or groups, with resulting maps shared to grow understanding and empathy for other system stakeholders in terms of the responsibilities/activities they undertake within a given scope of work being mapped, their critical needs for completing each, resources available/used (and a description of how useful they are) and what they wish for to be better supported in this work. System support maps can illuminate the complexity and diversity involved in achieving or maintaining health among diverse or vulnerable patients. They can also be used by stakeholders with a role in population health to uncover and clarify responsibilities, highlight gaps or redundancies, and illuminate opportunities to strengthen relationships within systems. While individual stakeholders are often asked to make their own maps, we often integrate findings into team, program, organizational, or full system maps that clarify who does what and how resources align to needs at higher levels. System support maps are focused on the two lowest levels of the iceberg—describing system structure in terms of connected roles and responsibilities and illuminating stakeholder goals (what they are trying to do and why) and knowledge (e.g., of available resources, others' potential to support their work, etc.). In one project, system support maps were appended to note outcomes associated with patients' actions/responsibilities—helping researchers understand what meaningful change would look like (the tip of the iceberg).[31]

9.5. RELEVANT BEST PRACTICES TO INFORM DEVELOPMENT AND TESTING OF SYSTEMATIC APPROACHES TO ENGAGING STAKEHOLDERS IN MAPPING AND MODELING SYSTEM STRUCTURE

There is tremendous value in meaningfully engaging stakeholder to understand complex population health outcomes and how to change them. While SD-GMB is well established, there is always room for improvement. And, other complexity science methods would benefit from practical, systematic approaches to facilitate such bidirectional collaboration between stakeholders and methodologists. We would like to close this chapter by reflecting on two best practices to inspire the reader in such methodological innovation—boundary objects and community-based participatory research.

9.5.1. Boundary Objects and Collaborative Learning

When a group of diverse stakeholders are working to understand and address a complex problem and differing perspectives inhibit their alignment for action, the use of system maps and models with facilitated discussion has been observed to be useful in supporting groups in having productive dialogue.[33] The models ground the stakeholders' perspectives in concrete representations (e.g., graphs over time, causal loop or stock and flow diagrams, simulation models, documented Five Rs, process flow diagrams, or system support maps), and by doing that, allow stakeholders to express their perspectives more precisely and feel "heard" in the process.

Black and Andersen[34p195] identified that when the visual representations or artifacts used in SD-GMB "turn situations of disagreement, tension, and conflict into collaborative problem-solving discussions," those representations are functioning as "boundary objects." The term *boundary object* is a construct from sociology that refers to a tangible representation (of a problem, building, system, organization, etc.) that enables a diverse group of individuals (with different perspectives, knowledge, goals, experiences, etc.) to work together across the boundaries that are a result of that diversity. Boundary objects can effectively support groups to arrive at a shared understanding of a problem when the group's members can transform them to reflect their goals and their understanding of related and relevant interdependencies.[34-36] Thus, the successful practice of GMB and collaborative system mapping—in whatever form—striving to promote collaborative learning requires the explicit management of boundary objects over the course of the project, more specifically, ensuring that the visual representations used in the project maintain three characteristics: They are tangible/concrete, reflect interdependencies among stakeholder participants, and are transformable by all involved.[37] These characteristics are of particular importance for developing participatory practices drawing on other complexity science approaches that may not already have rich visuals to draw on as SD does.

9.5.2. Community-Based Participatory Research

Minkler[38pS81] has stated that community-based participatory research (CBPR) "is not a research method, but an orientation to research." It is designed to improve the partnership between academic and community partners engaging in research, with two objectives being to ensure research properly accounts for real world realities and that research be used to strengthen communities, given their critically important impact on health. The approach has transformed population health research over the past decades, growing community capacity to partner in research, improving the quality of research, and increasing translation/use of research findings.[39] Particularly exciting is the extent to which these strengths extend to vulnerable communities and impact health disparities.[39] CBPR calls for engaging diverse stakeholders meaningfully in research and action, and holds the following 11 principles: (1) recognize centrality of community as a unity of identity; (2) leverage strengths and assets in the community; (3) maintain a collaborative and equitable partnership in all stages of research; (4) invest in co-learning and community capacity building; (5) create a balance between learning and action that benefits all participants; (6) focus on locally relevant problems, mindful of multilevel determinants; (7) invest in systems development supporting health and future research and action through a cyclical and iterative CBPR process; (8) involve all partners in broader dissemination and use of research findings; (9) commit to long-term sustainability of the partnership; (10) openly and actively address issues of race and racism, with an environment of cultural humility; and (11) invest in rigorous research that is generalizable to the full diversity within the community.

Synergies between CBPR and complexity science methods have been noted around five dimensions: recognizing the role of context and connections in research (e.g., eschewing a reductionist paradigm), bringing a socioecological perspective to research and action, investment in co-learning, actively supporting action grounded in co-learning, and building local capacity to partner in future learning and systemic action.[40] The GMB process further leverages these synergies and accentuates others. Most important, it guides respectful co-learning, moving down the iceberg (Figure 9.1), having been designed to support difficult and critical conversations. In this regard, GMB can enhance CBPR initiatives—bringing a needed structured approach to identifying and illuminating complex health outcomes.[40-42] In the other direction, CBPR's rich guidance on navigating power disparities can bolster GMB initiatives. To this list of synergies, we add that both approaches prioritize a balance of learning (moving down the iceberg) and action (moving back up, using insight about system structure to create desirable outcomes). For example, action was documented in 23% of peer-reviewed manuscripts describing use of SD-GMB with cross-sector collaborations to improve health outcomes[18]—well above the rate at which general science is translated into action.[1] In 71% of these initiatives, researchers reported collective learning, decisions, and/or action.

9.6. PUTTING IT TOGETHER TO ADVANCE COLLABORATIVE MAPPING AND MODEL BUILDING IN POPULATION HEALTH

Facilitating evidence-based use of boundary objects and emphasizing CBPR principles in stakeholder-engaged system mapping and modeling efforts will strengthen our research and practice-based impacts *while accommodating* the complexity inherent in so many population health challenges. We will close with several insights we have about synergies between SD-GMB and the other system mapping methods highlighted in this chapter, boundary objects, and CBPR.

A holistic systems approach, crossing socioecological levels when appropriate to explain and/or create change in problematic outcomes is fundamental to GMB. As well, when issues of race and racism contribute to trends, their mechanisms will need to be discussed and integrated in maps and models. In our GMB experience, the need to do so requires GMB participants to directly address key issues—however hard—moving beyond calling out racism to describing it mechanistically. The role of maps and models as boundary objects facilitates this happening, as participants can point to and correct error in the models rather than in each other. CBPR best practices can inform collaborative modeling processes around sensitive issues.[43] Other system mapping methods, such as system support mapping provide a vehicle for sharing intent on the part of stakeholders providing services, while they give voice to individuals experiencing systematic racism around the ways in which resources do not adequately meet their needs in their pursuit of health.

There is tremendous promise and power in building stakeholder capacity to lead systems thinking, enhancing their communication skills, and—through systems mapping and modeling—making better use of their limited resources. Hovmand's work to build local capacity within GMB initiatives (CBSD) is a good example of meaningfully engaging community stakeholders in GMB *while* building their capacity to use the approach to improve complex outcomes over time. We have trained public health workforce and their cross-sector partners in all of the other system mapping methods presented in Section 9.4.3 and see them used, repeatedly, thereafter. In our experience, system mapping and modeling boundary objects, if truly owned by participants, can help them communicate key insights and advocate for change (aligned with CBPR principle 9) and iterate them over time, supporting long-term co-learning and system-strengthening (CBPR principles 4 and 7). Furthermore, the Five Rs and system support mapping (see Section 9.4.3) are both designed to identify resources and assets that are/can be better leveraged to improve outcomes (CBPR principle 2). We have found using these approaches together with SD-GMB results in better integration of resources and their characteristics in system structure diagrams. For example, GMB could inform the group's understanding of potential consequence to leveraging specific resources, including reinforcing or balancing feedback loops that might affect their sustained presence or limits to their impact.

We encourage the reader to think about and test approaches to using and adapting system mapping and modeling approaches described in this chapter or elsewhere, drawing inspiration from best practices we have described. The best way to learn how to effectively facilitate complexity-aware and collaborative system mapping is by doing it regularly and experimenting. Take the time to work with experts around you, and remember to bring science (hypothesis testing, careful experimentation and evaluation) to your efforts as this emerging and expanding (though, to date, quite fragmented) field advances.

REFERENCES

1. Balas EA, Boren SA. Managing clinical knowledge for health care improvement. In: Bemmel J, McCray AT, eds. *Yearbook of Medical Informatics 2000: Patient-Centered Systems.* Stuttgart, Germany: Schattauer Verlagsgesellschaft mbH; 2000: 65–70.

2. Williams B, van 't Hof S. *Wicked Solutions: A Systems Approach to Complex Problems.* 2nd ed. Wellington, New Zealand: Bob Williams; 2016.

3. Barrett S. Why cooperate? The incentive to supply global public goods reply. *Perspect Polit.* Mar 2009;7(1):156–157.

4. Cronin MA, Gonzalez C, Sterman JD. Why don't well-educated adults understand accumulation? A challenge to researchers, educators, and citizens. *Org Behav Hum Decision Proc.* 2009;108(1):116–130.

5. Sterman JD. *Business Dynamics: Systems Thinking and Modeling for a Complex World.* Boston: Irwin/McGraw-Hill; 2000.

6. Sweeney LB, Sterman JD. Bathtub dynamics: Initial results of a systems thinking inventory. *Syst Dynam Rev.* 2000;16(4):249–286.

7. Epstein JM. *Generative Social Science: Studies in Agent-Based Computational Modeling.* Princeton, NJ: Princeton University Press; 2006.

8. Rouwette EAJA, Vennix JAM, van Mullekom T. Group model building effectiveness: A review of assessment studies. *Syst Dynam Rev.* 2002;18(1):5–45.

9. Hovmand PS. *Community Based System Dynamics.* New York: Springer; 2014.

10. Andersen DF, Vennix JAM, Richardson GP, Rouwette EAJA. Group model building: Problem structuring, policy simulation and decision support. *J Oper Res Soc.* 2007;58(5):691–694.

11. Vennix JAM, Akkermans HA, Rouwette EAJA. Group model-building to facilitate organizational change: An exploratory study. *Syst Dynam Rev.* 1996;12(1):39–58.

12. Stave K. Participatory system dynamics modeling for sustainable environmental management. *Sustainability.* 2010;2(9):2762–2784.

13. Kiraly G, Miskolczi P. Dynamics of participation: system dynamics and participation: An empirical review. *Syst Res Behav Sci.* 2019;36(2):199–210.

14. Hovmand PS, Andersen DF, Rouwette E, Richardson GP, Rux K, Calhoun A. Group model-building "scripts" as a collaborative planning tool. *Syst Res Behav Sci.* 2012;29(2):179–193.

15. Huz S, Andersen DF, Richardson GP, Boothroyd R. A framework for evaluating systems thinking interventions: An experimental approach to mental health system change. *Syst Dynam Rev.* 1997;13(2):149–169.

16. Richardson GP, Andersen DF. Teamwork in group model-building. *Syst Dynam Rev.* 1995;11(2):113–137.

17. Richardson GP. Reflections on the foundations of system dynamics. *Syst Dynam Rev.* 2011;27(3):219–243.

18. Cilenti D, Issel M, Wells R, Link S, Lich KH. System dynamics approaches and collective action for community health: An integrative review. *Am J Community Psychol.* 2019;63(3-4):527–545.

19. Scott RJ, Cavana RY, Cameron D. Recent evidence on the effectiveness of group model building. *Eur J Oper Res.* 2016;249(3):908–918.

20. Goodman M. *The Iceberg Model.* Hopkinton, MA: Innovation Associates Organizational Learning; 2002.

21. Lich KH, Urban JB, Frerichs L, Dave G. Extending systems thinking in planning and evaluation using group concept mapping and system dynamics to tackle complex problems. *Eval Progr Plan.* 2017;60:254–264.

22. Calancie L, Anderson S, Branscomb J, Apostolico AA, Lich KH. Using behavior over time graphs to spur systems thinking among public health practitioners. *Prev Chronic Dis.* 2018;15:E16.

23. Homa L, Rose J, Hovmand PS, et al. A participatory model of the paradox of primary care. *Ann Fam Med.* 2015;13(5):456–465.

24. Koh K, Reno R, Hyder A. Designing an agent-based model using group model building: Application to food insecurity patterns in a U.S. midwestern metropolitan city. *J Urban Health.* Apr 2018;95(2):278–289.

25. USAID. *Local Systems: A Framework for Supporting Sustained Development.* Washington, DC: USAID;2014.

26. Colligan L, Anderson JE, Potts HW, Berman J. Does the process map influence the outcome of quality improvement work? A comparison of a sequential flow diagram and a hierarchical task analysis diagram. *BMC Health Serv Res.* 2010;10:7.

27. Zhang B, Youngblood L, Murphy GD, Ramsay M, Xiao Y. System engineering approach to documentation: An evaluation of the documentation process in a gastroenterology laboratory. *J Biomed Inform.* Jun 2012;45(3):591–597.

28. Aleem S, Torrey WC, Duncan MS, Hort SJ, Mecchella JN. Depression screening optimization in an academic rural setting. *Int J Health Care Qual Assur.* 2015;28(7):709–725.

29. Johnson K, Burkett GS, Nelson D, et al. Automated e-mail reminders linked to electronic health records to improve medication reconciliation on admission. *Ped Qual Safe.* 2018;3(5):e109.

30. Jun GT, Ward J, Morris Z, Clarkson J. Health care process modelling: Which method when? *Int J Qual Health Care.* 2009;21(3):214–224.

31. Befus DR, Hassmiller Lich K, Kneipp SM, Bettger JP, Coeytaux RR, Humphreys JC. A qualitative, systems thinking approach to study self-management in women with migraine. *Nurs Res.*2018;67(5):395–403.

32. Calancie L, Margolis L, Chall SA, Mullenix A, Chaudhry A, Hassmiller Lich K. System support mapping: A novel systems thinking tool applied to assess the needs of maternal and child health title v professionals and their partners. *J Public Health Manag Pract.* 2019. doi:10.1097/PHH.0000000000000941. [Epub ahead of print]

33. Zagonel A. Model conceptualization in group model-building: a review of the literature exploring the tension between representing reality and negotiating a social order. In *Proceedings of the 2002 International System Dynamics Conference*, System Dynamics Society; 2002; Palermo, Italy.

34. Black LJ, Andersen DF. Using visual representations as boundary objects to resolve conflict in collaborative model-building approaches. *Syst Res Behav Sci.* 2012;29(2):194–208.

35. Luna-Reyes LF, Black LJ, Ran WJ, et al. Modeling and simulation as boundary objects to facilitate interdisciplinary research. *Syst Res Behav Sci.* 2019;36(4):494–513.

36. Black LJ. When visuals are boundary objects in system dynamics work. *Syst Dynam Rev.* 2013;29(2):70–86.

37. Carlile PR. A pragmatic view of knowledge and boundaries: Boundary objects in new product development. *Organ Sci.* 2002;13(4):442–455.

38. Minkler M. Linking science and policy through community-based participatory research to study and address health disparities. *Am J Public Health*. 2010;100(Suppl 1):S81–87.

39. Viswanathan M, Ammerman A, Eng E, et al. Community-based participatory research: assessing the evidence. *Evid Rep Technol Assess (Summ)*. 2004(99):1–8.

40. Frerichs L, Lich KH, Dave G, Corbie-Smith G. Integrating systems science and community-based participatory research to achieve health equity. *Am J Public Health*. 2016;106(2):215–222.

41. BeLue R, Carmack C, Myers KR, Weinreb-Welch L, Lengerich EJ. Systems thinking tools as applied to community-based participatory research: a case study. *Health Educ Behav*. 2012;39(6):745–751.

42. Davis MM, Lindberg P, Cross S, Lowe S, Gunn R; Dillon K. Aligning systems science and community-based participatory research: A case example of the Community Health Advocacy and Research Alliance (CHARA). *J Clin Transl Sci*. 2018;2(5):280–288.

43. Frerichs L, Lich KH, Funchess M, et al. Applying critical race theory to group model building methods to address community violence. *Prog Comm Health Partnersh*. 2016;10(3):443–459.

Is It Time to Rethink "Normal" in Population Health Research?

NEAL V. DAWSON AND PIERPAOLO ANDRIANI

10.1. CAN WE SIMPLIFY COMPLEXITY?

Since the 1800s, the Gaussian (normal) distribution has become a dominant method for displaying and making inferences about biological and social phenomena in human populations. This symmetrical pattern of measured values emerges when one sums many values of an independent random process. This pattern was noted by Gauss in his summarization of multiple measurements of the same phenomenon (e.g., length of an object) and by Quetelet in his analyses of single measurements of many entities (e.g., men's heights). The Gaussian distribution is a generatively entrenched concept in modern statistical methods,[1] as it has become fundamental to much of statistical inference about characteristics important to the health of human populations.

However, many population health and medical phenomena do not have Gaussian distributions because the processes that produce them are neither independent nor randomly generated. These phenomena come from one or more complex adaptive and interacting systems (see Chapter 3 of the volume) in which system purposes are manifested through reinforcing and balancing feedback relationships and rife with other aspects of complexity (see Chapter 2 of this volume).

An excellent example of such a set of adaptive interacting systems is cardiac rhythm. At the individual cardiac cellular level, charge flow across the cellular membrane initiates intracellular changes linked to cellular contractile processes. The quantity of charge flow across cellular membranes is controlled by ion channel proteins. Ion channel gating processes are influenced by multilevel feedback

Neal V. Dawson and Pierpaolo Andriani, *Is It Time to Rethink "Normal" in Population Health Research?* In: *Complex Systems and Population Health*. Edited by: Yorghos Apostolopoulos, Kristen Hassmiller Lich, and Michael Kenneth Lemke, Oxford University Press (2020). © Oxford University Press. DOI: 10.1093/oso/9780190880743.003.0010 loops, such as triggers to cell signaling (transmitters and hormones) and epige-netic control.[2] Adaptive interacting systems need to be considered as the interplay among all components. As noted by Noble,[2p58] "The sequence of events, including the feedback between the cell potential and the activity of proteins simply *is* car-diac rhythm. It is a property of the interactions between all components of the system. It does not even make sense to talk of cardiac rhythm at the levels of proteins and DNA." And, it does not make sense to boil cardiac rhythm down to a summary measure. To support the health of individuals, clinicians study car-diac rhythm as a set of connected observations. If some aspect of the system is behaving in an undesirable manner, understanding of the other aspects of the system is needed to uncover the problem in system functioning—and thus the best treatment approach.

This begs the question: How do we *attempt to* simplify complexity?

10.2. HOW USEFUL ARE NON-GAUSSIAN DISTRIBUTIONS?

Kindig and Stoddart[3p380] defined population health as "the health outcomes of a group of individuals, including the distribution of such outcomes within the group," the study of which "includes health outcomes, patterns of health determinants, and policies and interventions that link the two." This notion of describing *distributions of outcomes and contributing factors* is so common that it's even included in definitions of population health! And a collection of data sampled from and striving to generalize to a population needs an appropriate (i.e., meaningful) summarization to be understood at that level. As entrenched as the normal distribution is, population health researchers do often use other non-Gaussian distributions to summarize outcomes of interest when such distributions provide a better fit to data or are theoretically appropriate—for ex-ample, the lognormal distribution is often used to characterize right-skewed cost distributions and the exponential distribution to characterize interarrival times in a queueing system. Non-Gaussian distributions are frequently a better fit to, or aid in the meaningful summarization of, outcomes affected by complex systems. One example that we will explore in more detail later in this chapter involves power law distributions, which are known to be produced by a variety of complex adap-tive systems.[4]

Too often, however, researchers will identify a distribution as non-Gaussian, try to transform it to become normally distributed, and then use common statistical (e.g., generalized linear modeling) methods founded on the assumptions of nor-mality. This fundamentally misses the opportunity to learn about why the normal distribution is not a good fit—what aspects of complex adaptive systems involving this outcome are producing these observations?

Let's illustrate this point with an example. It is not uncommon to characterize length of stay (LOS; e.g., in an intensive care unit of a hospital) according to a single distribution. While doing so allows us to describe the distribution with a few descriptive statistics, it also misses potentially important indicators of what is actually going on. Seeking to avoid this, Marrie and colleagues[5] used quantile regression and restricted cubic splines to uncover important differences among a population of patients staying in an intensive care unit. Looking at the relationship between disease severity and LOS, they identified meaningfully different subpopulations. In the bottom three quartiles of LOS, they found an inverted U-shaped relationship in which the shortest LOS was among the least severe patients (who recover quickly) and the most severe patients (who die quickly). The longest stay quartile had a fundamentally different story—severity and LOS were more linearly related, but these patients were fundamentally different, needing specialized services and less likely to die.

10.3. WHAT WE CAN LEARN THROUGH COMPLEX SYSTEMS SCIENCE?

The principles of complex systems science (see Chapters 1 to 5 of this volume) can be productively applied to the studies of population health that investigate patterns of health determinants and health outcomes as well as the relationships between the two across time, place, and subparts of the population studied. Important to these efforts are studies that have investigated the relationships among networks of persons within populations[6,7] or among disease diagnoses,[8,9] cellular networks,[10] interactome networks,[11,12] and relationships between environmental and genetic factors—the etiome.[13]

Although important to determining the higher-level general descriptors of population characteristics, coarse-grained, average, or general relationships often leave important aspects of relationships obscured or unexplained.[14] This phenomenon is particularly apt to occur with the evaluation of complex biological and social systems, which often display heterogeneity (from adaptation, plasticity, and evolution[15]) within and among the involved complex adaptive systems. Useful constructs to evaluate heterogeneity should be consistent with assessment goals (e.g., explaining and improving population health) and should be predictive of the likelihood of important health-related states and outcomes.

Let's consider another example. Is the relationship between income and health linear? Would we expect it to be? Let's start by thinking about the distribution of income. Is income independent and randomly distributed? Figure 10.1, using a log-log scale, presents a classic example of the income distribution in Italy (and observed in many other times and places).[16] Income levels vary from a low on the left side of the distribution, where persons are likely to be dependent on a single source of income (living paycheck to paycheck); to those with more than a single source of income (central part of Figure 10.1); to those with the highest incomes (right hand part of Figure 10.1), where the income levels are likely to be interdependently related to both financially important information availability and social and business relationships.[16] That is to say, income for individuals on the tail of the distribution *is not independent or random*—individuals with high

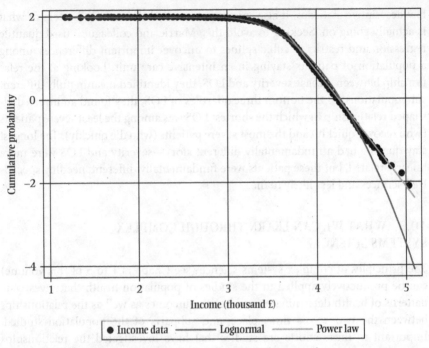

Figure 10.1 The Italian income distribution in 1998.[16] The vertical axis represents cumulative probability of an income equal or larger than x. The horizontal axis reports income.
SOURCE: Clementi F, Gallegati M. Power law tails in the Italian personal income distribution. *Physica A*. 2005;350:427–438. Reproduced courtesy of Elsevier.

income are more able, and often do, work together to increase their income. With these interdependencies among the extremely wealthy, why would we expect health to be independent and randomly distributed? With wealth comes the opportunity to have better education, better diet, opportunities for regular exercise, access to specialists, etc.

Complex systems science can guide us in recognizing signs of complexity and uncovering fundamental system mechanisms. But as should be obvious in this book by now, it requires a broad lens—focusing not on key factors in a single level, but all the relevant system components. Case in point here, population health is more than health care. Focusing only on healthcare aimed at treatment of and recovery from illness misses many processes that are associated with health promotion and disease prevention. Estimates of the effects of processes that affect population health reveal that healthcare services influence only about 10% of the variation in health outcomes and premature death.[17] Other influences include processes acting at multiple levels: genetic heritage, biology, educational attainment, personal behaviors (including diet and exercise), and social factors including social support and socioeconomic status (SES) as well as environmental exposures.[18]

10.4. THE IMPORTANCE OF HETEROGENEITY

One of the prominent challenges in biological systems science today is understanding how diversity in cellular behaviors is influenced by processes outside of the genome, including environmental influences, broadly conceived. Recently, investigators have begun to address some of the limitations of early studies such as the assumption of a higher degree of homogeneity of cellular function (based on ensemble results of populations of cells) than actually exist at the individual cellular level.[19] Recent work has found unexpected heterogeneity in biomolecules[20] and functional diversity of topological modules in protein–protein interaction networks.[21]

At the level of intact persons, concerns about heterogeneity in the response to clinical treatments have been expressed.[14,22] As previously discussed, an important source of heterogeneity of health outcomes among intact humans observed consistently across time within and across diverse countries is variation in income/wealth, and SES, more broadly.[23,24] SES is a spectral phenomenon, in which qualitative changes in relationships important to health outcomes vary in concert with changes in magnitude or level of SES. For health outcomes, SES is strongly contextualizing. For example, as previously described, the presence and effects of factors that influence health outcomes co-vary with SES (e.g., educational attainment, diet, exercise patterns, environmental exposures, access to health care, and many others).[25,26] Taken together, heterogeneous patterns of health risk structure at the whole-person level are associated with heterogeneity at the cellular level and at higher levels (i.e., multilevel heterogeneity). It is not enough to consider SES a variable that moderates the relationship between some exposure and a health outcome. In much the same way as boiling a complex outcome down to a distribution (and stopping there) oversimplifies complexity, treating a spectral variable as a moderator in a linear model fails to illuminate how these variables co-evolve and influence one another. As we move across the spectrum of income, so much moves along with it—life circumstances, opportunities (or lack thereof), skills, knowledge, and much, much more.

At the level of a national population, such as that of the United States, several additional sources of heterogeneity must be assessed. The consideration of age (how old someone is), time period (what point in time we are studying the system), and birth cohort effects contribute to our understanding of how the aggregate (average) risk structure of a population for a given disease changes over time in concert with differential selection pressures (e.g., mortality pressure) that produce differential types and effects of risk factors (such as SES) for disease and health outcomes. This kind of heterogeneity necessitates longitudinal data to illuminate key causal associations.[27]

A recent example of time period effects comes from the observations made by two separate sets of investigators regarding the decrease in the incidence and prevalence of dementia over the past 40 years. The first used data from the Framingham Heart Study to determine that from the 1970s through the early 2000s, the incidence of dementia, including Alzheimer's disease, has decreased in every decade.[28] The most pronounced decline was among dementias caused by vascular disease such as stroke. In this study, the decline in dementia incidence was limited to persons with a high school education or above.

The second set of investigators[29] used data from the Health and Retirement Study of persons 65 or older to estimate the prevalence of dementia in the United States. They found a decrease in prevalence of dementia between 2000 and 2012. In this study, more years of education were associated with lower levels of risk for dementia. Educational attainment increased among persons 65 and older between 2000 and 2012 (a cohort effect).

Smoking[30] and hypertension[31] are known risk factors for stroke and dementia. The diminished incidence rates of dementia are temporally associated with decreasing smoking rates in the United States (42% in 1965, 17% in 2014), which have been more prominent among persons of higher educational attainment (43% with GED, 17% with an associate degree, 5.4% with a graduate degree) and higher SES (25% below the poverty level, 15% overall).[32] Between 1999 and 2014, rates of recognition and treatment of hypertension increased for all age groups in the United States.[33] Longitudinal studies that are able to measure and keep track of changes in risk phenomena across the entire spectrum of socioeconomic position (SEP; a measure of aggregate SES at the neighborhood level) are critical to generating credible insights.

A step in the direction of illuminating spectral phenomena was recently published by Dalton and colleagues.[34] The goal of this study was to determine whether the prognostic performance (accuracy) of a state-of-the-art risk calculating tool was similar among patients who came from neighborhoods with varying levels of SEP. The tool, the Pooled Cohort Equation (an updated version of the Framingham risk model for cardiovascular diseases [CVD]: heart attack, stroke, cardiovascular death), assessed commonly used cardiovascular risk indicators (age, sex, race, total cholesterol, high density lipoprotein cholesterol, systolic blood pressure, treatment for hypertension, presence of diabetes, and smoking).[35] Patients (n=109,793) from a large North East Ohio hospital system who did not have diagnosis of CVD at baseline were assessed again during a five-year follow-up as part of a retrospective cohort. SEP was assessed by a neighborhood deprivation index developed using census data. Conditional autoregressive models were used to explain census tract level variation in CVD event rates for the Pooled Cohort Equation and neighborhood deprivation index, separately and in combination. The Pooled Cohort Equation explained 10% of the variation in census tract level CVD event rates, the neighborhood deprivation index explained 32%, and both together explained 39%. The relationship between the Pooled Cohort Equation estimates of risk and event rates varied by level of neighborhood deprivation. Estimates of risk were best (most accurate) among patients who came from more affluent neighborhoods (c-statistic = .80 with very good calibration for the upper 10th percentile of SEP) but were much less accurate for patients from least affluent neighborhoods (lowest 10th percentile, c-statistic = .70 with miscalibration that led to many estimates of risk being half of the actual event rates).

The lack of accuracy of a standard, biologically informed, guideline-based CVD risk calculation tool provides an opportunity to explore potential reasons contributing to the variation of population health outcomes by SES and SEP. Among the numerous nonbiological differences that co-vary with SEP and are associated with variation in health risks are the social gradient, stress levels, early-life experiences, educational opportunities, social exclusion, job types, unemployment rates, social support, transportation types and availability, addiction, serious mental illness, environmental exposures, and others.[36] Individual genetic predispositions with the physical, social, and cultural environments within which individuals live can lead to variation in health risks and health-related outcomes. Specific examples of individual predispositions and environmental features that may influence population health outcomes include differences in housing stock, exposure levels to heavy metals (e.g., lead) and air pollution, epigenetic effects associated with persistent poverty, untoward prenatal and early life exposures, chronic stress levels, noise levels, prevalence of serious mental illness, and more.

Differential mortality pressures can influence the prevalence of risk factors, and thus the risk structure of birth cohorts. Consider two birth cohorts as they reach Medicare eligibility at age 65: those born in 1920 and those born in 1950. These two cohorts were exposed to different mortality risks, changing the characteristics of the population surviving to 65. The 1920 cohort lived through disease epidemics, years without some of the most effective antibiotics, the great depression, and World War II. Those born in 1950 did not. Furthermore, those who survive to 65 in each cohort were exposed to different foods, environmental exposures, risk and protective factors (e.g., different experiences of community/social cohesion, tobacco exposure). Aging can take on different risk characteristics in different birth cohorts—as was previously described around dementia.[28,29] Time period effects can affect groups of birth cohorts differently. A recent study of susceptibility to bird flu in Asia and the Middle East[37] found that persons born before 1968 had a lower risk of serious illness or death from H5N1 influenza but a higher risk from H7N9. The opposite effect was found for persons born after 1968. H5N1 flu was more prominent prior to 1968 and H7N9 was more prominent after 1968. Those who survived their infection in each time period tended to have better immunity for subsequent exposure to the most prominent strains in that time period.

Differences in mortality pressure, and thus risk structure over time, induced by contextualizing variables such as SES/SEP suggest the potential for differential contributions of subgroups along the SES/SEP spectrum to the overall population average. Discovering how age, time period, cohort effects, and spectral relationships contribute to heterogeneity and influence risk structure for population health outcomes will be a fertile area for investigation of the complex, adaptive, and dynamic features of health states and diseases across hierarchical levels of population structure.[38] Incorporating deeper insights into the interplay between social and biological phenomena as they relate to health outcomes provides an opportunity to positively influence health policy, disease prevention, and clinical treatment decisions to enhance population health.

10.5. POWER LAW DISTRIBUTIONS: RECOGNIZING HALLMARKS OF COMPLEXITY

There are notable exceptions where researchers intrigued by non-Gaussian distributions, dig in to learn more. Toward the end of the 19th century and the beginning of the 20th, scientists including Pareto,[39] Auerbach,[40] Zipf,[41] and others in different domains, observed scientific, economic, and social phenomena that deviated significantly from the normal distribution. Their work demonstrated a "Kuhnian anomaly" that, with time, would contribute to generating a new approach to science grounded in complex systems science.[42] They identified and studied a variety of outcomes that follow a power law distribution.

Figure 10.2 shows the power law and Gaussian (normal) distributions; for simplicity, both distributions are centered on zero. A Gaussian distribution is expressed by an exponential equation (the variable is in the exponent), whereby in the power law the exponent is a constant. Therefore, a power law distribution shown on a double logarithmic axis graph becomes a straight line. On linear axes, one easily notices that a Gaussian distribution tends rapidly toward the zero, whereby power laws are characterized by long and (often) fat tails.[43]

Power laws are distributions characterized by unstable or nonexistent moment and by an extreme variability that spans several orders of magnitudes.[43] Consequently, the concept of the mean and variance, so important in how we all too often describe an outcome of interest, become meaningless. The main parameter defining power laws is the exponent. For negatively inclined power laws (negative exponent), the lower the exponent, the longer the tail of the distribution and consequently the higher the variance.

An interesting feature, power law–distributed phenomena exhibit the property of self-similarity, which in turn gives rise to scalability (also known as scale invariance). Self-similarity occurs when the same (or similar) set of relationships occurs

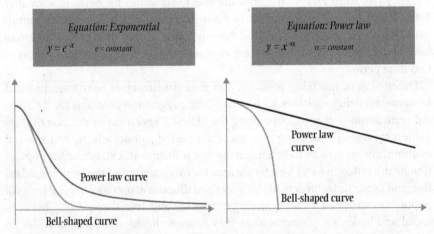

Figure 10.2 Power law versus Gaussian distribution. Left-side graph: linear axes; right-side: logarithmic axes.

among the parts of an entity across multiple scales.[44] Scale invariance implies that the shape or other properties of an entity do not change when multiplied by a common factor. In the socioeconomic area, scalability refers to the capability of business models or organizational structures (or other relevant variable) to accommodate rapid growth without change. For instance, Facebook's structure can accommodate dramatic changes in adoption just by linearly adding more servers. Brock[45p30] observes that the study of complexity "tries to understand the forces that underlie the patterns or scaling laws that develop" as newly ordered systems emerge.

Essentially, Gaussian and power law distributions represent the two extremes of a large family of distributions[42,46] based on radically different assumptions. As described in the beginning of this chapter, normal distributions describe situations in which the data points are assumed to be independent and additive. However, when events become interdependent (a complex adaptive system), normality in distributions is *not* the norm.

In practice, and aligned with the description of complex phenomena underlying distributions in the first part of this chapter (Section 10.2), it is relatively rare to find a pure power law distribution.[43] It is common, instead, to find data sets that show a mix of different distributions, which may span from the Gaussian to the power law. The transition from one extreme to the other is due to variable interdependence among the data points along the dynamical range of the phenomenon, as for instance in the case of the Italian income distribution shown in Figure 10.1 and as previously described.[16] This curve was observed by Pareto himself and is still debated by economists. Let's now consider this distribution as an illustration of a power law. The segment on the left-hand side represents the poor and much of the working class. These data points fit economists' assumptions about independence very well. Workers in this section of the graph are completely dependent on their wages (which mostly go into basic necessities) and unable to accumulate any savings. Their salaries do not depend on each other and, at least in the short term, are nearly completely detached from the evolution of the economy. The central part of Figure 10.1 shows a tendency toward a power law: Workers here still depend mainly on their wages. However, a fraction of their wages can be injected into the multiplicative system of credit. Wealth now depends on two components: additive salary plus interest-bearing investments. They begin to show the independent-multiplicative requirement for the lognormal distribution. Finally, the right part of Figure 10.1 shows the signature of power law distribution: As the wealth and status of the people increases, their wealth becomes dependent of the amount of information they get about investment possibilities: They meet each other at boards together; have common lawyers, financial advisors, and political contacts; can invest and or co-own each other's wealth-producing assets; and so on. Now the data points form a collective system of interdependencies. Interdependence engenders positive feedback dynamics that results in cascades of correlated extreme events that shift the whole distributions toward long and fat tails.

Power laws seem ubiquitous.[47] They apply to word usage, papers published, book sales, and web hits.[43] Cities follow a power law distribution when ranked by population, as does the structure of the Internet.[48] Until Watts and Strogatz's[49] seminal paper most scientists studying networks (from societal to metabolic networks) assumed that randomness was a realistic (or at least useful) representation of the network's underlying structure. The assumption of randomness (i.e., that links were randomly distributed among nodes) led naturally to the emergence of a Gaussian distribution of links, wherein the mean and the variance sufficed to describe the network's statistical properties. It turns out that many real-world networks (most "small-world" networks) are scale-free[50] and fractal.[51] The impact of this emerging science of networks has been profound.[52]

While the demonstration of outcomes following a power law in population health are few, they do exist. For example, patterns of urgent care use have been found to follow a power law[53] as have persistent microbials "lag phase" in the face of antibiotic treatment (e.g., E. coli).[54]

10.6. POWER LAW DISTRIBUTIONS: WHAT LIES BENEATH?

One may ask what the presence of a power laws signifies. Sornette,[55] Newman,[43] and Andriani and McKelvey[47] show that there are multiple mechanisms that generate power laws. In general, power law distributions emerge when the agents of a system are free to self-organize around a set of fundamental constraints subject to some sort of tensions and/or selecting mechanisms.

The variety of generative mechanisms and the variety of situations in which power laws emerge have engendered different interpretations: Simon[56p425] took a rather reductive stance: "Its appearance is so frequent, and the phenomena in which it appears so diverse, that one is led to the conjecture that if these phenomena have any property in common, it can only be a similarity in the structure of the underlying probability mechanism." Barabási,[57p19] instead, saw a different type of unity underlying the variety of mechanisms and situations: "Then power laws emerge—nature's unmistakable sign that chaos is departing in favor of order. The theory of phase transitions told us loud and clear that the road from disorder to order is maintained by the powerful forces of self-organization and is paved by power laws. It told us that power laws are the patent signatures of self-organization in complex systems."

We observe that all generative mechanisms (with the exception of the random walk with a barrier[58] share similar characteristics: (a) they are all based on historical processes, therefore indicating a path-dependent evolutionary dynamic; (b) they demand interdependence among data points; and (c) they generate self-similar nested structures, i.e. fractal structures. In practice, path dependency, interdependence, and self-similarity interact. Path-dependent evolutionary processes give rise to interconnected self-similar nested structures. In turn, distributed connectivity within and across levels together with the extreme variability of infinite variance scale-free mechanisms create the potential for tiny-initiating events to trigger self-organizing patterns that may escalate into extreme events. While documented power law in population health are few and far between, the underlying mechanisms are even less well understood. It is clear, however, that recognizing power law distributed outcomes is important in supporting population health.[47,53,59,60]

10.7. CONCLUSIONS

In this chapter, we describe the conditions under which normally distributed phenomena arise. And we argue that this distribution—and the statistical infrastructure built upon this distribution—is often inappropriate. At best, its use misses important heterogeneities in the population of which outcomes are aggregated. At worst, it fundamentally mischaracterizes phenomena embedded within complex adaptive systems. We hope that health researchers and practitioners will increase the extent to which they embrace opportunities to study the complex and uncover more explanatory mechanisms for population health. Such insights are the foundation for more powerful action.

REFERENCES

1. Wimsatt WC. Re-engineering philosophy for limited beings—piecewise approximations to reality. Cambridge, MA: Harvard University Press; 2007.
2. Noble D. A theory of biological relativity: no privileged level of causation. Interface Focus. 2012;2(1):55–64.
3. Kindig D, Stoddart G. What is population health? American Journal of Public Health. 2003;93(3):380–383.
4. West GB. Scale: the universal laws of growth, innovation, sustainability, and the pace of life in organisms, cities, economies, and companies. New York: Penguin Press; 2017.
5. Marrie RA, Dawson NV, Garland A. Quantile regression and restricted cubic splines are useful for exploring relationships between continuous variables. Journal of Clinical Epidemiology. 2009;62(5):511–517 e511.
6. Christakis NA, Fowler JH. The spread of obesity in a large social network over 32 years. The New England Journal of Medicine. 2007;357(4):370–379.
7. Christakis NA, Fowler JH. The collective dynamics of smoking in a large social network. The New England Journal of Medicine.2008;358(21):2249–2258.
8. Hidalgo CA, Blumm N, Barabasi AL, Christakis NA. A dynamic network approach for the study of human phenotypes. PLoS Computational Biology. 2009;5(4):e1000353.
9. Loscalzo J, Barabasi AL. Systems biology and the future of medicine. Wiley Interdisciplinary Reviews: Systems Biology and Medicine. 2011;3(6):619–627.
10. Barabasi AL, Gulbahce N, Loscalzo J. Network medicine: a network-based approach to human disease. Nature Reviews: Genetics. 2011;12(1):56–68.
11. Caldera M, Buphamalai P, Muller F, Menche J. Interactome-based approaches to human disease. Current Opinion in Systems Biology. 2017;3:88–94.
12. Vidal M, Cusick ME, Barabasi AL. Interactome networks and human disease. Cell. 2011;144(6):986–998.
13. Liu YI, Wise PH, Butte AJ. The "etiome": identification and clustering of human disease etiological factors. BMC Bioinformatics.2009;10 Suppl 2:S14.

14. Kravitz RL, Duan N, Braslow J. Evidence-based medicine, heterogeneity of treatment effects, and the trouble with averages. The Milbank Quarterly. 2004;82(4):661–687.

15. Gluckman PD, Hanson MA, Bateson P, et al. Towards a new developmental synthesis: Adaptive developmental plasticity and human disease. Lancet. 2009;373(9675):1654–1657.

16. Clementi F, Gallegati M. Power law tails in the Italian personal income distribution. Physica A. 2005;350:427–438.

17. Schroeder SA. Shattuck lecture.: We can do better—improving the health of the American people. The New England Journal of Medicine. 2007;357(12):1221–1228.

18. Healthy People 2020. HealthyPeople.gov. https://www.healthypeople.gov/2020/topics-objectives. Accessed August 22, 2019.

19. Altschuler SJ, Wu LF. Cellular heterogeneity: do differences make a difference? Cell. 2010;141(4):559–563.

20. Hinczewski M, Hyeon C, Thirumalai D. Directly measuring single-molecule heterogeneity using force spectroscopy. Proceedings of the National Academy of Sciences of the United States of America. 2016;113(27):E3852–3861.

21. Liu G, Wang H, Chu H, Yu J, Zhou X. Functional diversity of topological modules in human protein–protein interaction networks. Scientific Reports. 23 2017;7(1):16199.

22. Hayward RA, Kent DM, Vijan S, Hofer TP. Reporting clinical trial results to inform providers, payers, and consumers. Health Affairs. 2005;24(6):1571–1581.

23. Chetty R, Stepner M, Abraham S, et al. The association between income and life expectancy in the United States, 2001–2014. JAMA. 2016;315(16):1750–1766.

24. Deaton A. On death and money: History, facts, and explanations. JAMA. 2016;315(16):1703–1705.

25. Cutler D, Lleras-Muney A. Education and health: Evaluating theories and evidence. NBER Working Paper Series. http://www.nber.org/papers/w12352.

26. Woolf SH, Purnell JQ. The good life: Working together to promote opportunity and improve population health and well-being. JAMA. 2016;315(16):1706–1708.

27. Gunzler DD, Perzynski AT, Dawson NV, Kauffman K, Liu J, Dalton JE. Risk-period-cohort approach for averting identification problems in longitudinal models. PloS One. 2019;14(7):e0219399.

28. Satizabal CL, Beiser AS, Chouraki V, Chene G, Dufouil C, Seshadri S. Incidence of dementia over three decades in the Framingham Heart Study. The New England Journal of Medicine. 2016;374(6):523–532.

29. Langa KM, Larson EB, Crimmins EM, et al. A comparison of the prevalence of dementia in the United States in 2000 and 2012. JAMA Internal Medicine. 2017;177(1):51–58.

30. Ott A, Slooter AJ, Hofman A, et al. Smoking and risk of dementia and Alzheimer's disease in a population-based cohort study: The Rotterdam Study. Lancet. 1998;351(9119):1840–1843.

31. Benjamin EJ, Blaha MJ, Chiuve SE, et al. Heart disease and stroke statistics-2017 update: A report from the American Heart Association. Circulation. 2017;135(10):e146–e603.

32. Trends in Current cigarette smoking among high school students and adults, United States, 1965–2014 https://www.cdc.gov/tobacco/data_statistics/tables/trends/cig_smoking/index.htm Accessed August 22, 2019.

33. Zhang Y, Moran AE. Trends in the prevalence, awareness, treatment, and control of hypertension among young adults in the United States, 1999 to 2014. Hypertension. 2017;70(4):736–742.

34. Dalton JE, Perzynski AT, Zidar DA, et al. Accuracy of cardiovascular risk prediction varies by neighborhood socioeconomic position: A retrospective cohort study. Annals of Internal Medicine. 2017;167(7):456–464.

35. Goff DC, Jr., Lloyd-Jones DM, Bennett G, et al. 2013 ACC/AHA guideline on the assessment of cardiovascular risk: A report of the American College of Cardiology/ American Heart Association Task Force on Practice Guidelines. Journal of the American College of Cardiology. 2014;63(25 Pt B):2935–2959.

36. World Health Organization. Social determinants of health: The solid facts. http://www.euro.who.int/__data/assets/pdf_file/0005/98438/e81384.pdf. Published 2003. Accessed August 22, 2019.

37. Gostic KM, Ambrose M, Worobey M, Lloyd-Smith JO. Potent protection against H5N1 and H7N9 influenza via childhood hemagglutinin imprinting. Science. 2016;354(6313):722–726.

38. Glass TA, McAtee MJ. Behavioral science at the crossroads in public health: extending horizons, envisioning the future. Social Science and Medicine. 2006;62(7):1650–1671.

39. Pareto V. Cours d'economie politique. Paris: Rouge; 1897.

40. Auerbach F. Das gesetz der bevolkerungskoncentration. Petermanns Geographische Mitteilungen. 1913;59:74–76.

41. Zipf GK. Human behavior and the principle of least effort. New York: Hafner; 1949.

42. West BJ, Deering B. The lure of modern science: Fractal thinking. Singapore: World Scientific; 1995.

43. Newman MEJ. Power laws, Pareto distributions and Zipf's law. http://arxiv.org/PS_cache/cond-mat/pdf/0412/0412004. Published 2005.

44. Mandelbrot BB. The fractal geometry of nature. New York: Freeman; 1983.

45. Brock WA. Some Santa Fe scenery. In: Colander D, ed. The complexity vision and the teaching of economics. Cheltenham, UK: Edward Elgar; 2000:29–49.

46. Kleiber C, Kotz S. Statistical size distributions in economics and actuarial sciences. New York: Wiley; 2003.

47. Andriani P, McKelvey B. From Gaussian to Paretian thinking: Causes and implications of power laws in organizations. Organizational Science. 2009;20(6). doi:10.1287/orsc.1090.0481

48. Réka A, Jeong H, Barabási A-L. Diameter of the world wide web. Nature. 1999;401:130–131.

49. Watts DJ, Strogatz SH. Collective dynamics of "small-world" networks. Nature. 1998;393(6684):440–442.

50. Ball P. Critical mass: How one thing leads to another. New York: Ferrar, Straus and Giroux; 2004.

51. Song C, Havlin S, Makse HA. Self-similarity of complex networks. Nature. 2005;433(7024):392–395.

52. Newman MEJ, Barabasi AL, Watts DJ. The structure and dynamics of networks. Princeton, NJ: Princeton University Press; 2006.

53. Burton C, Elliott A, Cochran A, Love T. Do healthcare services behave as complex systems? Analysis of patterns of attendance and implications for service delivery. BMC Medicine. 2018;16(1):138.

54. Simsek E, Kim M. Power-law tail in lag time distribution underlies bacterial persistence. Proceedings of the National Academy of Sciences of the United States of America. August 19, 2019.

55. Sornette D. Critical phenomena in natural sciences: chaos, fractals, self organization, and disorder: Concepts and tools. Berlin: Springer; 2000.

56. Simon H. On a class of skewed distribution functions. Biometrika. 1955;42(3/4):425–440.

57. Barabasi AL. Linked: the new science of networks. Cambridge, MA: Perseus; 2002.

58. Sornette D. Why stock markets crash: critical events in complex financial systems. Princeton, NJ: Princeton University Press; 2003.

59. Andriani P, McKelvey B. From skew distributions to power-law science. In: Allen P, Maguire S, McKelvey B, eds. Sage handbook of complexity and management. Los Angeles: SAGE; 2011:254–273.

60. Whittles LK, White PJ, Didelot X. A dynamic power-law sexual network model of gonorrhea outbreaks. PLoS Computational Biology. 2019;15(3):e1006748.

TAKE-HOME MESSAGES

Designing and conducting complex-systems–grounded research is not necessarily a dramatic departure from how traditional research in population health is done—many of the same steps are followed, but with new thinking and tools within each step. However, as delineated in this section, designing and conducting complex-systems–grounded research is much more than that. To meaningfully engage in this type of research requires digging deeper to evaluate the underlying mental models that shape how we think about research and action and strive to clarify them after appreciating and integrating the complex realities of population health through the use of system mapping and complex systems modeling. It requires thinking more inclusively to strategically and meaningfully engage key stakeholders as we conceptualize and conduct research and to do so in complex systems-aware ways. And it requires challenging and better integrating the diverse assumptions that are the foundation of population health science and practice, including better accommodating the consideration of non-normality and other complex characteristics of the population health systems we wish to understand and improve. We need to invest in learning about and designing action to address "the whole"—complex system structures producing undesirable population health outcomes.

Although there are differences, it is important to remember that complex-systems–grounded research approaches are not intended to wholly replace traditional research tools. Instead, the choice of research design should be contingent on the early steps in the design process, at which point the research questions and objectives will inform the choice of design—and system complexity must be considered. Any methodology has inherent strengths and limitations, and the key is matching objectives and context within which the objectives will be addressed with appropriate methods. Sometimes mental models can be reconciled using a simple approach (e.g., surveys), stakeholders can be meaningfully engaged in a traditional research study (e.g., semi-structured interview or focus group), and a normal distribution can be wholly appropriate for a population health outcome of interest. But when the outcome of interest is complex, care should be taken to select methods capable of accommodating this complexity—or conclusions could be incorrect or insufficient for meaningful improvements to population health. Complex systems and traditional approaches are complementary, and studies have combined the strengths of each to maximize the value of a given research endeavor. Furthermore, more traditional methods can—and are—being adapted to better respond to complexity.

RESOURCES FOR FURTHER READING

Andersson C, Törnberg A, Törnberg P. Societal systems: Complex or worse? *Futures.* 2014;63:145–157.

Axelrod R. Advancing the art of simulation in the social sciences. In: Rennard J-P, ed. *Handbook on Research on Nature Inspired Computing for Economy and Management.* Hershey, PA: Idea Group; 2005.

Diez-Roux AV. Complex systems thinking and current impasses in health disparities research. *Am J Public Health.* 2011;101(9):1627–1634.

Epstein JM. Why model? *JASSS.* 2008;11(4):12–16.

Frerichs L, Hassmiller Lich K, Dave G, Corbie-Smith G. Integrating systems science and community-based participatory research to achieve health equity. *Am J Public Health.* 2016;106(2):215–222.

Galea S, Riddle M, Kaplan GA. Causal thinking and complex system approaches in epidemiology. *Int J Epidemiol.* 2010;39(1):97–106.

Glass TA, Goodman SN, Hernán MA, Samet JM. Causal inference in public health. *Annu Rev Public Health.* 2013;34:61–75.

Hassmiller Lich K, Ginexi EM, Osgood ND, Mabry PL. A call to address complexity in prevention science research. *Prevention Science.* 2013;14(3):279–289.

Hassmiller Lich K, Urban JB, Frerichs L, Dave G. Extending systems thinking in planning and evaluation using group concept mapping and system dynamics to tackle complex problems. *Eval Program Plann.* 2017;60:254–264.

Hovmand PS. *Community Based System Dynamics.* New York, NY: Springer; 2014.

Hovmand PS, Andersen DF, Rouwette E, Richardson GP, Rux K, Calhoun A. Group model-building "scripts" as a collaborative planning tool. *Sys Res Behav Sci.* 2012;29(2):179–193.

Leischow SJ, Best A, Trochim WM, et al. Systems thinking to improve the public's health. *Am J Prev Med.* 2008;35(2):S196–S203.

Leischow SJ, Milstein B. Systems thinking and modeling for public health practice. *Am J Public Health.* 2006;96(3):403–405.

Louth J. From Newton to Newtonianism: Reductionism and the development of the social sciences. *Emerg Complex Org.* 2011;13(4):63–83.

Luna-Reyes LF, Martinez-Moyano IJ, Pardo TA, Cresswell AM, Andersen DF, Richardson GP. Anatomy of a group model-building intervention: Building dynamic theory from case study research. *Syst Dynam Rev.* 2006;22(4):291–320.

Meadows DH, Wright D. *Thinking in Systems: A Primer.* White River Junction, VT: Chelsea Green; 2008.

Newman M. Power laws, Pareto distributions and Zipf's law. *Contemp Physics.* 2005;46(5):323–351.

Olaya C. Cows, agency, and the significance of operational thinking. *Syst Dynam Rev.* 2015;31:183–219.

Page SE. *The Model Thinker.* New York, NY: Basic Books; 2018.

Richardson GP. Concept models in group model building. *Syst Dynam Rev.* 2013;29(1):42–55.

Richardson GP, Andersen DF. Teamwork in group model building. *Syst Dynam Rev.* 1995;11(2):113–137.

Sterman JD. *Business Dynamics: Systems Thinking and Modeling for a Complex World.* Boston, MA: Irwin/McGraw-Hill; 2000.

Sterman JD. Learning from evidence in a complex world. *Am J Public Health.* 2006;96(3):505–514.

Sterman JD. Sustaining sustainability: Creating a systems science in a fragmented academy and polarized world. In: Weinstein MP, Turner RE, eds. *Sustainability Science: The Emerging Paradigm and the Urban Environment.* New York, NY: Springer; 2012:21–58.

Complex Systems and Analytical Techniques in Population Health Science

Introductory Material: Preview and Objectives

PREVIEW

Analytical methods for studying complex population health challenges are the focus of Part IV of this book. In Chapters 11 to 18, an array of analytical techniques, primarily grounded in mathematical and computational modeling (simulation) and analysis, are described. Several chapters focus on specific approaches; for these chapters, thematic population health examples are provided to demonstrate the value of these analytical methods for advancing understanding and guiding decision-making in population health science.

Chapter 11 describes mathematical modeling, which is the use of mathematical notation and techniques to describe, represent, and/or analyze diverse phenomena. These approaches provide means to parsimoniously describe, test representations of, and study elements of complex systems. In this chapter, several types of mathematical modeling used in population health are described, including statistical modeling (highlighting more complexity-aware approaches such as structural equation modeling), infectious disease modeling, cost-effectiveness analysis, and the use of operations research methods in population health.

Chapter 12 introduces dynamic simulation modeling—an extension of mathematical modeling of dynamic systems typically used when equations cannot easily or adequately capture system complexity or when their analysis is not possible and computation (computer simulation) is necessary. This chapter discusses fundamental characteristics, attributes, and assumptions of dynamic simulation models; in particular, the ability of dynamic models to allow users to operationally express their "dynamic hypotheses" (their precise theories about the underlying causal structure of real-world phenomena) and seek to understand the "generative mechanisms" underlying the complex system. In this chapter, three key types of simulation modeling approaches are reviewed—system dynamics modeling, agent-based modeling, and discrete event simulation. These analytical methods are compared and contrasted, in the context of in-depth discussion about the general purpose of simulation models as a whole.

Chapter 13 explicates system dynamics modeling by demonstrating its application in the U.S. healthcare system. Using the Rethink Health Dynamics Model, which is a system dynamics model that represents the complex dynamics of a regional health system in the United States, the value of this modeling approach is demonstrated by showing how simulation can be used to aid decision-making. Here, four common pitfalls and possible ways to overcome each pitfall with additional intervention are demonstrated using system dynamics tools, including causal feedback diagrams and simulation output graphs. This chapter also goes "under the hood" of the model to see how it can explain, in clear structural terms, why well-intended interventions sometimes fall short.

Chapter 14 describes agent-based modeling by showing how it can be applied to drug use epidemics. As is described in this chapter, drug use epidemics have characteristics that require complex-systems–grounded approaches: They have features of infectious diseases and chronic diseases, and effectively understanding them requires considering multiple connected and interacting system components and outcomes. Agent-based modeling provides a way to include and combine data from different domains into a single analytical framework. Further, this modeling approach allows researchers to combine neurobiological, decisional, and environmental components inherent to drug use epidemics in models that can be used to simulate their nonlinear dynamics and emergent outcomes. The agent-based model PainTown is described to demonstrate the value of this modeling approach in drug use epidemics.

Chapter 15 explores the use of hybrid simulation, in which aspects of different approaches to modeling are combined. Using case studies from the United Kingdom, this chapter presents the foundational concepts of hybrid simulation modeling and describes how the various stages in developing a single-method model can be adapted for hybrid simulation. Additionally, a set of guidelines is provided for modelers that show how an integrated, multiscale simulation modeling framework can be developed, validated, and exploited for population health problems.

Chapter 16 discusses validation of simulation models—defined here as determining whether a model is sufficiently credible, accurate, and reliable to be used for its intended applications—in population health. This chapter describes some of the common considerations that can be used to gauge the extent to which a model is validated for a given application. Although focusing on microsimulation models that simulate the life histories of individual agents in discrete time, the considerations discussed in this chapter are also relevant for system dynamics modeling, agent-based modeling, discrete event simulation, and other approaches to simulation modeling.

Chapter 17 describes, compares, and contrasts five simulation models developed and used in population health research and practice. These applications are sequenced from abstract and/or relatively small (in terms of lines of code; often described as generic, archetypical, conceptual or stylized) to more detailed and intended for data-driven, context-specific policy analysis. For each model, its various objectives—what it sought to achieve—are described. Each application is used to illuminate "model thinking," as introduced in Chapter 8 of this volume.

Chapter 18 illustrates the study of noncommunicable diseases using statistical physics tools. As discussed in the chapter, heterogeneity and complexity in human disease suggests new methodological and analytical ways in which the physical sciences can play a role in population health research. The author argues that the system of individuals constitutes an example of a complex system in statistical physics, meaning that these tools can be brought to bear. The fundamental concepts and methods in statistical physics that can be applied to population health research are reviewed, which can help to improve our understanding of how noncommunicable diseases (and other population health-relevant phenomena) emerge.

OBJECTIVES

The objectives of this section are as follows:

1. Appreciate the diverse application of mathematical modeling to population health—and the broader conventions used to develop analyze such models, as well as the opportunity to further extend these methods to better accommodate complexity inherent to population health systems.
2. Describe the overarching approach to dynamic simulation modeling, as well as three common specific approaches—agent-based modeling, system dynamics modeling, and discrete event simulation—including their unique modeling goals and norms.
3. Appreciate the strengths, weaknesses, and tradeoffs among agent-based modeling, system dynamics modeling, and discrete event simulation.
4. Demonstrate how system dynamics modeling can be used as a research and decision-making tool to avoid pitfalls in policy decision-making that are particularly likely in the context of dynamic complexity.
5. Illustrate how agent-based modeling can be used to combine and model the multiple components and complex dynamics of population health phenomena (e.g., drug use epidemics) to test mechanistic assumptions about the complex system structure capable of producing observed "emergent" outcomes.
6. Understand the foundational concepts of hybrid simulation modeling—what it is, and why and how to do it.
7. Present a set of guidelines for modelers that show how an integrated, multiscale simulation modeling framework can be developed, validated, and exploited for population health problems.
8. Examine common factors and considerations that can collectively be used to gauge the extent to which a model is validated for a given application.
9. Provide and compare diverse applied examples of simulation models in population health and healthcare that demonstrate "model thinking" with different objectives in motivating the work.
10. Describe how statistical physics and nonlinear dynamics can contribute to the delineation and control of an array of population health problems.

11

Mathematical Modeling in Population Health Research

KAREN HICKLIN AND KRISTEN HASSMILLER LICH

11.1. INTRODUCTION

Mathematical modeling is the use of mathematical notation and techniques to describe, represent, and/or analyze real-world phenomena. Mathematical models are fundamental tools used in diverse disciplines and research domains such as engineering, the physical sciences, social sciences, and medicine/population health. Mathematical models provide stakeholders, including researchers, population health practitioners and policymakers, a way to efficiently describe, test representations of, and study elements of society or complex systems in a low-stakes environment—the many benefits of which are described in more detail in Chapters 8 and 9 of this volume.

Mathematical modeling has unique strengths—and limitations—among the set of complex systems methods. It is the oldest of these methods, typically used to predict system behavior (outcomes) or to test mechanistic assumptions underlying outcomes. Mathematical equations provide powerful and parsimonious means for describing complex systems. Advances in population health have been driven through mathematical analysis of equations—for example, solving for steady-state behavior or conditions maximizing/minimizing outcomes. One example is the "reproductive number"—the mathematically derived equation for the tipping point determining whether and under what conditions a given disease outbreak will die out or reach an endemic level.[1-4] Another example is the "steady state equations" for a queueing system, for example, representing a health clinic and estimating how long the average patient will wait for service, how many

Karen Hicklin and Kristen Hassmiller Lich, *Mathematical Modeling in Population Health Research* In: *Complex Systems and Population Health*. Edited by: Yorghos Apostolopoulos, Kristen Hassmiller Lich, and Michael Kenneth Lemke, Oxford University Press (2020). © Oxford University Press. DOI: 10.1093/oso/9780190880743.003.0011 people will be waiting at a given time, and the percentage of time each doctor is providing care.[5-7]

While there is a long history of mathematical modeling in population health, its use is often advanced within siloes; rarely are researchers or practitioners taught about the breadth of applications. This gap and illuminate the diversity of applications of mathematical modeling to inform complex problems in population health is addressed in this chapter. The objective is to help readers appreciate similarities and differences across applications. We begin with a brief overview of mathematical modeling basics and then discuss four common classes of applications—biological modeling, statistical modeling, cost-effectiveness analysis (CEA), and operations research.

11.2. MATHEMATICAL MODELING BASICS

Mathematical modeling refers to the "set of assumptions together with implications drawn from them by mathematical reasoning."[8pv] Here, *assumptions* take the form of one or more mathematical equations that describe the nature of the relationships between the values of input variables and the outcomes they determine. The level of detail within mathematical models can vary. On one end, *mechanistic models* explicitly represent the detailed mechanisms that translate inputs to outputs. On the other extreme, *black box models* relate inputs to outputs, but without specifying the mechanisms underlying these relationships. So, what do we mean by "mathematical reasoning" producing insights? This refers to any sense-making analysis done using the model, and can include studying how outputs change as inputs vary (e.g., in different contexts, for different individuals) or change over time (whether desired/controlled or not) or determining the most critical components of system (model) structure. Throughout this chapter a spectrum of sense-making activities are described. The implications drawn from mathematical models include enhanced understanding of how systems function (as just described) or predicted outcomes based on input variable values. Models vary based on their objectives. For example, if careful prediction is the goal, more specific and detailed models are typically used. If, instead, more generalizable understanding is sought, more abstract models are often used.

Several types of variables are commonly distinguished within mathematical modeling. As just described, *input variables* (sometimes referred to as explanatory variables) are the variables that, when parameterized (i.e., given values), determine the outputs/outcomes of interest. *Output variables* are defined through model equations. Some input parameters can be controlled through decisions or intervention and, as such, are referred to as *decision variables*. Other input variables are not controllable and are estimated and fed into model calculations and described as *exogenous variables*. Another set of input variables are described as *intermediate or endogenous variables*—calculated or updated by the mathematical model and a function of other model variables. Sometimes the goal is to estimate outputs given inputs, other times we might use observed outputs to estimate unobservable input parameter values (e.g., cancer progression rates or the impact exposure to an educational campaign has on behavior). Some input parameters are *stochastic* (i.e., random). We often describe patterns in stochastic variables, typically in the form of a *probability distribution* defining the likelihood the variable will take on different values. When input parameters are stochastic and endogenous, the outcome variables they affect are also stochastic.

11.3. MODELING BIOLOGICAL SYSTEMS

One common use of mathematical modeling, relevant to population health, is the description, quantification, and study of complex biological systems. Here, mathematical modeling of infectious disease progression/spread and human physiology are highlighted.

11.3.1. Infections Disease Development and Spread

One of the oldest and most prominent examples of mathematical modeling in health is infectious disease modeling. Often described as compartmental modeling, it is used to study the progression, spread, and control of infectious diseases. A relatively simple foundational example is the SIR model. Each letter represents a different and mutually exclusive compartment, or subset of individuals within the population. Let S represent the number of individuals who are susceptible to a given disease; I, the number currently infected; and R, the number who had the disease but are now recovered. The choice of compartments depends on the characteristics of the particular disease being modeled. Variations on the theme allow for revisiting compartments over time (e.g., SIRs in which recovered individuals become susceptible after some delay) and additional compartments added for exposed (E) individuals and individuals with passive immunity (M) or under quarantine (Q).[9-13] The transition (flow) of individuals from one compartment to another is proportional to the number present in the compartment, multiplied by the rate of leaving, that might be a function of time (e.g., a constant rate), or based on more complex assumptions. For example, the mass action principle finds the rate of infection proportional to the density of susceptible and infectious individuals.[1]

What do the mathematical formulae look like for the SIR model? Let $S(t)$ be the number of susceptible individuals at time t, $I(t)$ be the number of infected individuals at time t, $R(t)$ be the number of recovered individuals with immunity at time t. The total population size is N and therefore $S(t) + I(t) + R(t) = N(t)$. "Force of infection" is represented as $\beta c > 0$, which is equal to the average number of contacts a susceptible individual makes in a fixed unit of time (c) multiplied by the probability any one of those contacts, if made with an infectious individual (the case with probability I/N) will transmit infection (β). With the recovery rate represented by $\gamma > 0$, the classic epidemic model is described by the following set of nonlinear ordinary differential equations:

$$dS/dt = -\beta IS/N,$$

$$dI/dt = \beta IS/N - \gamma I,$$

$$dR/dt = \gamma I,$$

with initial values such that $S(0), I(0), R(0) \geq 0$. This simple example assumes no birth or death, though death (and other transitions) could be added to these equations. For example, if the death rate in all compartments is constant, d, then $d*$ each compartment size could be subtracted from each equation. This type of modeling structure has been applied to a variety of infectious diseases such as influenza, HIV, Ebola, and hepatitis C. Extensions of these models incorporate additional complexities, such as assortment (nonrandom mixing), delays, vaccination (with perfect or imperfect protection), seasonality (varied rates of β across months or seasons of the year).[1-4,10,11] Infectious disease models have been used as inspiration for modeling other transmittable phenomena, such as the diffusion of information or influence through social networks.

Model analysis (mathematical reasoning) is used to understand disease trajectories and phase transitions or to mathematically solve for threshold conditions—the equations for which we refer to as the reproductive number, above which outbreaks become epi/endemic and below which they die out.[9-13] In the previously described SIR model, the first two equations for change in S and I are only considered, as knowing these determines R. Then, if the right-hand sides of these equations are set equal to zero (no change), the condition(s) under which the compartments will stabilize can be solved for. Depending on the complexity of the modeled system, this may be done by solving a series of equations for closed form solutions or equations for stability (e.g., using linear algebra or solving by matrix inversion if the equations are/can be made linear) and determining the asymptotic stability of each stabilizing condition.[1,2] The latter means that we need to determine whether all/which initial conditions will trend toward that equilibrium. While solving for closed form solutions is very helpful, allowing ready calculation and analysis as input parameter values are estimated and an appreciation of which model parameters affect where the disease stabilizes, it is often not possible and numerical analysis or simulation is required.

11.3.2. Other Physiological Models

The health literature is full of diverse applications of mathematical modeling to explain and predict a variety of other physiological phenomenon, such as tumor growth and mechanisms of treatment response[14,15] and a variety of cardiovascular and respiratory phenomena.[16] Mathematical modeling has been used to develop and test coherent and quantitative descriptions of dynamical systems, such as "the interplay between gene expression, metabolite concentrations, and metabolic fluxes" affecting how *E. coli* responds to oxygen levels.[17] For a more general discussion of how to build sufficiently complex mathematical models capable of obeying physical laws and producing observed patterns of outcomes, see the seminal work of Hoppensteadt and Peskin.[18]

11.4. STATISTICAL MODELING

Perhaps the most common application of mathematical modeling in population health research is statistical modeling. Statistical modeling typically involves approaches to learn about whether a model or some aspect of it is a good representation of reality, using statistical analysis to estimate model parameters given sample data and/or to evaluate the accuracy/goodness of fit of the model itself.

11.4.1. Regression

Regression analysis is a prominent statistical method used to approximate and quantify relationships between input and output variables. An equation or set of equations are used to represent the relationship between independent (input) and dependent (output) variables. Since dependent variables are a function of independent variables (often times referred to as "predictors"), regression models can be used to quantify the expected dependent variable value given a set of independent variable particular values—or to estimate the "elasticity" or change in the dependent variable expected to correspond to a specified change in independent parameter values. In population health, regression can be used to estimate the association between costs, treatment effectiveness, and a variety of other outcomes and key explanatory variables, while also controlling for confounding factors such as prior health care utilization, levels of access to care, and demographic characteristics.[19] The basis of regression analysis is correlation between independent and dependent variables with the goal of estimating a line derived as the best fit from a set of data points relating independent and dependent variable values. A simple linear regression model takes on the following structure,

$$Y = \alpha + \beta X + \varepsilon,$$

where Y is the dependent variable, X is the independent variable or a vector of variables, α is the intercept or constant, β is the slope coefficient corresponding to each independent variable, and ε is the error term for the equation. Linear regression models such as this have been used to study many population health outcomes and to inform or evaluate the impact of interventions.

Not all regression models are as simple, or linear, with model structure varied based on characteristics of variables (e.g., continuous or discrete) or the nature of their relationships. For example, logistic or multinomial regression is used when the dependent variable is binary or categorical, respectively. Nonlinear terms (e.g., X^2) can be included if it is a more appropriate way to describe the nature of the relationship. Cox regression (often referred to as proportional hazards modeling) is a variant on regression used to estimate the impact of independent variables (X) on the hazard of a given event (e.g., death) at time t ($H(t)$) with the form $H(t) = H_0(t) \cdot \exp(\beta X)$, where $H_0(t)$ is the baseline hazard at time t for an individual with a value of 0 for all independent variables X. Where meta-analysis methods are long used to pool estimates across studies, meta-regression uses regression to estimate the relationship between effect estimates and characteristics varied across studies.[20]

11.4.2. More Complexity-Aware Statistical Modeling Methods

As researchers are becoming more aware of and needing to address the complexity of population health challenges, statistical modeling approaches are being advanced to accommodate this complexity. Several simple adaptations in the previous paragraph were described. Recently, the sophistication of statistical modeling has grown rapidly while the objectives motivating this work have largely remained the same—to understand relationships between variables and to test and compare the accuracy (goodness of fit) of competing models (either a model compared to a null hypothesis of no effect or more sophisticated models to each other).[21]

Disciplinary differences in approaches are emerging. It is beyond the scope of this chapter to comprehensively review and compare all approaches, though we briefly highlight two of the more innovative statistical modeling approaches being used within population health research—structural equation modeling and directed acyclic graphs (DAGs).

Structural equation modeling is a flexible and typically (though not always) linear and cross-sectional set of statistical modeling techniques used to analyze structural relationships. Four common approaches include the following.

- Path analysis allows for the inclusion of direct and indirect relationships among independent (or predictor) variables. Path analysis is often used in mediation modeling—for example, to illuminate diverse factors and pathways linking pregnancy in adolescence and early child undernutrition[22] or the factors differentially affecting women's and men's social capital over time.[23]
- Exploratory and confirmatory factor analysis is a lot like path analysis, but include paths between observed and latent variables—variables that are not directly observed but are critical constructs inferred from a set of observed variables (e.g., overall health or substance use onset). As an example, confirmatory factor analysis was used to illuminate the links between obstructive sleep apnea syndrome and metabolic syndrome.[24]

- Latent variable structural models include latent variables within the path analysis approach. In one application of this approach, researchers tested the hypothesis that reinforcing characteristics of electronic cigarettes are linked to individual's propensity to quit smoking—among dual electronic and combustible users.[25]
- Growth curve models (similar approaches are referred to as trajectory analysis, latent curve analysis, or latent trajectory analysis) seek to explain variation in intra-individual change over time (trajectories) in terms of both fixed and time-varying factors in a bottom–up (individual-centric) approach using data across individuals. As an example, researchers used this approach to understand the effects of physical and neuropsychiatric medical comorbidities on functional outcomes and life satisfaction within the ten years after traumatic brain injury.[26]

DAGs use network conventions to depict complex interrelationships (edges) between variables (nodes). "Directed" means that the direction of the relationship is one-way and clearly indicated. "Acyclic" means there are no closed loops. DAGs are a powerful tool to support researchers in hypothesizing the complex structural relationships between variables involved in causal research questions (e.g., causal inference) to inform the bias-minimizing analytical strategy."[27] Austin and colleagues[27p78] introduce and illustrate the value of DAGs in child maltreatment research, supporting the identification of "confounders, mediators, and colliders, detailing the manner in which each type of variable can be used to inform study design and analysis." While DAGs in and of themselves are not statistical models, they are an approach for carefully reflecting on complexity when formulating statistical models. While DAGs prohibit closed loops, feedback loops can be depicted by including multiple variables (nodes) corresponding to a single variable at different time points.

11.5. MODELING IN COST-EFFECTIVENESS ANALYSIS

CEA has a long history in health services research, with foundations in mathematical modeling. A decision tree, the format of many such decision support models, consists in its simplest form of a decision node, chance nodes, and outcome nodes (which may include utility and/or costs). Using algebra, probability theory, and logic, decision trees are used to evaluate the tradeoff of one or more decision alternatives versus another related to cost, effectiveness (impact), and potentially other outcomes of interest. A decision node represents decision points. For each outcome of interest, potential states of nature under each decision alternative are represented by chance nodes, with associated probabilities of occurrence. Each outcome has an associated reward or cost. By evaluating all the probabilistic events that may occur from each decision alternative, which can include adverse side effects or secondary positive outcomes along with all associated costs and primary health benefits, modelers can learn whether/when one decision alternative dominates another. CEA typically calculates the incremental cost-effectiveness ratio (ICER)—the ratio of the difference in costs between two decision alternatives and the difference in health outcomes. Quality-adjusted life years are often used to bring together, in a single measure, impacts the decision alternatives have on saving lives, adding length to life, and/or improving the quality of life lived.[28,29]

Incorporating more uncertainty (stochasticity) into the chance nodes (i.e., using probability distributions instead of point estimates), the decision maker is able to conduct further analysis regarding the probability one decision is more cost-effective than another. This analysis can provide additional insight into the robustness of decision recommendations through reviewing the range of possible ICER values across modeled scenarios in "ICER planes" or identifying the most cost-effective decision alternatives for various levels of willingness to pay for an addition unit of the primary outcome.

A simple example to illustrate how decision trees are utilized is the consideration of whether to treat a patient with a new drug therapy A instead of the more common drug therapy B. This decision can be made complicated when the new drug therapy is more expensive but could be more beneficial for a patient. For each drug therapy, there are various outcomes a decision maker may be concerned with. For instance, the efficacy of drug A versus drug B, the severity of the side effects for either treatment plan, or short- and long-term costs associated with the drug alternatives. If the objective is defined as minimizing long-term complications, then the decision problem becomes a minimization problem. If we assume each new therapy is associated with two primary outcomes (O_1 and O_2), the costs for drug therapy A and B are C_A and C_B, respectively, and treatment cost for the outcomes are C_1 for O_1 and C_2 for O_2, then the problem takes on the following form:

$$\min\{\Pr\left(O_1 \mid \text{drug therapy } A\right)*\left(C_A - C_1\right) + \Pr\left(O_2 \mid \text{drug therapy } A\right)*\left(C_A - C_2\right),$$

$$\Pr\left(O_1 \mid \text{drug therapy } B\right)*\left(C_B - C_1\right) + \Pr\left(O_2 \mid \text{drug therapy } B\right)*\left(C_B - C_2\right)\}.$$

An example of a more complex problem is the decision about type of hysterectomy (e.g. laparoscopic with morcellation versus abdominal) to perform for women who undergo the surgery for treatment of uterine fibroids. The first alternative allows for the uterus to be removed laparoscopically by cutting it into pieces that fit through small incisions and is associated with a shorter hospital stay, less pain, and lower rates of wound infection. However, there is a chance that benign or malignant tissue may unintentionally spread throughout the body if morcellation is not contained in a bag. Although the second option of an abdominal surgery prevents the potential tissue spreading, the outcomes overall are reported to be better for laparoscopic removal. A decision tree model was used to estimate the likelihood that one alternative is better than the other.[30]

Decision trees are useful for evaluating the trade-off between alternatives at a specified point in time (e.g., 1 year or 10 years after the initial decision) based on the probability of occurrences associated with each decision. Such models can accommodate substantial complexity, including, for example, many-stage decisions (do X, then if Y, do Z) and heterogeneity in effects across subpopulations or the lag time between change and consequences.

Another complex structure often built into CEA models when decision alternatives affect disease state transitions over time is Markov state-transition structure. So-called Markov models make use of Markov chains and are named after Russian mathematician Andrei Markov.[31] A Markov chain is a representation of states in one time period that have a probability of transitioning to another state in the next time period (much like compartmental models described above, but with some differences in conventions used, such as the inclusion of an absorbing death state). As an example, we might characterize HIV+ individuals as in one of four categories based on CD4 count, which is the count of a type of white blood cell in the blood and a measure of disease progression.[32] If the four categories (known as states) are CD4<200, 200≤CD4<350, 350≤CD4<500, and CD4≥500, the probability that an individual moves from one category to another within a given time period can be represented as a Markov model as long as the probability of being in the current state depends only on the last state visited. That is, there must be enough information to credibly predict the probability of transitioning to each other state (or remaining in the same state) for individuals based solely on their current state. This assumption is often referred to as "memoryless"—no "memory" is needed beyond current state to predict next state. Understanding how CD4 counts change over time is useful, not only in understanding the underlying disease structure and its effect on white blood cells over time, but also in developing treatment plans. A Markov model was used to model the cost-effectiveness of a particular drug combination therapy on HIV infection, a dynamic outcome over time.[33] Outcomes of the model include annual costs per patient, patient survival curves for each drug therapy, and the ICER describing the novel treatment alternatives to standard practice. Markov models, like decision trees, can accommodate more complexity when appropriate—for example, building in more memory (e.g., disease state across multiple time points) or different assumptions about the time to transition across disease states. As CEA models have become more complex, modelers are better supported through the use of software to support careful projects and sense-making analysis.

11.6. MODELING IN OPERATIONS RESEARCH

Operations research is a multidisciplinary field that uses analytical modeling to study systems, improve processes, and aid in decision-making. Methods rooted in operations research have been applied to a broad variety of fields including healthcare. We highlight two relevant mathematical modeling tools from operations research—the study of stochastic processes and constrained optimization.

11.6.1. Stochastic Processes

A collection of random variables used to represent systems that change randomly over time are referred to as stochastic processes, for which methods to represent and analyze system behavior have been developed. Examples of a stochastic process include the number of people who arrive in the emergency department each day, the length of time a patient spends with his or her primary care provider, or the way cancerous tumors may grow in size over time before diagnosis and treatment. Two common health-related topics for which stochastic processes are studied involve queuing and discrete/continuous Markov processes and chains (similar to those previously discussed and used within CEA).

Queuing theory is the study of waiting through a sequential series of events. Historically, queuing theory is rooted in telecommunication systems where a consumer would make a call and be placed in a queue to wait for the operator. In this simple example, all calls must go through the operator they have been directed to, and the amount of time spent waiting and being served are represented by random input variables while the total time in the system is a random output variable. Stochastic process models are built up to describe realistic distributions of time between events (e.g., time between arrivals, time until each unit of service ends) and rules about queues (e.g., how many people can be accommodated in a queue, how long people are willing to wait before leaving, how people are served from a queue).

These models can become quite complex, requiring computational modeling. When possible, tremendous power comes from analytical (closed-form) solution of their steady-state behavior—just as was described for infectious disease models and their steady state conditions. For example, the steady-state behavior of a queueing system with a first-in/first-out queue with no maximum capacity and from which no one leaves without being served, a single unit of service, and Markovian (i.e., exponentially distributed or memoryless) inter-arrival and service times, is well characterized as an "M/M/s" model, where the first M represents the inter-arrival time (λ), the second M represents the service time (μ), and s represents number of equivalent servers available.[5-7] The simplest queuing system is the M/M/1. For this system, a series of equations characterize system outputs once the system warms up and hits its equilibrium behavior ("steady state"). The following equation can be used to estimate the expected wait time in the system:

$W = \dfrac{1}{\mu(1-\rho)}$, where $\rho = \lambda / \mu$ and represents the server utilization (an approx-

imation of the fraction of time a server is busy). The wait time in the queue is

estimated by $W_q = W - \dfrac{1}{\mu} = \dfrac{\rho}{\mu(1-\rho)}$. And the following equations estimates the

number of people waiting in the queue and number of people in the system, re-

spectively: $L_q = \dfrac{\rho^2}{1-\rho}$ and $L = \lambda W$.

Queuing theory has been used to model healthcare systems and their impact on population health. Common motivating objectives focus on making health facility operations more effective (better outcomes) or more efficient (equivalent outcomes at lower cost), estimating requisite staff or capacity to achieve a service objective, informing triaging rules (e.g., rules for how to prioritize individuals from a queue), or learning where to target change to most substantially improve system outcomes. Queueing theory is extensively used to improve Emergency Department outcomes,[34,35] to inform approaches to address mass-casualty incidents,[36] or to inform state-investment to improve mental health services systems.[37]

11.6.2. Constrained Optimization

In constrained optimization models, the goal is to optimize an objective function subject to a set of constraints. An objective function is a mathematical representation of the goal of interest, which is either maximized (e.g., health or profit) or minimized (e.g., life lost, incident cancer, time in hospital, or service system cost). Equations for each of a set of goals can be weighted and included in a single objective function (e.g., to balance overall quality-adjusted life years across distinct subpopulations or to balance cost reduction and health promotion objectives).

Constraints represents bounds, limits, or relationships between variables within the problem. Constraints may reflect elements of the system itself, such as the number of nurses available during a particular shift within the emergency room, or may represent desired guidelines, such as limiting the amount of time a patient waits before being triaged in an emergency room. The previously described maximization problem may have the following structure.

$$\min\ expected\ time\ a\ patient\ is\ in\ the\ hosptial\ for\ outpatient\ procedure$$

$$subject\ to$$

$$(1)\ number\ of\ procedures\ needed\ constraint$$

$$(2)\ time\ needed\ for\ each\ procedure\ constraint$$

$$(3)\ staffing\ constraint$$

The modeler seeks to identify the values of decision variables (e.g., the order of procedures scheduled across the hospital stay) that optimize the objective function. Each of the previous constraints(1–3) is a separate equation, limiting the space of decision variable values that are feasible. Constrained optimization models can be formulated using linear programming, nonlinear programming, integer programming, stochastic programming, and Markov decision processes—and have been used in organ donation allocation, infectious disease treatment, workforce planning, and hospital facility location decision-making.[38,39]

11.7. CONCLUSIONS

Mathematical models provide a powerful and parsimonious way to describe complex systems and inform their control. In healthcare, this can be very useful. From understanding how infectious disease spreads to making better decisions regarding healthcare management, mathematical modeling provides insight into various systems and phenomena in a low-stakes (virtual) setting. This chapter highlights a variety of forms and uses of mathematical modeling, all of which derive from a rich foundation of common analytic approaches, notational conventions, and best practices. As the level of complexity in the models increases, it is less likely that closed-form (analytical) solutions can be obtained—and the benefits of computational approaches and simulation increase. However, when model simplification can produce robust closed-form representations of complex phenomena to inform real-time decision-making, it can be a tremendous support to decision makers through guiding their intuition about system behavior and informing their decisions.

REFERENCES

1. Anderson RM, May RM. *Infectious diseases of humans: dynamics and control.* Oxford: Oxford University Press; 1991.
2. Castillo-Chávez C. *Mathematical approaches for emerging and reemerging infectious diseases: an introduction.* New York: Springer; 2002.
3. Diekmann O, Heesterbeek JAP. *Mathematical epidemiology of infectious diseases: model building, analysis, and interpretation.* New York: Wiley; 2000.
4. Keeling MJ, Rohani P. *Modeling infectious diseases in humans and animals.* Princeton, NJ: Princeton University Press; 2008.
5. Allen AO. *Probability, statistics, and queueing theory: with computer science applications.* 2nd ed. Boston: Academic Press: Harcourt Brace Jovanovich; 1990.
6. Kendall DG. Stochastic processes occurring in the theory of queues and their analysis by the method of the imbedded Markov chain. *The Annals of Mathematical Statistics.* 1953;24(3):338–354.
7. Shortle JF, Thompson JM, Gross D, Harris CM. *Fundamentals of queueing theory.* 5th ed. Hoboken, NJ: Wiley; 2018.
8. Neimark ED, Estes WK. *Stimulus sampling theory.* San Francisco, CA: Holden-Day; 1967.
9. Wearing HJ, Rohani P, Keeling MJ. Appropriate models for the management of infectious diseases. *PLoS Medicine.* 2005;2(7):e174.
10. Hethcote H, Zhien M, Shengbing L. Effects of quarantine in six endemic models for infectious diseases. *Mathematical Biosciences.* 2002;180:141–160.
11. Hethcote HW, van den Driessche P. Two SIS epidemiologic models with delays. *Journal of Mathematical Biology.* 2000;40(1):3–26.

12. Gao LQ, Mena-Lorca J, Hethcote HW. Four SEI endemic models with periodicity and separatrices. *Mathematical Biosciences.* 1995;128(1-2):157–184.

13. Gao LQ, Hethcote HW. Disease transmission models with density-dependent demographics. *Journal of Mathematical Biology.* 1992;30(7):717–731.

14. Xu S, Wei X, Zhang F. A time-delayed mathematical model for tumor growth with the effect of a periodic therapy. *Computational and Mathematical Methods in Medicine.* 2016;2016:3643019.

15. Magni P, Simeoni M, Poggesi I, Rocchetti M, De Nicolao G. A mathematical model to study the effects of drugs administration on tumor growth dynamics. *Mathematical Biosciences.* 2006;200(2):127–151.

16. Ottensen JT, Olufsen MS, Larsen JK. *Applied mathematical models in human physiology.* Philadelphia: Society for Industrial and Applied Mathematics; 2006.

17. Ederer M, Steinsiek S, Stagge S, et al. A mathematical model of metabolism and regulation provides a systems-level view of how Escherichia coli responds to oxygen. *Frontiers in Microbiology.* 2014;5:124.

18. Hoppensteadt FC, Peskin CS. *Mathematics in medicine and the life sciences.* Vol. 10. New York: Springer Verlag; 1992.

19. Skrepnek GH. Regression methods in the empiric analysis of health care data. *Journal of Managed Care Pharmacy.* 2005;11(3):240–251.

20. Stanley TD, Doucouliagos H. *Meta-regression analysis in economics and business.* New York: Routledge; 2012.

21. Rodgers JL. The epistemology of mathematical and statistical modeling: a quiet methodological revolution.*American Psychologist.* 2010;65(1):1–12.

22. Nguyen PH, Scott S, Neupane S, Tran LM, Menon P. Social, biological, and programmatic factors linking adolescent pregnancy and early childhood undernutrition: a path analysis of India's 2016 National Family and Health Survey. *The Lancet: Child & Adolescent Health.* 2019;3(7):463–473.

23. Moore S, Carpiano RM. Measures of personal social capital over time: A path analysis assessing longitudinal associations among cognitive, structural, and network elements of social capital in women and men separately. *Social Science & Medicine.* 2019. doi:10.1016/j.socscimed.2019.02.023. [Epub ahead of print]

24. Wang F, Xiong X, Xu H, et al. The association between obstructive sleep apnea syndrome and metabolic syndrome: a confirmatory factor analysis. *Sleep & Breathing.* 2019;23(3):1011–1019.

25. Brandon KO, Simmons VN, Meltzer LR, et al. Vaping characteristics and expectancies are associated with smoking cessation propensity among dual users of combustible and electronic cigarettes. *Addiction.* 2019;114(5):896–906.

26. Malec JF, Ketchum JM, Hammond FM, et al. Longitudinal effects of medical comorbidities on functional outcome and life satisfaction after traumatic brain injury: An individual growth curve analysis of NIDILRR traumatic brain injury model system data. *Journal of Head Trauma Rehabilitation.* 2019;34(5):E24–E35.

27. Austin AE, Desrosiers TA, Shanahan ME. Directed acyclic graphs: An underutilized tool for child maltreatment research. *Child Abuse & Neglect.* 2019;91:78–87.

28. Gold MR. *Cost-effectiveness in health and medicine.* New York: Oxford University Press; 1996.

29. Neumann PJ, Sanders GD, Russell LB, Siegel JE, Ganiats TG. *Cost effectiveness in health and medicine.* 2nd ed. New York: Oxford University Press; 2017.

30. Siedhoff MT, Rutstein SE, Wheeler SB, et al. Cost-effectiveness of laparoscopic hysterectomy with morcellation compared to abdominal hysterectomy for presumed benign leiomyomata. *Journal of Minimally INVASIVE gynecology*. 2015;22(6S):S78.

31. Gagniuc PA. *Markov chains: From theory to implementation and experimentation*. Hoboken, NJ: Wiley; 2017.

32. Ford N, Ball A, Baggaley R, et al. The WHO public health approach to HIV treatment and care: looking back and looking ahead. *The Lancet: Infectious Diseases*. 2018;18(3):e76–e86.

33. Chancellor JV, Hill AM, Sabin CA, Simpson KN, Youle M. Modeling the cost effectiveness of lamivudine/zidovudine combination therapy in HIV infection. *PharmacoEconomics*. 1997;12(1):54–66.

34. Liu N, Stone PW, Schnall R. Impact of mandatory HIV screening in the Emergency Department: A queuing study. *Res Nurs Health*. 2016;39(2):121–127.

35. Tachfouti N. Application of the queuing analytic theory in emergency department. *Arch Trauma Res*. 2014;3(2):e10526.

36. Lodree EJ, Altay N, Cook RA. Staff assignment policies for a mass casualty event queuing network. *Annals of Operations Research*. 2019;283(1), 411–442.

37. La EM, Lich KH, Wells R, et al. Increasing access to state psychiatric hospital beds: Exploring supply-side solutions. *Psychiatric Services*. 2016;67(5):523–528.

38. Crown W, Buyukkaramikli N, Sir MY, et al. Application of constrained optimization methods in health services research: Report 2 of the ISPOR Optimization Methods Emerging Good Practices Task Force. *Value Health*. 2018;21(9):1019–1028.

39. Crown W, Buyukkaramikli N, Thokala P, et al. Constrained optimization methods in health services research—An introduction: Report 1 of the ISPOR Optimization Methods Emerging Good Practices Task Force. *Value Health*. 2017;20(3):310–319.

12

Computational Simulation Modeling in Population Health Research and Policy

NATHANIEL OSGOOD

12.1. DYNAMIC MODELING

Inspired by policy resistance in and difficulties in understanding diverse complex health challenges, the growing "Complexity Science" or "Systems Science" movement in the health sciences seeks to confront the challenges of complexity head on. Dynamic (simulation) models constitute a central tool in the arsenal of this "science of the whole." Such models go by many designations—simulation models, dynamic models, mechanistic models, mathematical models, "models of the physics of the system," etc., and names specific to various simulation traditions. While this chapter highlights several such particular traditions, it is to be emphasized that *these traditions have more similarities than differences*. Most notably, they share certain characteristics to help investigators reason consistently about the implications of hypotheses concerning "how things work" within a system, with many modelers taking a generative perspective[1] that we do not truly understand a phenomenon until we can generate it out of (until it *emerges from*) a mechanistic (causal) explanation that does not presuppose it.

Modelers exhibit a diversity of viewpoints on the role of models; the particular perspective that we adopt here views these models as operationally expressing dynamic hypotheses—precise theories regarding "what's going on" in a system in terms of the underlying processes. In so doing, the model posits a causal structure hypothesized to underlie observed patterns. To use terms familiar to readers acquainted with the important cognate philosophy of Critical Realism,[2] we are seeking to understand here the *generative mechanisms* underlying the system. In this enterprise, we often seek to have a means of representing a hypothesis

Nathaniel Osgood, *Computational Simulation Modeling in Population Health Research and Policy* In: *Complex Systems and Population Health*. Edited by: Yorghos Apostolopoulos, Kristen Hassmiller Lich, and Michael Kenneth Lemke, Oxford University Press (2020). © Oxford University Press. DOI: 10.1093/oso/9780190880743.003.0012 concerning the causal structure of a system—not out of a desire to privilege that hypothesis, but because this representation allows us to secure understanding and critique from others, to more quickly test the consistency of our working hypothesis with what is observed from the system and reason consistently and rigorously about what that hypothesis would imply about the tradeoffs obtaining between policies or interventions. To enable the latter two benefits, modelers characterize such dynamic hypotheses in an operational manner—sufficiently precisely to use a computer to understand the behavior over time that is logically entailed by each hypothesis. By allowing us to characterize the hypothesized structure of the underlying system, to test it against empirical data, and to then investigate the consequences of counterfactuals in light of that hypothesized structure, dynamic modeling allow us to understand and investigate system vulnerabilities and leverage points—areas where a given investment will have little to no impact versus areas where it could secure great improvements in cost-effectiveness, cost, health outcomes, etc. Such methods can further clue us into ways of changing system structure and improving ways for stakeholders in different areas of the system to work together.

There are many distinct frameworks for specifying simulation models capturing such dynamic hypotheses; below, we review three—system dynamics (SD), agent-based modeling (ABM), and discrete event simulation (DES). These frameworks differ not only in terms of the formalisms they use—the particulars of how modelers specify the structure and rules they hypothesize to govern the processes depicted in the model—but often also in the goals of modeling.

Regardless of the particular system science modeling framework employed, by representing dynamic hypotheses, we benefit by taking our understanding of that posited set of causal relationships out of our head and placing it in a public sphere, where it can be understood, scrutinized, critiqued, and refined by others. By so doing, the resulting model will often integrate together a wide variety of knowledge and data concerning the system being characterized. While possession of the models that emerge from this process often confers great utility, the *modeling process itself* also offers great benefit by bringing together many stakeholders for ongoing reflection on their understanding regarding the underlying system, related sources of evidence, and the linkages between their contributions.

Across modeling traditions, dynamic models focus on precisely specifying hypotheses as to how the *system state (i.e., the current situation of that system) will evolve over time*. Regardless of tradition, when a modeler precisely specifies assumptions about the model in terms of causal relationships, the dynamic hypotheses specified are generally couched in a way that indicates how, *given the current situation of the system (i.e., the current state of the system), the state of that system changes*. The specific details of how the different modeling approaches characterize this will differ: For example, in SD, one specifies rates of change in the form of the values of the flows; for ABM—which routinely includes stochastics—often one will specify the hazard rates of transitioning from one state to the other, or the residence time in that state, or conditions under which the transition will be transited. DES models specify resource dependencies for distributions over the time required to undertake certain tasks.

As a result of the previous specifications, we ask the software to run these models, and we see behavior that emerges from them that is emergent and often surprising, in that it cannot be reduced to any one piece of the system (as represented by the model), but rather it results from the interaction for broad set of factors tangled in the model in a way that broadly reflects their entangling in the real world.

We are dealing here with the sphere of human activity and understanding. While models are tools that help us learn more quickly and advance that understanding, as with other ways in which might characterize hypotheses—for example, in prose—they are subject to shortcomings and misunderstandings. Inasmuch as they are depicting features of the world, we can analogize models to maps. This analogy is more than a superficial one—models, like maps, represent abstractions of features in the world; they hide much detail, not as a shortcoming, but to make them useful and feasible to work with. So, it is with models—we omit detail so that we can reason with greater clarity about the system being characterized. With a simpler model, we can pursue a description of the system more quickly and we can speed learning by running that model much more quickly as well. A key related point is that, as with maps, it is a model's *purpose* that shapes what detail is omitted. Sterman[3] speaks about model purpose being used as a logical knife to excise away unnecessary complexity—which details we omit depends on what types of insights we seek from the model.

There is a widespread misconception that dynamic models represent a sort of crystal ball—an attempt to predict the world. Models are, in fact, much better viewed as *learning prostheses*[a]. A prosthesis is something that helps us be fully functional, despite some pronounced limitations. So, it is with simulation models— but unlike a crutch or cane, models are designed to address *cognitive* rather than *physical* limitations. Diverse studies have shown that even the most technically astute individuals have difficulties in reasoning through the consequences of event simple dynamic hypotheses.[4] Given how handicapped humans are in terms of consistently understanding the implications of even simple dynamic hypotheses, we use simulation models in a way similar to a prosthetic limb—to allow us to achieve full functionality despite our (cognitive) limitations.

When considering such processes, it is important to keep the attention on *modeling*, rather than a particular *model*, and to recognize that the success of modeling as an endeavor is not imperiled by inaccuracy in a given model. It is not that any given model is necessarily highly effective; rather, the process of modeling speeds us toward better understanding. Having *some* model in place allows us to think through the dynamic implications of possible hypothesis more consistently, quickly, and reliably than we can unassisted, thereby allowing us to more quickly spot inconsistencies between what that hypothesis suggests (as captured by model output) and what empirical evidence suggests. This process uses models not as a

a. https://healthmodeling.org/bundles/view/6330. Accessed September 1, 2019.

crystal ball, but as a tool to allow us to think more effectively and to spot more quickly our blind spots, oversimplifications, and misplaced assumptions—and thus as a means of learning more quickly, deeply, and robustly in a complex and uncertain world.

12.2. SYSTEM DYNAMICS MODELING

SD originated as a tradition in the 1950s, in Forrester's cybernetics contributions at MIT. While different in its origins, it has a cognate in the form of compartmental modeling—modeling using ordinary differential equations, a tradition whose health applications date back to the 1910s and 1920s with the pioneering of work of Ross[5] on malaria and that of Kermack and McKendrick[6] on person-to-person communicable diseases, respectively. Understanding from such compartmental modeling now plays a foundational role in infectious disease epidemiology, in concepts such as herd immunity, basic reproductive constants, and critical immunization thresholds.[7]

SD modeling draws on the same mathematical foundation as compartmental modeling but approaches system understanding from a distinctive perspective— one focusing on accumulation and feedback processes and which recognizes the importance of supporting changes to mental models using simple graphical depictions of models. The focus on feedback and accumulation reflects Forrester's cybernetics work and a personal commitment to broader application of such understanding, in what he termed "Industrial Dynamics." Drawing on his seminal contributions to digital computing, The 1960s witnessed Forrester's development means of concisely specifying and simulating SD models, and of a growing diversity of models of industrial and societal concerns.[8] The 1970s saw SD thrust into the public spotlight and weathering fierce criticism due to models highlighting the sustainability crisis,[9] as well as a flowering of contributions, notably including application of SD to a variety of health issues such as smoking[10] and heroin addiction,[11] and emergence of causal loop diagrams as a simple way to depict feedbacks governing a system. The 1980s led to Richmond's impactful vision of making SD models broadly accessible through graphical modeling software. While controversial at the time, model graphical depictions proved foundational for SD evolution. Recent decades have witnessed an explosion of applications of SD in health and diverse methodological advances.

SD is particularly notable among dynamic modeling traditions on account of several features. One lies in the value it places on model mapping. Figure 12.1 depicts a "causal loop diagram," which posits relationships between a set of different factors that, while not fully quantified, captures polarities and associations and supports some understanding of the entailed dynamic behavior. The immediate accessibility of such causal loop diagrams to a wide variety of stakeholders facilitates elicitation of stakeholder understanding.

A second distinctive feature of SD lies in its focus on feedbacks as a fundamental shaper of behavior and our ability to manage it. As Forrester exploited in his cybernetics innovations, feedbacks exert profound effect on system evolution.

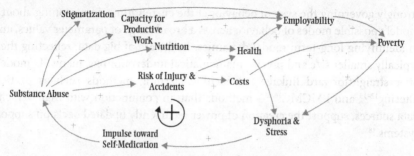

Figure 12.1 Example causal loop diagram used in system mapping for SD.

Reinforcing (positive) feedbacks tend to engender instability, while balancing (or negative) feedbacks can lead to great system stability. Taken in combination, feedbacks can lead to unexpected system behavior that—in the absence of understanding—can thwart our ability to manage the system. SD further focuses on *accumulations* as a critical cause for inertia, delay, and disequilibria and captures them through one of the key building blocks of SD models—stocks.

A third factor distinguishing the SD approach from other dynamic modeling traditions is its central focus on sharpening stakeholder mental models, so as to improve the quality and reliability of decision-making. This focus on shifting stakeholder's mental models has many ramifications, including a widespread commitment use of participatory processes and purposefully smaller models.

SD quantitative modeling characterizes systems in terms of stocks and flows. Stocks (depicted as rectangles) represent accumulations; flows drive the rates of change of such accumulations. Thus, for an aggregate SD model in the area of diabetes, for instance, we might have a stock associated with the count of people who suffer from diabetes without complications, another stock for diabetes with complications, and a flow between them representing development of complications amongst diabetics. Another flow *into* the stock of diabetes with diabetes without complications could represent those developing diabetes from a prediabetic state. The state of the system at any one time is completely specified by the value of the stocks. That state determines the value of flows; for example, the number of people with diabetes without complications (a stock) will naturally influence how many people develop complications—for example, if there is no-body with diabetes without complications, there will be no such complications developed. While the values of the stocks determine the rate of the flows over the next bit of time, the net value of the flows for a stock dictates the rate at which that stock changes over time. While SD models applied within health have tended to focus on high-level aggregate models, it bears emphasis that the method can be applied at many different levels of granularity, including in highly stratified models, and (separately) with stocks characterizing dynamics of associated continuous variables in particular system actors.

The unified mathematical basis underlying SD enables powerful model analysis—for example, in identifying what causal linkages or feedbacks are most strongly governing the system behavior at the current time, in reasoning about a model's possible modes of behavior across a broad range of parameter values, and in identifying long-term model dynamics. In the era of big data, reflecting their typically smaller size and precise mathematical underpinnings, many SD models offer straightforward linkage to machine learning methods such as particle filtering[12-15] and PMCMC[16,17]—methods that, in conjunction with high-velocity data sources, support the creation of power recurrently updated decision support systems.[18]

12.3. AGENT-BASED MODELING

Like SD, ABM is a tradition dating back to the mid-20th century, with the foundational cellular automata contributions of von Neumann and Ulam in the 1940s. Following these contributions, and partly reflecting limitations in access to high-speed computers essential for nimble ABM, the methodology remained underexplored until contribution of seminal models in the 1970s. Economist Schelling introduced a model demonstrating emergence of spatial patterns disconcertingly reminiscent of segregated neighborhoods from extremely simple rules positing that individuals hold even slight preferences for living near people like them. Gardner's *Scientific American* column highlighting Conway's Game of Life spurred popular imagination and launched countless hours of exploratory simulation worldwide.[19] Axelrod used ABMs to investigate the performance of different strategies involving multiple rounds of engagement in the so-called prisoner's dilemma.[20] Los Alamos National Labs performed pioneering work, with the 1980s witnessing the emergence of the nearby Santa Fe Institute and computational management organizational theory as an interdisciplinary field. The 1990s saw the emergence of ABM platforms such as StarLogo, SWARM, Repast, and even specialized hardware support for cellular automata.[21] The 2000s witnessed an explosion in the level and diversity of work, including in health[22]—a trend that has continued thereafter.

ABMs depict one or more populations of individual agents. In health models, agents most commonly represent people, but sometimes other types of actors (e.g., community organizations, service dogs). Each population is composed of individual agents of a given type, each of whom is endowed with a set of characteristics according to a simplified "theory of agenthood" captured by the model for that type of agent. Parameters are properties considered constant within the scope of this model—for example, an agent's ethnicity, self-identified gender, and income. Running the simulation creates a set of particular people, each associated with a specific value for each such parameter—here, each person would have a particular ethnicity, gender, and income. Beyond parameters, agents are typically endowed with an evolving state, which can have multiple—continuous, discrete, or relational—components. Agents are further endowed with actions evolving that state, and rules dictating situations under which such actions apply. A popular way of capturing an aspect of state and the rules and actions governing its evolution is with UML statecharts (see Figure 12.2),[23] which depict possible categorical

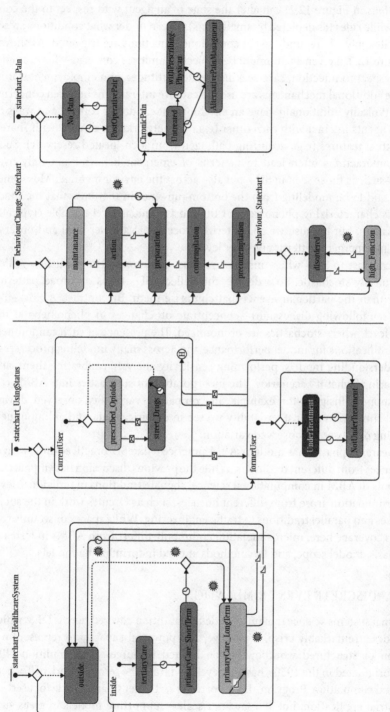

Figure 12.2 ABM statecharts.

states of an agent with respect to a particular concern. Actions (associated with *transitions* in Figure 12.2) can alter the state of an agent with respect to the concern, while rules (as depicted by small icons) govern under what conditions an action will apply—here, under what conditions transitions are triggered. As shown in Figure 12.2, a given agent might be subject to multiple concerns—for example, with respect to infection, care-seeking–related attitudes, and employment status. Simple additional mechanisms are used to capture interactions between concerns. ABM typically additionally have an environment capturing context and ways in which agents interact with each other (e.g., via networks) or directly with shared contextual features (e.g., acquiring pathogen from a co-located reservoir). Such agent interactions often lead to patterns of emergent behavior not only over time—such as those seen in SD—but also across the environment. ABM is sometimes said to be modeling from the bottom–up—not in the sense that the modeling is characterizing phenomena at the most granular level possible (typically impossible), but because we characterize processes at a lower level and observe resulting emergent patterns at higher levels.

In contrast to SD—where models are most commonly deterministic—ABMs are typically stochastic. To a degree, this reflects SD's focus on broad patterns, rather than the particular events that comprise them. By contrast, ABMs—like DES (see following discussion)—concentrate on changes to phenomena at the event level, where stochastics are pronounced. The presence of such randomness has ramifications for model performance and across many modeling processes—in understanding models, performing sensitivity analysis, calibrating them, and comparing "what if" scenarios. The incorporation of stochastics into ABMs can also support insight—for example, in comparing variability observed during model simulation against variability we see in empirical data and aiding understanding of causes for observed variation.

It bears emphasis that modern ABM practice—like SD practice—interweaves influences from different traditions. While the previous discussion has emphasized the roots of ABM in computational science, cognate traditions of individual-level microsimulation arose from different lineages, such as Orcutt's work in the social sciences and parallel traditions in traffic engineering. While space constraints rule out its coverage here, microsimulation commonly differs from ABMs in terms of emphasis, model scope, and the methods applied in formulating models.

12.4. DISCRETE EVENT SIMULATION

The final systems science dynamic modeling tradition covered here is DES, which provides a remarkably crisp, expressive, and powerful capacity to represent operation of structured workflows given limited resources. This tradition—like SD—originated in the 1950s, having developed from the seminal work of Tocher's General Simulation Program. Like Forrester's, Tocher's early work focused on industrial application, but at a far finer scale—supporting models in areas such as industrial scheduling and job planning that highlighted the role of individual events and workflows rather than the patterns, feedbacks, and accumulations that serve as the focus in SD. The 1960s witnessed a proliferation of applied DES simulation work, including initial health applications, as well as early work on higher-level computer languages to specify DES models. In the 1970s, Conway, Johnson, and Maxwell put into place a richer foundational theory of DES, and the field witnessed a strong expansion in health and other applications, with a 1978 review already highlighting 92 healthcare applications of DES.

DES remains a central contributor of applications of system science to health; such applications are notable for emphasis on *healthcare*—particularly subfields such as health service delivery—rather than across the broader spectrum of health subfields addressed by SD and ABM. This concentration reflects DES's focus on systems amenable to characterization in terms of a structured workflow—that is, where entities (e.g., patients, vials of vaccine, etc.) flow through a defined set of tasks, being operated upon by successive processes whose operation is often contingent on resource availability (Figure 12.3). There is typically a capacity imposed on resource pools, reflecting the fact that only a certain amount that resource can be in use at any one time. Commonly, entities can only proceed through a task—say, a patient can only undergo a computed tomography scan—if the appropriate resource (here, a computer tomography scanner) is available for use. If a resource is not available for use, the entity awaits that resource in a queue. The interest in DES projects often lies in studying the impact of resourcing levels, coordination, or placement on system performance measures—for example, the length of waiting times or queues, system throughput (e.g., patients per day served), and other (often domain-specific) quality of service measures. It is further notable that this field—like the previously described microsimulation—tends to draw heavily on the tradition of statistical grounding of models. This sort of modeling is often applied in facilities that admit to a detailed representation of room layout and where resource placement may have a significant impact on factors such as movement times. DES modelers in health are generally interested in a more fine-grained understanding of dynamics than is typical in SD health models—dynamics such as that associated with the length of waiting queues, the distribution of time patients spend traversing certain processes, or utilization rates for or waiting time to make use of particular resources. As these descriptions suggest, DES modelers also tend to be more focused on resource constraints, limits, structured workflows, and associated process indicators than are typically considered in ABM. While both DES and ABM admit to individual level representation, a particular difference from ABM in this area lies in the character of the flow of entities through the system: While ABM traditionally focuses much attention on active interactions by agent, DES entities are typically somewhat passive, being operated upon by the workflow, and with agent–agent interaction typically limited to keeping each other waiting for resources. Conversely, ABMs often do not provide the rich characterization of resource dependencies lying at the heart of DES.

DES's focus on lower-level workflows familiar to system stakeholders' aids in their engagement in mapping system processes based on their experience. By contrast, stakeholders immersed in work with individuals and resources can

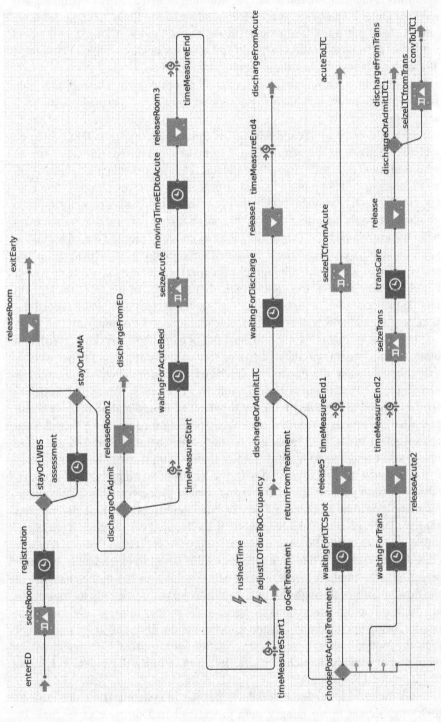

Figure 12.3 Example of DES workflow.

find disorienting the higher level of abstraction associated with an aggregate SD model. DES is more reliably articulated in a visually parseable way than is traditionally the case in ABM. The capacity to show both a model workflow and simulation results to stakeholders to elicit their understanding and critique supports models as learning tools and is of great value in building stakeholder confidence, buy-in, and ownership in a model.

12.5. CHOICE OF MODELING METHOD

In closing, we offer some basic comments regarding the relationships between the methods discussed in this chapter. When considering the place of different dynamic modeling traditions, three points bear emphasis. First, these methodologies are less in competition than they are complementary: Each brings unique strengths and focuses on different questions. A given projects can therefore often use multiple methods to great effect. Despite claims to the contrary—coming almost exclusively from those with practical experience largely confined to a single modeling tradition—no one systems science methodology offers a replacement for the others. Second, within a growing number of software platforms, multiple approaches can be interwoven within a given model in a fashion playing to the comparative advantages of each approach. For example, the rise in the computational power offered by affordable computing resources makes feasible flexible, performant and insightful models incorporating phenomena at multiple scales using mixtures of different dynamic modeling methods.[24-26] Third, the learning that takes place in modeling projects (e.g., via sensitivity analysis and stakeholder engagement) typically informs improved understanding of modeling needs. Using hybrid models throughout this process can allow the boundary between methods to evolve over time, based on such learning, stakeholder preferences, and resource availability.[18]

As previously noted, while all three methods serve as close cousins of one another, there are features that recommend each to certain types of modeling problems or subproblems and certain areas within a hybrid model. As the author has argued elsewhere,[27] the most salient distinctions in this area lie not between the methods per se, but between individual-level (IBMs) and aggregate-level representations, regardless of formalism in which they are characterized. It is to be emphasized that while aggregate modeling is strongly associated with SD and cognates, IBMs are well-supported not only in cognate traditions such as ABM and microsimulation modeling, but also the distinctive DES approach.

Due to the need to both simulate large number of agents per realization and to run many such realizations, IBMs suffer from substantial computational cost; by contrast, the simulation time of aggregate models is invariant with population size. However, such scaling advantages are reversed for heterogeneity: Within SD aggregate models, capturing heterogeneity along multiple dimensions (e.g., age, sex, region) entails model stratification—introduction of a subscript for each such dimension—and an overall model size grows geometrically with the count of heterogeneity dimensions. In addition, continuous dimensions must be quantized (e.g., age divided into age categories). The result is a model that often is conceptually simple but of a marked size and detail complexity. By contrast, within an IBM, additional heterogeneity dimensions—both continuous and discrete—are readily accommodated as parameters of a given agent, with no such combinatorial explosion.

Another key advantage of IBMs with broad ramifications relates to their ability to capture individual-level trajectories—and thus parameterize, compare, and calibrate against individual level longitudinal statistics. The ability for individual-based models to capture individual context (in a network or spatial/geographic space) is also of formidable importance for many models, including in terms of representing situated decision-making. Moreover, for models that contain multiple levels of context—for example, children nested within schools, within regions—an individual-based model will often mirror such nesting, with each individual agent being nested inside an agent characterizing school, nested, in turn, in its associated region; an aggregate SD model offers no similarly natural nesting or structure. While it is accompanied by substantial computational costs, IBM's representation of stochastics can also support comparison against statistical variability in the world.

The deeper issue here, however, concerns model purpose: Models across different traditions often seek to investigate different types of questions or address different types of problems. As a result, the problem framing is different, and the focus of analysis is different. For example, SD has traditionally tended to focus on higher-level dynamic patterns, is traditionally focused more fundamentally on bringing stakeholders together in a way that shifts their mental models and broadening narrow understanding. As such, it has tended to focus on simpler, higher-level models whose depiction is readily accessible to stakeholders. It is critical that comparisons between modeling approaches consider the different model goals that typically motivate them.

REFERENCES

1. Epstein JM. *Generative Social Science: Studies in Agent-Based Computational Modeling.* Princeton University Press; 2006.
2. Pawson R, Tilley N, Tilley N. *Realistic Evaluation.* SAGE; 1997.
3. Sterman JD, et al. A skeptic's guide to computer models. In: Barney GO, Kreutzer WB, Garrett MJ, eds., *Managing a Nation: The Microcomputer Software Catalog,* 2nd ed. Boulder, CO: Westview; 1991:209–229.
4. Sterman JD. Modeling managerial behavior: Misperceptions of feedback in a dynamic decision making experiment. *Manage Sci.* 1989;35(3):321–339.
5. Ross R. An application of the theory of probabilities to the study of a priori pathometry. Part I. *Proc R Soc A Math Phys Eng Sci.* 1916. doi:10.1098/rspa.1916.0007
6. Kermack WO, McKendrick AG. A contribution to the mathematical theory of epidemics. *Proc R Soc A Math Phys Eng Sci.* 1927;115(772). doi:10.1098/rspa.1927.0118

7. Anderson RM, Anderson B, May RM. *Infectious Diseases of Humans: Dynamics and Control*. Oxford University Press; 1991.

8. Forrester JW. Urban dynamics. *Manag Rev*. 1970;11(3):67.

9. Behrens W, Meadows DH, Meadows DL, Randers J. *The Limits to Growth*. Universe Books; 1972.

10. Roberts EB, Homer J, Kasabian A, Varrell M. A systems view of the smoking problem: Perspective and limitations of the role of science in decision-making. *Int J Biomed Comput*. 1982;13(1):69–86.

11. Levin G, Roberts EB, Hirsch GB. *The Persistent Poppy: A Computer-Aided Search for Heroin Policy*. Ballinger; 1975.

12. Safarishahrbijari A, Osgood ND. Social media surveillance for outbreak projection via transmission models: Longitudinal observational study. *JMIR Public Heal Surveill*. 2019;5(2):e11615.

13. Safarishahrbijari A, Teyhouee A, Waldner C, Liu J, Osgood ND. Predictive accuracy of particle filtering in dynamic models supporting outbreak projections. *BMC Infect Dis*. 2017;17(1):648. doi:10.1186/s12879-017-2726-9

14. Li X, Doroshenko A, Osgood ND. Applying particle filtering in both aggregated and age-structured population compartmental models of pre-vaccination measles. *PLoS One*. 2018;13(11):e0206529.

15. Ong JBS, Mark I, Chen C, et al. Real-time epidemic monitoring and forecasting of H1N1-2009 using influenza-like illness from general practice and family doctor clinics in Singapore. *PLoS One*. 2010;5(4):e10036.

16. Andrieu C, Doucet A, Holenstein R. Particle Markov chain Monte Carlo methods. *J R Stat Soc Ser B* 2010;72(3):269–342.

17. Li X, Keeler B, Zahan R, et al. *Illuminating the hidden elements and future evolution of opioid abuse using dynamic modeling, big data and particle Markov chain Monte Carlo*. International Conference on Social Computing, Behavioral-Cultural Modeling, & Prediction and Behavior Representation in Modeling and Simulation, Washington DC; 2018.

18. Osgood N. Frontiers in health modeling. *Syst Sci Popul Heal*. 2017;191:191–215.

19. Gardener M. Mathematical games: The fantastic combinations of John Conway's new solitaire game "life." *Sci Am*. 1970;223:120–123.

20. Axelrod R, Hamilton WD. The evolution of cooperation. *Science* (80-). 1981;211(4489):1390–1396.

21. Toffoli T, Margolus N. Programmable matter: concepts and realization. *Phys D, Nonlinear Phenom*. 1991;47(1–2):263–272.

22. Axtell R, Durlauf S, Epstein JM, et al. Social influences and smoking behavior: Final report to the American Legacy Foundation. Brookings Institution. https://www.brookings.edu/wp-content/uploads/2016/06/02dynamics_social.pdf. Published 2006.

23. Fowler M, Scott K. *UML Distilled: A Brief Guide to the Standard Object Modeling Language*. Addison-Wesley Professional; 2004.

24. Freebairn L, Atkinson J-A, Osgood ND, Kelly PM, McDonnell G, Rychetnik L. Turning conceptual systems maps into dynamic simulation models: An Australian case study for diabetes in pregnancy. *PLoS One*. 2019;14(6):e0218875.

25. Qin Y, Freebairn L, Atkinson J-A, Qian W, Safarishahrbijari A, Osgood ND. Multiscale simulation modeling for prevention and public health management of diabetes

in pregnancy and sequelae. In: *International Conference on Social Computing, Behavioral-Cultural Modeling and Prediction and Behavior Representation in Modeling and Simulation*. Springer; 2019:256–265.

26. Vickers DM, Osgood ND. The arrested immunity hypothesis in an immunoepidemiological model of Chlamydia transmission. *Theor Popul Biol*. 2014;93:52–62.

27. Osgood N. Using traditional and agent based toolsets for system dynamics: present tradeoffs and future evolution. In: *Proceedings from The 25th International Conference of the System Dynamics Society*; July 2007, Boston. 19pp.

13

System Dynamics Modeling to Rethink Health System Reform

JACK HOMER, BOBBY MILSTEIN, AND GARY B. HIRSCH

13.1. INTRODUCTION

The US health system has repeatedly resisted attempts at improvement. Compared with other high-income countries, US health spending per capita—and as a percentage of gross domestic product—remains much higher than the average (and the highest in the world),[1] while the rate of preventable mortality is worse.[2] A large fraction of Americans are still uninsured or underinsured.[3] Obesity keeps rising.[4] Physicians continue to overprescribe antibiotics, despite the knowledge that antibiotic resistance is a major threat.[5] Long-standing racial, ethnic, and geographical disparities in healthcare quality and life expectancy persist.[6,7] These problems continue unabated, despite the fact they have been around for decades and that plentiful recommendations and investments have been made to reverse them.[8]

Such policy resistance is the hallmark of a dynamically complex system involving the interplay of feedback loops, time delays, resource constraints, and conflicting goals. System dynamics modeling is a qualitative and quantitative approach designed to improve policymaking in systems with these complexities.[9–12]

The Rippel Foundation supported development of the Rethink Health Dynamics Model (hereafter, Rethink Health model). This system dynamics model focuses on health reform within any designated region of the United States and is a descendant of the Centers for Disease Control and Prevention's (CDC) "HealthBound" model of national health reform.[13] It also incorporates elements from a model of the health economy that explains and reproduces 40-plus years of US historical trends.[14]

Jack Homer, Bobby Milstein, and Gary B. Hirsch, *System Dynamics Modeling to Rethink Health System Reform* In: *Complex Systems and Population Health*. Edited by: Yorghos Apostolopoulos, Kristen Hassmiller Lich, and Michael Kenneth Lemke, Oxford University Press (2020). © Oxford University Press. DOI: 10.1093/oso/9780190880743.003.0013

We have previously described how the Rethink Health model can be used for policy analysis, learning, and helping local leaders in their collective endeavors.[15-17] But we have not shown how its dynamic structure can be used to diagnose and suggest solutions to various kinds of policy resistance. In this chapter, we go "under the hood" of the model to see how it can explain, in clear structural terms, why well-intended interventions sometimes fall short, as well as what more can be done to overcome those pitfalls and improve system performance.

13.2. AN OVERVIEW OF THE SIMULATION MODEL AND ITS COMPONENTS

Figure 13.1 presents an overview of the Rethink Health model's logical structure. Like other system dynamics models, this model represents stocks, flows, nonlinearities, and feedback loops through interlocked differential and algebraic equations and is run deterministically under various possible scenarios and interventions, including tests of its sensitivity to numerical or structural assumptions. The model starts in 2000 and runs to 2040 with a time step of one-quarter year. The simulated population is divided into subgroups differentiated by age (youth, working age, seniors), income status (advantaged or disadvantaged, based on household income above or below 200% of the US federal poverty level), and health insurance status (yes or no).

A reference guide to the simulation model[18] presents its full code, which includes about 1,000 input parameters and 4,400 calculated output elements, as well as 27 data series for model validation at the US national level. These include data on subgroup population growth, births, deaths, migration, and hospital profits, as well as all seven major categories of personal healthcare costs in the Center

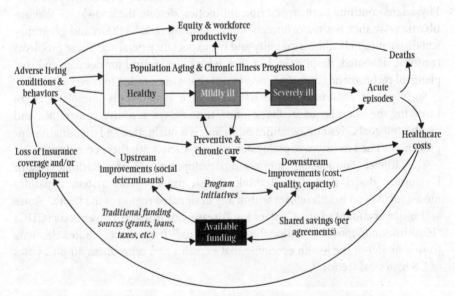

Figure 13.1 Basic logical structure of the Rethink Health Dynamics model.

for Medicare and Medicaid Services' National Health Expenditures Accounts. The model closely reproduces all of these data at the national level. Many other data sources and studies helped in building and calibrating the model, including information on behavioral risks, environmental risks, quality of care, health status, ambulatory visits, hospital stays, provider capacity and income, medical bankruptcies, underinsurance, economic productivity (as affected by physical and mental health status), and the costs of interventions named in the model.

The model has been calibrated to represent more than 10 specific regions of the country and examine their possible intervention strategies,[16] but for the analysis here we use the "Anytown" version of the model, which reflects the demographic and health system characteristics of the nation as a whole.[15,17,18]

As seen in Figure 13.1, the model's main logical flow runs (left to right) from health risks to illness, then to acute episodes, and then to healthcare costs and deaths. The model simulates changes in health states as they are shaped by risky behaviors, crime, environmental hazards, poverty, lack of insurance, aging, and the adequacy of preventive and chronic care. The health states include chronic physical illness (none, mild, severe) and chronic mental illness (no, yes). The acute episodes may be urgent or nonurgent. Health status and acute episodes, in turn, drive the demand for routine and episodic office visits, outpatient procedures and tests, hospital emergency department and inpatient stays, as well as postacute and extended care in skilled nursing facilities and through home health and hospice.

Figure 13.1 also shows two adverse feedback effects that can become significant under some scenarios. One (represented by a leftward arrow from the population box back to adverse living conditions) reflects the fact that, when working age people become severely ill or disabled, they may suffer a loss of income. This loss of income can affect an entire household by exposing family members to a higher risk of illness as a result of their reduced economic status. The second adverse effect involves the link from healthcare costs (following all the way downward to the left) to a possible loss of insurance coverage and/or employment. A household may thereby lose the ability to afford routine care or fall into economic disadvantage, both of which lead to greater risk of illness. At a societal level, these feedbacks lead to reduced health equity and economic productivity, as seen at the top of Figure 13.1.

The model contains more than 20 options for simulating interventions to improve healthcare ("downstream" initiatives), reduce health risks ("upstream" initiatives), or support continued financing of these program initiatives. The downstream initiatives include a variety of demonstrated approaches for reducing cost, improving quality, or improving primary care capacity. They typically involve direct initiative-specific funding to physicians and hospitals but may also be supplemented by broader changes in how providers are paid by insurers.[19-21]

The upstream initiatives include those that reduce environmental risks, lower crime, enable healthy behaviors, or lift people out of economic disadvantage. Multiple cost-effective interventions have been documented in each of these areas.[22-25]

The Rethink Health model allows for multiple ways in which downstream or upstream initiatives may be financed. These include typical means, such as grants, loans, taxes, tax credits, and bonds, as well as the newer mechanism of shared savings, where a health insurer agrees to return to a provider institution within the community (often a hospital or a provider network) a specified fraction of the reimbursed costs that institution has saved against a cost benchmark.[26] When the arrangement is broad, encompassing all key stakeholders in the community and most major insurers, it has been called an Accountable Community for Health.[27] The hope is that this sort of broad shared savings arrangement could facilitate substantial, sustainable improvements in population health.[28]

13.3. INTERVENTION PITFALLS IN THE MODEL—AND POSSIBLE CORRECTIONS

Testing the Rethink Health model's interventions, we find that the simulated improvement in system performance along one or more dimensions—healthcare cost, quality of care, population health, health equity, or workforce productivity— is often less than we had expected. By looking closely at model outputs and experimenting with combinations of interventions, we have been able to identify recurring reasons for underperformance that we call intervention pitfalls. In this section, we present four common pitfalls and discuss illustrative simulations with the aid of focused causal feedback diagrams and output graphs. We start in each case with a specific underperforming intervention strategy and then discuss one or more additional interventions that can offset the negatives and allow for improved performance. All interventions here are assumed to start in 2017, and results are compared to those of the model's baseline (or base) run.

13.3.1. Pitfall 1: Trying to Cut Costs without Changing Provider Incentives

Some of the model's downstream initiatives aim to reduce healthcare costs by keeping patients at the primary care level when appropriate, limiting the number of referrals to specialists who are more prone to do costly testing and procedures and to admit patients for elective inpatient stays. These initiatives include investments in coordination of care, pre-visit screening, or primary care "medical homes."

Figure 13.2 shows what happens in the model when one of these initiatives, expanded care coordination, is implemented. The diagram indicates that fewer referrals to specialists should lead to lower specialist income and, thus, to lower healthcare costs overall. And, indeed, this does happen to some extent. As seen in the right-hand graph, healthcare costs in the "Coord" run are 5% lower than those in the base run. (Costs are shown in this chapter in constant 2010 healthcare dollars, without price inflation; hence, "deflated.")

But this cost reduction is less than it could be. Specialists operating in a fee-for-service payment environment have the ability, and indeed have shown the tendency, to offset threats to their income by doing more income-generating tests and procedures or, sometimes, "upcoding" or "unbundling" billed charges to produce the same effect.[29] The result is a strong compensating feedback loop that has

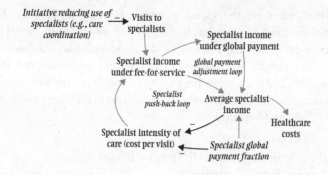

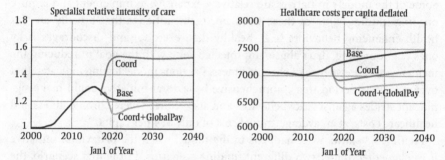

Figure 13.2 Care coordination intervention: specialist pushback corrected by global payment.

been described as "supply push" behavior,[30] shown in Figure 13.2 as the "specialist push-back" loop.

The result of the push-back loop may be seen in the left-hand graph of Figure 13.2, which shows specialist intensity of care relative to 2000. Even in the base run (absent care coordination), some push-back occurs, first in response to the economic recession of the late 2000s, and also because hospitals acquire more specialty group practices and facilities and insist on greater "production" from them. The relative intensity of care rises to 1.28 in the base run and then settles to 1.21 as the economy recovers. But in the "Coord" run, the relative intensity of care does not settle back but rather rises to 1.52—more than 25% above its base run value.

To counteract the push-back loop, the payment scheme for specialists can be changed, replacing fee-for-service with global (or capitated) payment, as well as value-based payment (based on meeting targets for cost-effective care). About 25% of specialists are already paid through a salary,[31] though many (if not most) of these specialists still receive bonuses for doing more, not less. However, insurers have expressed a desire to move away from conventional fee-for-service, and it seems likely they will be driving hospitals and specialists more toward global and value-based payment in the years to come.[21]

In the base run, we assume that the fraction of specialists receiving global payment reaches 15% by 2015 and increases no further. In the run labeled

"Coord+GlobalPay," we raise the global payment fraction to 80% by 2020. Specialist incomes continue to grow, but in a controlled way (see the "global payment adjustment" loop in the diagram; Figure 13.2), and with the push-back loop much diminished in strength. The relative intensity of care now settles at 1.18, far below the "Coord" run and even below the base run. Healthcare costs now decline further than under coordination alone: about 7% relative to the base run by 2020, and nearly 8% by 2030 and beyond.

13.3.2. Pitfall 2: Depleting Available Funds without Arranging for Longer-Term Financing

Some of the model's initiatives are relatively expensive to implement and require ongoing funding. One of these is an upstream initiative that broadly enables health-enhancing behaviors (e.g., healthy diet, exercise) and discourages risky ones (e.g., smoking, drug abuse, unprotected sex), with the goal of reducing the incidence and prevalence of chronic illness. Previous model testing indicated that over a 25-year period this comprehensive behavioral initiative could make significant strides against risky behaviors and also reduce severe chronic illness and healthcare costs, at an average annual cost of only $34 per capita.[15]

Figure 13.3 shows what happens in the model when the behavioral initiative is implemented under two different funding scenarios. In the first scenario, the initiative is financed by a five-year grant of $75 per capita per year, with any unused funds rolled over and available in subsequent years. The prevalence of risky behaviors is reduced by 17% relative to the base run during these first five years, leading to a 2% reduction in total healthcare costs. The reduction in high-risk behavior prevalence also reduces the cost of running the initiative, from $62 to $51 per capita per year; see the "reduce-the-need" loop in Figure 13.3.

But even with the somewhat reduced cost, the rolled over funds are insufficient to finance the initiative fully beyond the first five years, and the funds are virtually exhausted within a few more years; see the plunging Program Spending per Capita curve in Figure 13.3. Once the funds are exhausted and the initiative forced to discontinue, high risk behaviors start to rebound and by 2040 are only 6% below the base run. Consequently, healthcare costs also rebound and are only 1% below the base run by 2040.

In the second scenario, all insurers, both commercial and government, enter into a shared savings agreement that returns to the community half of any savings relative to established benchmarks for healthcare costs. These shared savings are enough to double the amount of funding available at the end of the five-year grant period and, with a steady inflow, allow the initiative to continue at full force through 2040; see the "reinvestment" loop in Figure 13.3. The prevalence of high-risk behaviors is reduced by 47% relative to the base run by 2040, and healthcare costs drop by more than 4%.

Why would a community pursue a purely grant-based initiative, like the one in the first scenario, knowing that the funding is insufficient for the long term? Health leaders are concerned about this problem, warning that the impacts of

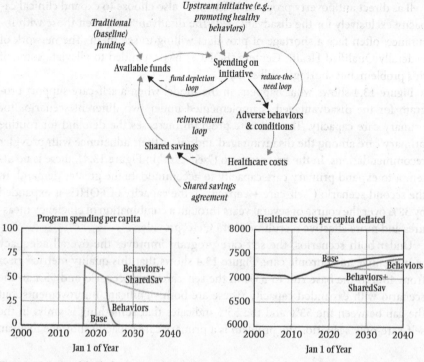

Figure 13.3 Healthy behaviors intervention: fund depletion corrected by shared savings reinvestment.

initiatives could be short-lived without sustainable financing.[32] Nonetheless, public health agencies continue to rely primarily on temporary grants for financing initiatives, perhaps hoping that the reduce-the-need loop in Figure 13.3 will be sufficiently strong to solve the problem before the fund depletion loop kicks in. But, in fact, persistent problems like high risk behaviors require persistent attention. History suggests that even when it is possible to largely eliminate one adverse behavior—for example, targeting a specific dangerous substance—there will always be other adverse behaviors available (e.g., other risky substances) to fuel a rebound. Thus, health agencies need to find sustainable sources of financing, such as shared savings, for initiatives that require a broad reach and long-term effort. [33]

13.3.3. Pitfall 3: Trying to Correct Health Inequities but Overloading Clinical Capacity

The model offers some initiatives aimed at helping economically disadvantaged people, who comprise about 33% of the US population, and who have significantly worse health than the advantaged do. The model offers the option to focus solely on the disadvantaged when selecting initiatives addressing self-care, mental health, health-related behaviors, crime, and environmental hazards (as well as direct antipoverty programs). One may also choose to expand clinical capacity exclusively for the disadvantaged. The disadvantaged, even those with insurance, often face a shortage of providers willing to see them. The network of Federally Qualified Health Centers (FQHCs) has expanded to alleviate some of this problem, but shortages still exist.[34,35]

Figure 13.4 shows what happens in the model when a self-care support program for the disadvantaged is implemented under two different scenarios for primary care capacity. The self-care program increases the demand for routine primary care among the disadvantaged and raises their adherence with provider recommendations. In the first scenario ("self-care" in Figure 13.4), there is no attempt to expand primary care capacity to accommodate the greater demand. In the second scenario ("self-care + capacity"), the capacity of FQHCs is expanded by 38% over the course of several years through a combination of efficiency measures and more effective recruitment of FQHC providers.

Under both scenarios, the self-care program improves the overall adequacy of preventive and chronic care. Figure 13.4 shows that this quality metric[36] rises from 48% in the base run to 53% in the self-care-only scenario and 55% in the scenario with expanded capacity. These are both significant improvements, but the gap between the 53% and the 55% indicates that something is amiss in the self-care-only scenario. The problem is a primary care capacity shortage that can

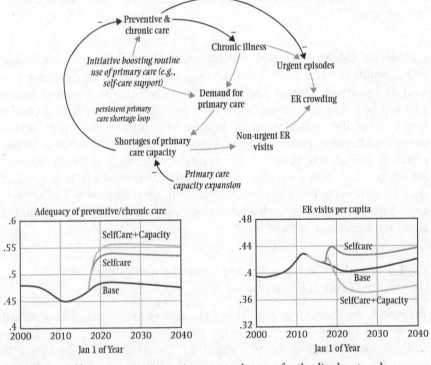

Figure 13.4 Self-care intervention: primary care shortage for the disadvantaged population corrected by boosting capacity.

undermine the provision of routine care and, in extreme cases, can result in a self-reinforcing loop of persistent primary care shortage, as seen in the diagram. Thus, without expansions of capacity, interventions to improve primary care quality for the disadvantaged may fall short of their potential. Because the disadvantaged population faces capacity shortages not faced by the advantaged, interventions to improve care quality for all could have the unintended effect of worsening health inequities.[37]

The problems of primary care capacity shortage, however, go beyond the fact that they limit improvements in healthcare quality for the disadvantaged. The second graph in Figure 13.4 shows that the emergency room (ER) visit rate (for the entire population) increases significantly relative to the base run under "self-care," while it decreases significantly under "self-care + capacity." This result is explained by the fact that a portion of ER visits are nonurgent or ambulatory sensitive, meaning that they could be handled by a primary care physician if one were available. If the shortage of primary care capacity becomes worse, as in the "self-care" scenario, nonurgent ER visits will go up. Conversely, to the extent the shortage is alleviated, as in the "self-care + capacity" scenario, nonurgent ER visits will go down.

Why is the increase in ER visits in the self-care-only scenario a concern? One might think the issue is greater healthcare costs, but in fact the two intervention scenarios end up costing about the same: "Self-care" has more ER visits, but "self-care + capacity" has more primary care visits with aggregate cost that is only slightly less. The real concern, rather, is the possibility of ER crowding, which can lead to hours of delays and reduced quality of care. ER crowding has been a problem in the United States for many years and is especially prevalent in more disadvantaged areas.[38,39]

In sum, trying to improve the quality of routine care for the disadvantaged, without also expanding their primary care capacity, can undermine health equity in two ways: First, it can effectively reduce their access to primary care, and second, it can worsen crowding in the ERs they use.

13.3.4. Pitfall 4: Failing to Address All Goals with a Balanced Mix of Interventions

We have discussed here three different initiatives that are likely to underperform without additional actions to compensate for their shortcomings. If the pitfalls are avoided, each of these three initiatives can achieve its *individual* potential: care coordination can quickly reduce healthcare costs, health-enhancing behaviors can improve health and gradually reduce healthcare costs, and self-care for the disadvantaged can improve health equity.

A fourth pitfall (one might say a meta-pitfall) is a failure to harness the full potential of combining these diverse initiatives to address multiple goals simultaneously. This ambition is reminiscent of the Triple Aim of better health, better care, and lower costs.[40] We have previously used the Rethink Health model to identify a comprehensive strategy with the potential to fulfill such a multipronged ambition.[15] That comprehensive strategy involved a large number of the interventions in the model.

Here we can demonstrate something similar with only six initiatives, combining the three previously presented pairs: care coordination plus global payment, health-enhancing behaviors plus shared savings, and self-care plus primary care capacity expansion for the disadvantaged. Figure 13.5 shows graphical results from each pair individually as well as the full combined scenario, compared with the base run.

The top-left graph (Figure 13.5) shows how the prevalence of severe chronic physical illness is reduced in the combined scenario in both the short term and the longer term. The moderate short-term contribution comes from the self-care (plus capacity) initiative, while a substantial longer-term contribution comes from the health-enhancing behaviors (plus shared savings) initiative.

The top-right graph (Figure 13.5) shows how health equity can be improved; the metric here is the fraction of the severely ill who are economically disadvantaged. The improvement in the combined scenario comes from the self-care and care coordination (plus global payment) initiatives starting in the short term, with some additional contribution in the longer term by the health-enhancing behaviors initiative.

The lower-right graph (Figure 13.5) shows how healthcare costs are improved in both the short term and the longer term in the combined scenario. Even though the self-care initiative raises healthcare costs by 1.5%, the combined scenario shows a net 6% reduction as of 2020, thanks mostly to care coordination

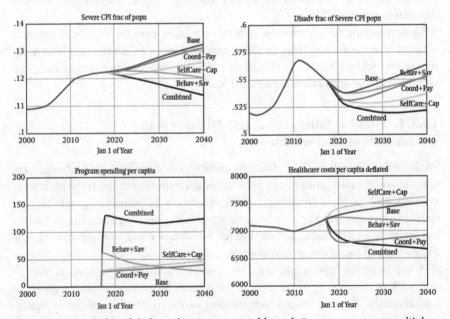

Figure 13.5 A combined, balanced strategy can yield steady improvements on multiple fronts and be affordable.

paired with global payment. By 2040, the combined scenario shows a net reduction of 12%, with about 70% of this still coming from care coordination and the other 30% coming from health-enhancing behaviors. These two interventions attack healthcare costs in two different, complementary ways: Care coordination makes care more cost-effective starting in the short term, while health-enhancing behaviors reduce illness and the need for care in the longer term.

The combined scenario could not achieve these successes unless it were affordable. As seen in the lower-left graph (Figure 13.5), the combined scenario costs an average of $120 per capita per year. The full package of initiatives is still funded by a grant of only $75 per year for first five years (as in Pitfall 2), and otherwise must rely on the reinvestment of shared savings. In the first year (2017), no shared savings have yet been generated, which means the initiatives (all six of them) can be funded at only about 65% of full strength. But even this somewhat restricted level of intervention activity in the first year is sufficient to generate significant cost savings, half of which are shared (per the shared-savings agreement) and reinvested. By the second year (2018) and beyond, these shared savings are sufficient to fully fund all of the initiatives through 2040 and beyond.

Although a significant investment is made in the combined scenario by both the community and the insurers involved in the shared-savings agreement, the purely financial return in terms of healthcare cost reductions (aside from the substantial health benefits) is impressive. The model calculates the cumulative return on investment (ROI) (discounted at 3% per year) from 2017 to 2040. The ROI on all investments (grants and shared savings) is 6.5 to 1, while the ROI on the kick-off grant funding alone is 10 times that: 65 to 1.

In sum, the combined scenario demonstrates that it is possible to achieve multiple goals for health system reform, in both the short term and the longer term, through a balanced combination of initiatives: some downstream and some upstream, some addressing the entire population while others focus on the disadvantaged. With a sustainable source of funding, such as shared savings, it becomes possible to pursue greater ambitions and avoid the pitfall of pursuing modest goals.

13.4. DISCUSSION

Here we have presented details of the Rethink Health Dynamics Model and have used it both to identify intervention pitfalls and to show how they might be overcome. We have also shown how, with a sustainable financing mechanism in place, one can combine diverse interventions to achieve improvements across multiple dimensions in the both the short and longer term.

Local health leaders who have used this model have experimented with a variety of intervention scenarios. They have also helped to create a list of general criteria to assess whether a strategy that seeks to reform a dynamically complex regional health system is sound and likely to yield the desired results. Several of those criteria have been demonstrated in this chapter, namely, that a sound intervention strategy should be ambitious, balanced, equitable, sustainable, and cost-effective. Other criteria include plausibility of the strategy, its consistency with a broad vision for regional transformation, and its ability to motivate and inspire commitment.

The systems approach described here is already more encompassing than most analyses of the US healthcare system. But we would like to extend it even further to consider place-based socioeconomics in greater depth, tying health to other sectors that affect population wellbeing. Building on previous work,[41] we are now developing a dynamic model that links health and safety to employment, housing, education, transportation, and the physical environment, as well as to civic involvement and discrimination.[42] We hope to make this model available to local leaders, as we have done with the existing model, to help them maximize the potential of their action strategies as stewards of a complex health system.

ACKNOWLEDGMENTS

Many thanks to the Rippel Foundation for financial support of the ReThink Health model since 2011, and to Rebecca Niles, Kristina Wile, Christina Ingersoll, and other colleagues at ReThink Health for their contributions to the ideas presented in this chapter.

REFERENCES

1. Sawyer B, Cox C. How does health spending in the U.S. compare to other countries? Peterson-Kaiser Health System Tracker. https://www.healthsystemtracker.org/chart-collection/health-spending-u-s-compare-countries. Published December 7, 2018. Accessed March 15, 2019.
2. Sawyer B, Gonzales S. How does the quality of the U.S. healthcare system compare to other countries? Peterson-Kaiser Health System Tracker. https://www.healthsystemtracker.org/chart-collection/quality-u-s-healthcare-system-compare-countries. Published May 22, 2017. Accessed March 15, 2019.
3. Collins SR, Rasmussen PW, Beutel S, Doty MM. The problem of underinsurance and how rising deductibles will make it worse: findings from the Commonwealth Fund Biennial Health Insurance Survey. Commonwealth Fund Pub. 1817, Vol. 13 (Issue Brief). https://www.commonwealthfund.org/sites/default/files/documents/___media_files_publications_issue_brief_2015_may_1817_collins_problem_of_underinsurance_ib.pdf. Published May 2015. Accessed March 15, 2019.
4. National Center for Health Statistics. *Health, United States, 2016: With Chartbook on Long-Term Trends in Health.* Hyattsville, MD: NCHS; 2017.
5. Centers for Disease Control and Prevention. *Antibiotic Use in the United States, 2017: Progress and Opportunities.* Atlanta, GA: CDC; 2017.
6. Institute of Medicine (Board on Health Sciences Policy). *Unequal Treatment: Confronting Racial and Ethnic Disparities in Health Care.* Washington, DC: National Academies Press; 2003.
7. Murray CJL, Kulkarni SC, Michaud C, Tomijima N, Bulzacchelli MT. Eight Americas: investigating mortality disparities across races, counties, and race-counties in the United States. *PLoS Med.* 2006;3(9):e260, 1513–1524.

8. Lee P, Paxman D. Reinventing public health. *Annu Rev Pub Health.* 1997;18:1–35.
9. Forrester JW. *Urban Dynamics.* Cambridge, MA: MIT Press; 1969.
10. Sterman JD. *Business Dynamics: Systems Thinking and Modeling for a Complex World.* Boston, MA: Irwin McGraw-Hill; 2000.
11. Homer J, Hirsch G. System dynamics modeling for public health: background and opportunities. *Am J Pub Health.* 2006;96(3):452–458.
12. Hirsch GB, Homer J. System dynamics applications to health care in the United States. In: Meyers RA, ed. *Encyclopedia of Complexity and Systems Science.* Berlin, Germany: Springer; 2016. doi:10.1007/978-3-642-27737-5_270-2
13. Milstein B, Homer J, Hirsch G. Analyzing national health reform strategies with a dynamic simulation model. *Am J Pub Health.* 2010;100(5):811–819.
14. Homer J, Hirsch G, Milstein B. Chronic illness in a complex health economy: the perils and promises of downstream and upstream reforms. *Sys Dynam Rev.* 2007;23(2–3):313–343.
15. Homer J, Milstein B, Hirsch GB, Fisher ES. Combined regional investments could substantially enhance health system performance and be financially affordable. *Health Aff.* 2016;35(8):1435–1443.
16. Milstein B, Hirsch G, Minyard K. County officials embark on new collective endeavors to ReThink their local health systems. *J County Admin.* March/April 2013; p. 1, 5–10.
17. McFarland L, Reineke E, Milstein B, Niles RD, Hirsch G, Cawvey E, Homer J, Desai A, Andersen D, MacDonald R, Irving R. The NASPAA student simulation competition: reforming the US health care system within a simulated environment. *J Pub Affairs Educ.* 2016;22(3):363–380.
18. Homer J. *Reference Guide for the ReThink Health Dynamics Simulation Model: A Tool for Regional Health System Transformation, Model Version 3v.* https://www.rethinkhealth.org/wp-content/uploads/2019/09/ReThink-Health-Dynamics-Reference-Guide-v3v-Nov-2018-1.pdf. Published June 2016. Accessed February 19, 2020.
19. Antos J, Baicker K, Chernew M, Crippen D, Cutler D, Daschle T and others. Bending the curve: person-centered health care reform—a framework for improving care and slowing health care cost growth. Washington, DC: Brookings Institution. http://www.brookings.edu/research/reports/2013/04/person-centered-health-care-reform. Published April 29, 2013. Accessed March 15, 2019.
20. Porter ME, Pabo EA, Lee TH. Redesigning primary care: a strategic vision to improve value by organizing around patients' needs. *Health Aff.* 2013;32(3):516–525.
21. Muhlestein D, Saunders RS, Richards R, McClellan MB. Recent progress in the value journey: growth of ACOs and value-based payment models in 2018. Health Affairs Blog. Bethesda, MD: Project HOPE. https://www.healthaffairs.org/do/10.1377/hblog20180810.481968/full Published August 14, 2018. Accessed March 15, 2019.
22. Truman BI, Smith-Akin CK, Hinman AR, et al.; Community Preventive Services Task Force. Developing the guide to community preventive services—Overview and Rationale. *Am J Prev Med.* 2000;18(1 Suppl):18–26.
23. Andrews NO, Erickson DJ, eds. *Investing in What Works for America's Communities: Essays on People, Place & Purpose.* San Francisco, CA: Federal Reserve Bank of San Francisco; 2012.

24. County Health Rankings and Roadmaps. What works for health? Madison, WI: University of Wisconsin Population Health Institute and Robert Wood Johnson Foundation. http://www.countyhealthrankings.org/take-action-to-improve-health/what-works-for-health Published 2018. Accessed March 15, 2019.

25. Center on Budget and Policy Priorities. What works to reduce poverty. Washington, DC: CBPP. http://www.cbpp.org/what-works-to-reduce-poverty. Multiple reports published 2013 to 2018. Accessed March 15, 2019.

26. Bailit M, Hughes C. Key design elements of shared-savings payment arrangements. New York, NY: Commonwealth Fund. https://www.commonwealthfund.org/publications/issue-briefs/2011/aug/key-design-elements-shared-savings-payment-arrangements. Published August 16, 2011. Accessed March 15, 2019.

27. Mongeon M, Levi J, Heinrich J. Elements of accountable communities for health: a review of the literature. Discussion paper. Washington, DC: National Academy of Medicine. https://nam.edu/elements-of-accountable-communities-for-health-a-review-of-the-literature. Published November 6, 2017. Accessed March 15, 2019.

28. Hester JA, Stange PV, Seeff LC, Davis JB, Craft CA. Toward sustainable improvements in population health: overview of community integration structures and emerging innovations in financing. CDC Health Policy Series, No. 2. Atlanta, GA: CDC. https://www.cdc.gov/policy/docs/financepaper.pdf. Published 2015. Accessed March 15, 2019.

29. Eckholm E and New York Times staff. Solving America's Health-Care Crisis. New York, NY: Times Books; 1993.

30. Wennberg JE. Tracking Medicine: A Researcher's Quest to Understand Health Care. New York, NY: Oxford University Press; 2010.

31. Rosenthal E. Apprehensive, many doctors shift to jobs with salaries. New York Times. A-14; February 14, 2014.

32. Institute of Medicine. For the Public's Health: Investing in a Healthier Future. Washington, DC: National Academies Press; 2012.

33. Alexander L, Becker S, Wright K, Farris-Berg K. Beyond the grant: A sustainable financing workbook. Morristown, NJ: Rippel Foundation. https://www.rethinkhealth.org/financingworkbook/ Published 2019. Accessed March 15, 2019.

34. National Association of Community Health Centers. Access Denied: A Look at America's Medically Disenfranchised. Washington, DC: NACHC; 2007.

35. Pear R. Shortage of doctors proves obstacle to Obama goals. New York Times. A-1; April 27, 2009.

36. Asch SM, Kerr EA, Keesey J, Adams JL, Setodji CM, and others. Who is at greatest risk for receiving poor-quality health care? N Engl J Med. 2006;354(11):1147–1156.

37. Mechanic D. Disadvantage, inequality, and social policy. Health Aff. 2002;21(2):48–59.

38. Institute of Medicine. Hospital-based Emergency Care: At the Breaking Point. Washington, DC: National Academies Press; 2006.

39. Barish RA, McGauly PL, Arnold TC. Emergency room crowding: a marker of hospital health. Trans Am Clin Climatol Assoc. 2012;123:304–310.

40. Whittington JW, Nolan K, Lewis N, Torres T. Pursuing the Triple Aim: The first 7 years. Milbank Q. 2015;93(2):263–300.

41. Mahamoud A, Roche B, Homer J. Modelling the social determinants of health and simulating short-term and long-term intervention impacts for the city of Toronto, Canada. *Soc Sci Med.* 2012;93:247–255. doi:10.1016/j.socscimed.2012.06.036.

42. Milstein B, Homer J. Which priorities for health and well-being stand out after accounting for tangled threats and costs? Simulating potential intervention portfolios in large urban counties. *Milbank Q* 2020. Early View available at: http://bit.ly/39kCGVB.

Agent-Based Modeling to Delineate Opioid and Other Drug Use Epidemics

GEORGIY V. BOBASHEV, LEE D. HOFFER,
AND FRANCOIS R. LAMY

14.1. BACKGROUND: MULTIPLICITY OF DRUG USE PROCESSES

14.1.1. Why Drug Epidemics Are Important?

A principal topic in population health involves understanding disease epidemics. While all epidemics present challenges to research, illicit drug-use epidemics present unique considerations. Waves of increased drug use recurrently happen in the United States, and many are routinely called epidemics. Examples include marijuana in the late 1960s and 1990s, heroin the early 1950s and 1970s, crack in the late 1980s, and the methamphetamine in late 2000s.[1,2] The latest opioid epidemic reached the level of a *National Public Health Emergency* in 2017. Drug epidemics have enormous costs that often persist years after the epidemic has declined. This is because they do not only affect individuals who are using drugs: they also destroy families and communities and affect the labor force. Unlike diseases with a clear symptomatic outcome, drug use and addiction produce mental and physical health problems, as well as broad societal challenges such as loss of child custody, potential overdose death, crime, and incarceration.[3]

A recent analysis has shown that the rate of drug overdose deaths in the United States has been growing exponentially for the last 37 years, although the specific drugs causing death have varied.[4] The recent opioid epidemic is an example of multiple waves.[5] As indicated by a Centers for Disease Control and Prevention (CDC) report, overdose deaths from prescription opioids (POs) are not decreasing, and

Georgiy V. Bobashev, Lee D. Hoffer, and Francois R. Lamy, *Agent-Based Modeling to Delineate Opioid and Other Drug Use Epidemics* In: *Complex Systems and Population Health*. Edited by: Yorghos Apostolopoulos, Kristen Hassmiller Lich, and Michael Kenneth Lemke, Oxford University Press (2020). © Oxford University Press.
DOI: 10.1093/oso/9780190880743.003.0014

heroin overdose deaths continue to increase exponentially.[6] Latest records show that deaths from fentanyl, fentanyl analogs, and nonpharmaceutical synthetic opioids are growing even faster than deaths involving heroin,[6] indicating a relatively new epidemic, which is now followed by the co-involvement of stimulants.[7]

14.1.2. How Are Drug Epidemics Defined?

The term *epidemic* has been well-defined for infectious diseases and often used to describe historical periods of increased drug use in the United States. While applied in the context of drug use, it has not been defined as clearly as for infectious diseases. Herein we describe some of the key issues arising with defining a drug use epidemic and discuss how these issues affect modeling the complexity of the process.

14.1.2.1. Variety of Technical Terms

Epidemiological terms such as endemic, trend, outbreak, epidemic, and pandemic reflect specific time trajectories, specifying different numbers of people being affected by a disease, and often locating where the problem is occurring. But these terms also reflect social norms. For example, despite a large increase in its prevalence of use over the last thirty years, few discussions of the "cannabis epidemic" in the United States could be found in the scientific literature. The same is true for scientific and public discussions about the "alcohol epidemic" or the "benzodiazepine epidemic." For these substances, the term *trend* appears to be more frequently employed. For other substances, such as "synthetic cannabinoids" (i.e., Spice, or K2), the term *outbreak* tends to be preferred. Specific terms are applied for a variety of reasons, such as the drugs are different (e.g., new vs. old), a perception of risk is different (e.g., with newer drugs and higher perceived risk), or simply to create a more dramatic narrative.

Unpacking these definitions, the baseline, or *endemic*, levels of drug use are often unknown, and measurement resources and capabilities are localized and highly variable. Notably, there are no places, geographically speaking, in which drug use does not occur, and that means a drug epidemic can potentially "start" anywhere. Usually an epidemic is defined as a sustained growth of incidence beyond a baseline level. In the presence of a "trend" baseline measures are shifting, which might mask a potential epidemic.

14.1.2.2. Multiplicity of Indicators

Unlike clear biomarker indications of infectious diseases, drug use outcomes can be difficult to identify because of the progressive nature of drug-using behaviors, discussed later in this chapter. Without markers, a number of common epidemiological *indicators* of drug use (e.g., drug treatment entry data, arrest data, insurance claims data, etc.) are used that *may* reflect the level of drug use in the population. Yet, because these are *indirect* measures of drug use, their reliability might vary. Some indicators (e.g., drug treatment admissions, arrest data) are also known to have long lag times; that is, they do not occur until a person has been using a drug for a significant period of time.

Counting overdoses and/or overdose deaths is a tangible way to address an epidemic, but it only represents one, highly visible consequence of drug use and might reflect something else. For instance, a localized outbreak of overdoses might indicate something other than an epidemic in drug use (e.g., a "bad" batch of drug or drug combination entering the market). Responding to the final and terminal manifestations of an epidemic may not lead to solving or reducing the drivers of it. For example, broad introduction of naloxone can avert a large number of overdose deaths, which is critically important, but it will not address issues associated with increased opioid use or reduce the damage it has on other domains of society.

14.1.2.3. VARYING TEMPORAL SCALE

Practically speaking, one should be able to estimate the rate of epidemic growth and classify the shape of population trends (e.g., constant, linear, quadratic, exponential, etc.). Based on the shape of the temporal relationship, the observed dynamics can then be classified as an outbreak (short term, large rate of increase), trend (long term, low rate of increase), or epidemic (long term, large rate of increase). In infectious diseases, an epidemic process is characterized by a basic reproductive rate, characterized in terms of how many susceptible individuals are likely to be infected by a single infective individual. Using this standard for drug epidemics is challenging because drug use is not an episodic disease, but it instead blends different types of use over varying time scales. The pool of "susceptible" individuals are people who have never used, occasional users who haven't used recently, and abstinent or former users, with each category having a different propensity to use.

14.1.2.4. THE ADAPTIVE (REACTIVE) NATURE OF DRUG USE

What is now called an "opioid" epidemic is a uniquely sequenced blend of a prescription opioid epidemic, heroin epidemic, and epidemic of synthetic opioids (e.g. fentanyl, U-47,700). But as drug users continue to adapt to this epidemic by using multiple different drugs (polydrug use), it becomes more complex to define. For example, some opioid users are moving to stimulant use (i.e., methamphetamine and cocaine) as observed by the National Drug Early Warning System. If the polydrug use trend continues to grow, it could further complicate the opioid epidemic.

A key difference in drug use from infectious or chronic diseases is the *drug seeking* behavior among users. It would be strange to expect someone willing to infect oneself with influenza; however, drug users are often purposely seeking drugs despite knowledge of their harms. But drug users also change the drugs that they use for many different reasons, and this can make assessing epidemics more challenging. For instance, under intense public and police pressure, methamphetamine users might switch to using heroin. These sorts of reactive elements of drug use are difficult to predict.

14.1.2.5. STIGMA, REPORTING, AND DATA QUALITY

Like HIV and some major mental health disorders, illicit drug use and substance use disorder evokes a strong social stigma. Drug users tend to hide their consumption from others. Stigma is enhanced as the substances being used are illicit or are used in an illicit or nonsanctioned way. This sociopolitical context cannot be ignored, as it has consequences on understanding epidemics of illegal drug use. For instance, even for popular drugs such as marijuana or, more recently, prescription pain medicine, the people who use may not self-report use to family, friends, employers, or health professionals. But self-report is also challenging because of the unregulated nature of the substances themselves. Sometimes users might not even *know* the drug(s) they are using (e.g., some opiate users think they are using heroin when they are, in fact, using heroin *combined* with fentanyl), which makes investigating epidemics of drug use more challenging.

14.2. COMPLEXITY OF DRUG EPIDEMICS

Illicit drug use is a complex social behavior that changes across temporal, environmental, and spatial contexts. In the following discussion, we consider the main components of this complexity and its challenges in thinking about drug epidemics.

14.2.1. Polydrug Use Is Prevalent and Cannot Be Ignored

Drugs that people use can be grouped in a number of ways based on their neurobiological effect (e.g., stimulants, sedatives), legal status (e.g., legal, illicit/scheduled), production (e.g., natural vs. synthetic), origin (e.g., domestic vs. imported), and so on. But people who use illicit drugs often use more than one drug.[8] This polydrug use can be independent (i.e., using multiple drugs separately) or constitute multiple drugs used together or in close succession. Drugs in combination can enhance the effect of each other (e.g., cigarettes and alcohol) or can be used in conjunction with each other to cure the negative effect of the first drug (e.g., methamphetamine in the evening to enhance physical performance in a night club, followed by benzodiazepine next day to relax and get sleep, or heroin, followed by marijuana to alleviate withdrawal symptoms).

Some of the joint drug combinations could be extremely dangerous, such as heroin and fentanyl that often leads to overdose, heroin and cocaine (speedball) that is known to be linked to self-induced injuries and death or heroin and benzodiazepine that is known to be linked with overdose.

14.2.2. The Natural History of Drug Use Is Adaptive

The natural history of drug use has components of both infectious (spread from one person to another) and chronic diseases (long-term progression within an individual). To start using drugs, especially injecting drugs, a person is usually introduced to the drug by someone else, such as friend, peer group, or family member. After initiation, individual drug use trajectories and patterns can vary and be nonlinear. As described in Figure 14.1, a common pattern is starting with "Never used," one can move to "Initiation of use," and then to "Recreational use or misuse." Recreational use and misuse (in the case of POs) might then escalate to "Heavy" use. Heavy use might then lead to treatment and "Recovery/Abstinence," which might potentially result in "Relapse" back to Light or Heavy use.[9,10] This potential cycle of abstinence and relapse is an important characteristic of the recovery process.

Unlike infectious diseases, where the course of the disease is affected by the pathogen biology, host immune response, and treatments, drug use involves numerous causal factors affecting each state transition. These factors could be grouped into three hierarchical domains: *neurobiological, decisional,* and *social/environmental.* These domains are interconnected and can produce the variety of observed behaviors as described in the following discussion.

At the *neurobiological domain level,* drug use and addiction are induced by a range of biological characteristics and mechanisms. Variations in the users *neurophysiology* can lead to low production of one or some neurotransmitters, altering brain functions.[11] This imbalance in the normal neurological process may induce drug abuse mediating the lack/excess of specific neurotransmitters—for example, a lack of dopamine receptors increases the chance to consume dopamine agonist substances (e.g., amphetamine-type or cocaine).[12] Repeated consumption induces gradual modifications of the brain structure through *synaptic plasticity.*[13,14] This gradual modification induces substance *tolerance,* causing users to consume higher doses to obtain desired effect(s).[15] The *withdrawal* inherent to neurotransmitters depletion partially explains the compulsion experience by users once drug effects are wearing off (e.g., opiate users actively seeking for opiates once they become "dope sick" due to depletion of their natural stocks of endorphins).

At the *individual decisional level,* drug use can be understood as a choice reflecting individuals' mindset. For example, the *motivational* model considers that individuals decide to consume drug(s) if the positive affective consequences

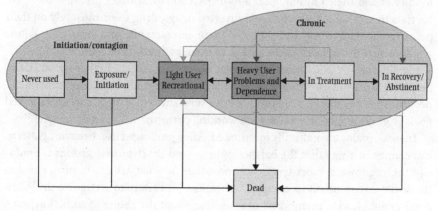

Figure 14.1 A natural history diagram of drug use process.

of using substance(s) outweigh the positive affective consequences of not con-suming.[16] In addition, because each substance acts differently on the brain (e.g., opiates mediating the endorphin receptors to regulate pain), users might be in-clined to *self-medicate* themselves by consuming drugs accordingly to their par-ticular situation (e.g., chronic back injury, desire to dance all night).[17] From a psycho-sociological perspective, choices are based on the information, beliefs, and meanings attached by users to substances.

The decision domain must also consider that people are not making decisions alone. Here, the concept of "agency" is challenged. The beliefs and meanings that users attribute to the drugs they use are shaped through social interactions with other users: Peer influence and the *social-familial environment* are common risk factors associated with substance initiation,[18,19] continuation,[19,20] and relapse.[21] From an economic standpoint, drugs have often been shown to be *inelastic*, which means that price increases are not necessarily linked to demand diminution, es-pecially among dependent users.[22] However, the increasing price of one drug can have repercussions on other drug consumption through *cross-price elasticity*, meaning that users switch from the costly drug to a cheaper one.[23]

The *environmental domain* comprises all external factors affecting decisions about initiation and specific use. Drug *production* and *availability* are particu-larly relevant here. Unlike a replicating virus, illegal drugs do not replicate; in-stead, someone has to produce a drug and deliver to the users. This could be done through legal prescription, illicit diversion of prescription meds, or illicit produc-tion by drug cartels and individuals. The dynamics of drug cartels and availability of drugs over the Internet can impact which drugs and their combinations could be used and co-used.

Legislation regarding legal substance *accessibility* (e.g., alcohol under 21 years old), *taxation*,[24] and drugs *availability* have a structural impact on users' selection. However, the *normalization* of drug use,[25-29] the constantly increasing number of new psychoactive substances,[30] combined to an increased availability of these substances due to the Internet (both Surface and Deep Webs),[31] generate a unique context where users can consume a large panel of psychoactive substances to modify at will their physiological and/or psychological states. Because there are barriers to accessing both illicit and diverted drugs, drug users must rely on their peers to facilitate drug availability.[32] These interactions, and how they define relationships, are important because they influence and pattern use.

Finally, *culture*, as expressed by social norms (e.g., attain higher social status, be successful, or live a "complete" life) may also potentially influence individuals' decisions to consume specific psychoactive substances to achieve socially accepted goals (e.g., amphetamine to increase working performance or study longer).[33,34]

These domains are naturally interlinked. After prolonged use, behavior patterns can change in a way that the balance of long- and short-term decisions is gradu-ally shifting toward short-term and immediate benefits, which, in turn, changes the social environment to change in response.[23,35] Failure to recognize this com-plexity could lead to many years of confusion about the nature of addiction being a disease or moral failure. A common argument against the disease model is that a person who uses drugs has made several bad choices—for example, pay money for a bottle of liquor, open the bottle, and drink the contents—each of which could be averted with the power of will. While this argument may seem reasonable, especially at the early stages of use (e.g., light use), it fails to consider the social and environmental factors noted previously. More important, this logic fails once the brain is affected to the point that using the substance becomes the new normal and the will power control is limited.

14.2.3. Drug Use Transitions Are Understudied

Understanding and measuring the transition between drug use and disorder remains a major research challenge. Large prevention efforts have targeted reducing drug initiation. Similarly, major efforts have sought to develop, expand, and implement drug treatment programs. However, a major gap in knowledge and the data remains when describing the pathway from initiation and recreational use to disorder. It is not part of prevention policy (the person has already initiated) or treatment (the person has not yet developed a disorder to treat). Unlike other chronic diseases (e.g., cancer, diabetes), there are no biological markers and too much nonlinearity in the course of disease progression. This complicates the studies of the transition from the early stages to the later stages of drug use.

14.3. COMPLEX SYSTEMS MODELING TO ADDRESS DRUG USE EPIDEMICS

Responses to complex health problems are often assisted by simulation models. For the opioid epidemic, for example, as many as 56 policy recommendations have been identified by the National Commission on Combating Drug Addiction.[36] These recommendations cover opioid prescribing practices, prevention, treatment, and law enforcement tactics. The commission emphasizes that "more complex models are needed to address whether prescribing policies result in time-dependent reductions in prescription opioid diversion or increase heroin/fentanyl use, who is at risk for transitioning to heroin or fentanyl, the incidence and prevalence of OUD [opioid use disorder], and others."[36] The complexity of the epidemic makes it challenging for health professionals and policymakers to evaluate the balance of multiple interventions. Policy simulation models have been successfully used to address complex health challenges, including, among others, social norms that users develop to avoid problems during recreational drug use. Perez and colleagues[37] simulated the impacts of the 2000 heroin drought in Melbourne, Australia, on the behaviors of both users and dealers.[37] SimUse, an agent-based model (ABM) mimicking the trajectory of polydrug users,[38,39] was developed as a complex adaptive system encompassing five subsystems interacting dynamically: substance, intra-individual, inter-individual, context, and society. The multilayered ontological structure, informed by theoretical concepts and qualitative findings, allowed SimUse to recreate numerous feedback loops generating the complexity involved in the polydrug use trajectory of the agents. This architecture also helps to describe the inner dynamics inherent to drug use and provide the possibility to test what-if scenarios relevant to population health. Similar models could be developed to simulate potential policy responses, such as the reduction of prescribed opioids and the increase availability of naloxone. As indicated by Dasgupta and colleagues,[40] the prescription dose is associated with the probability of the overdose, suggesting that a 90 mg morphine equivalent (MME) cap for prescribed opioids could potentially reduce the number of deaths. Similarly, the distribution of naloxone, a drug reversing the effects of opioids, can revive overdosed individuals. However, the responses to these interventions are difficult to predict due to the complexity inherent in the phenomenon.

The recently developed ABM PainTown[8] intends to simulate the opioid use pathways (Figure 14.2) of an individual from her first opioid prescription, considering the potential MME limitation and naloxone distribution to reverse opioid overdose. PainTown simulates a community of agents representing patients, physicians, drug dealers, Emergency Departments (EDs), and a pharmacy.

> PATIENT. If suffering from chronic pain, patients seek treatment from a physician. If prescribed opioids, the patient will buy them at the pharmacy and use over prescribed time. Patients can develop tolerance (i.e., larger dose needed to achieve the same effect) over time depending on the prescribed dose, and some will take a higher dose than prescribed. A patient can eventually choose to visit additional physicians, an ED, buy from another patient/friend or a dealer, or switch to heroin. A patient can accidentally overdose, based on the prescribed dose and type of opioid. Probabilities of overdose and death depend on the type of drug (e.g., heroin can contain fentanyl), Figure 14.2).
>
> PHYSICIAN: Can choose to prescribe opioids to patients. Before deciding whether to prescribe, a given physician has some likelihood of checking patients' purchase record in the prescription drug monitoring program (PDMP).
>
> DEALER: A dealer will give a patient the requested dose of opioids or heroin without a prescription.
>
> PHARMACY AND EDs: Can choose to give patients opioids. They can check patients' purchase record in the PDMP and have to record sale of opioids in PDMP.

Agents are connected via link relations—each patient has links to one or more physicians, one or more friends who may be other patients or nonpatient dealers, and a pharmacy. Social networks are key to sustain the use of the mix of legal and illicit drugs. As was shown in another ABM of heroin market in Denver, a drug market survives because a lot of drug distributions is done not by the "formal" dealer but through drug brokers, that is, individuals in the network who are connected to dealers but are not dealers per se.[41] Such networks allow drugs to penetrate the community without most members being directly connected to dealers.

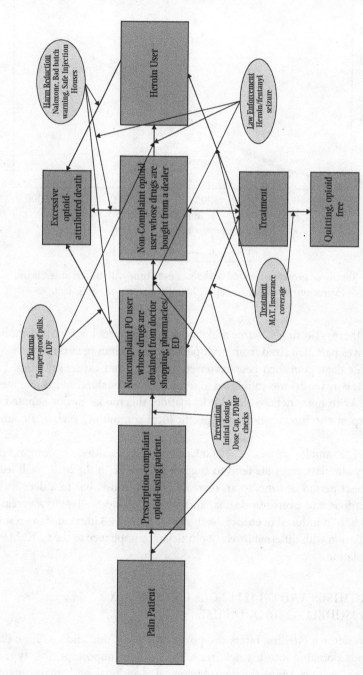

Figure 14.2 A diagram of patient's possible states and transitions between the states. Interventions impact specific transitions between the states.

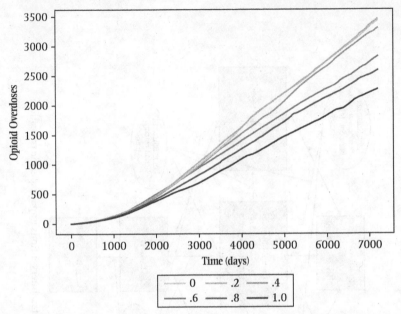

Figure 14.3 Simulated growth of opioid overdoses over time with different levels of compliance for the recommended dose cap of 90 mg of morphine equivalent.

Because there is no single source of data (e.g., a long-term longitudinal study), the model was parameterized from multiple sources, including national surveys, ethnographic data, published peer-reviewed literature, and expert opinions. For example, the core model was calibrated to reproduce national morbidity and mortality rates. With more detailed local information, this model can be adapted to forecast response to intervention in a specific local community such as a county or a town.

A model example simulates 10,000 agents representing a community. Preliminary simulation results tend to suggest a decrease in the MME will lead, within a short period of time, to an increase in heroin use, but to a decreasing rate of overdose and overdose deaths, and that naloxone availability decreases opioid and heroin induced overdose death rates. Figure 14.3 illustrates the results of the simulation with different levels of physician's compliance to the CDC MME recommendation.

14.4. PROMISES AND CHALLENGES OF COMPLEX SYSTEMS MODELING OF DRUG USE

Complex systems modelling offers the possibility to include and combine data from various domains into a single framework. More important, this type of modelling allows to combine the neurobiological, decisional, and environmental components inherent to drug epidemics to simulate their nonlinear dynamics and reproduce their emergence.

Several challenges arise in terms of building, analyzing, and interpreting of drug epidemic models. First, gathering all data required to design a simulation must consider that these data may exist across different disciplines and domains. Multiple data sources, (e.g., government surveys, private treatment data, hospital data, medical records, administrative data) are owned by various entities and are not commonly shared across agencies even for research purposes. As most of the modelling tools are computer-based, the second challenge is to "translate" these data into computational language. Quantitative data (from epidemiology, neurophysiology or economic) are mostly numerical and less complicated to address, but information gathered through ethnography, which detail social processes, are qualitative and need to be transformed into algorithms. Another challenge lies in the ratio between model complexity and computational performance needed to simulate such phenomena. Although synthetic populations allow us to link multiple datasets at the geographical scale, the computational power required exponentially increases. Simple models are easy to manage and efficient in running numerous simulations, but they are unable to encompass all aforementioned factors nor can they represent a large synthetic population. On the other hand, more complex models may be capable of integrating all needed elements in a large population of agents, but they are difficult to calibrate and manage, and they demand high computational performance. They can also be difficult to interpret. In our past research, we have shown how complex models could be simplified to capture the essence of drug use without losing accuracy.[42] Such approaches could be further expanded to more complex models. Finally, each drug epidemic has its own specificities (e.g., time period, substance, population), which rapidly changes in time. Careful calibration, validation, and generalization of such model will be difficult for any drug epidemic.

Despite great challenges that modeling drug epidemics meet, this area of population health research has been fast developing and is very promising. As we learn more about the nature of human neurobiology, the roles of the drugs and social environments on drug using behavior, the more rapidly and accurately models will be able to describe an adequate response to future challenges. With evolving drug markets, information sharing, and drug legalization and availability, the need for understanding the bigger picture of drug epidemics, even vaguely, will deem useful for population health and science in general.

REFERENCES

1. Hunt DE, Kuck S, Truitt L. *Methamphetamine use: Lessons learned.* Cambridge, MA: Abt Associates; 2005.
2. Nutt D, King LA, Saulsbury W, Blakemore C. Development of a rational scale to assess the harm of drugs of potential misuse. *Lancet.* 2007;369:1047–1053. http://dx.doi.org/10.1016/S0140-6736(07)60464-4
3. Galea S, Nandi A, Vlahov D. The social epidemiology of substance use. *Epidemiologic Review.* 2004;26:36–52.

4. Jalal H, Buchanich JM, Roberts MS, Balmert LC, Zhang K, Burke DS. Changing dynamics of the drug overdose epidemic in the United States from 1979 through 2016. *Science.* 2018;361:eaau1184. http://dx.doi.org/10.1126/science.aau1184

5. Ciccarone D. The triple wave epidemic: supply and demand drivers of the US opioid overdose crisis. *Int J Drug Policy.* 2019;72:183–188. http://dx.doi.org/10.1016/j.drugpo.2019.01.010

6. Hedegaard H, Warner M, Miniño AM. Drug overdose deaths in the United States, 1999-2016. US Department of Health and Human Services, Centers for Disease Control and Prevention, National Center for Health Statistics; 2017.

7. Kariisa M, Scholl L, Wilson N, Seth P, Hoots B. Drug overdose deaths involving cocaine and psychostimulants with abuse potential—United States, 2003-2017. *MMWR Morb Mortal Wkly Rep.* 2019;68:388–395. http://dx.doi.org/10.15585/mmwr.mm6817a3

8. Bobashev G, Goree S, Frank J, Zule W. Pain Town, an agent-based model of opioid use trajectories in a small community. In: Thomson R, Dancy C, Hyder A, Bisgin H, eds. *Social, Cultural, and Behavioral Modeling. SBP-BRiMS 2018.* Vol 10899. New York: Springer; 2018:274–285.

9. Rossi C. The role of dynamic modelling in drug abuse epidemiology. *Bull Narcotics, LIV.* 2002:54(1):33–44.

10. Behrens DA, Caulkins JP, Tragler G, Feichtinger G. Optimal control of drug epidemics: Prevent and treat –But not at the same time? *Manag Sci.* 2000;46:333–347.

11. Comings DE, Blum K. Reward deficiency syndrome: genetic aspects of behavioral disorders. *Prog Brain Res.* 2000;126:325–341. http://dx.doi.org/10.1016/S0079-6123(00)26022-6

12. Volkow ND, Chang L, Wang GJ, et al. Association of dopamine transporter reduction with psychomotor impairment in methamphetamine abusers. *Am J Psychiatry.* 2001;158:377–382. http://dx.doi.org/10.1176/appi.ajp.158.3.377

13. Malenka RC. Synaptic plasticity and AMPA receptor trafficking. *Ann N Y Acad Sci.* 2003;1003:1–11. http://dx.doi.org/10.1196/annals.1300.001

14. Kauer JA, Malenka RC. Synaptic plasticity and addiction. *Nat Rev Neurosci.* 2007;8:844–858. http://dx.doi.org/10.1038/nrn2234

15. Koob GF, LeMoal M. *Neurobiology of addiction.* Oxford: Elsevier; 2001.

16. Cooper ML, Kuntsche E, Levitt A, Barber LL, Wolf S. Motivational models of substance use: A review of theory and research on motives for using alcohol, marijuana, and tobacco. *Oxford handbook of substance use and substance use disorders.* Vol 1. Oxford: Oxford University Press; 2016:375–421.

17. Feldman RS, Meyer JS, Quenzer LF. *Principles of neuropsychopharmacology.* Sunderland, UK: Sinauer Associated; 1997.

18. Boyd CJ, Mieczkowski T. Drug use, health, family and social support in "crack" cocaine users. *Addict Behav.* 1990;15:481–485.

19. Levy SJ, Pierce JP. Predictors of marijuana use and uptake among teenagers in Sydney, Australia. *Int J Addict.* 1990;25:1179–1193.

20. Schroeder JR, Latkin CA, Hoover DR, Curry AD, Knowlton AR, Celentano DD. Illicit drug use in one's social network and in one's neighborhood predicts individual heroin and cocaine use. *Ann Epidemiol.* 2001;11:389–394. http://dx.doi.org/10.1016/s1047-2797(01)00225-3

21. Havassy BE, Wasserman DA, Hall SM. Social relationships and abstinence from co-caine in an American treatment sample. *Addiction.* 1995;90:699–710.

22. Chaloupka FJ, Grossman M, Tauras JA. The demand for cocaine and marijuana by youth. In: Grossman M, Hsieh C-R, eds. *The economic analysis of substance use and abuse: An integration of econometrics and behavioral economic research.* Chicago: University of Chicago Press; 1999: 133–156.

23. Bickel WK, DeGrandpre RJ, Higgins ST. The behavioral economics of concur-rent drug reinforcers: a review and reanalysis of drug self-administration re-search. *Psychopharmacology (Berl).* 1995;118:250–259. http://dx.doi.org/10.1007/bf02245952

24. Lewit EM. U.S. tobacco taxes: behavioural effects and policy implications. *Br J Addict.* 1989;84:1217–1234.

25. Parker H, Williams L, Aldridge J. The normalization of 'sensible' recreational drug use: Further evidence from the North West England Longitudinal Study. *Sociology.* 2002;36: 345–367.

26. Parker H, Williams L. Intoxicated weekends: Young adults' work hard–play hard lifestyles, public health and public disorder. *Drugs Ed Prevent Pol.* 2003;10:345–367.

27. Parker H, Aldridge J, Measham F. *Illegal leisure: The normalization of adolescent drug use.* New York: Routledge; 1998.

28. Parker H. Normalization as a barometer: Recreational drug use and the consump-tion of leisure by younger Britons. *Addict Res Theory.* 2005;13:205–215.

29. Parker H. Pathology or modernity? Rethinking risks factors analyses of young drug users. *Addict Res Theory.* 2003;11:141–144.

30. European Monitoring Centre for Drugs and Drug Addiction (EMCDDA). *European Drug Report 2016: Trends and Developments.* Luxembourg: Publications Office of the European Union; 2016.

31. European Monitoring Centre for Drugs and Drug Addiction. *Drugs and the darknet: Perspectives for enforcement, research and policy.* Luxembourg: EMCDDA–Europol Joint Publications; 2017.

32. Hoffer LD. *Junkie business: The evolution and operation of a heroin dealing network.* London: Thomson/Wadsworth; 2006.

33. Ehrenberg A. *L'individu incertain.* Paris: Hachette; 1996.

34. Ehrenberg A. *La société du malaise.* Paris: Odile Jacob; 2012.

35. Bickel WK, Johnson MW, Koffarnus MN, MacKillop J, Murphy JG. The behavioral economics of substance use disorders: reinforcement pathologies and their repair. *Annu Rev Clin Psychol.* 2014;10:641–677.

36. Christie C, Baker C, Cooper R, Kennedy PJ, Madras B, Bondi P. *The President's Commission on combating drug addiction and the opioid crisis.* Washington, DC: National Commission on Combating Drug Addiction; 2017. Available from https://www.whitehouse.gov/sites/whitehouse.gov/files/images/Final_Report_Draft_11-1-2017.pdf.

37. Perez P, Dray A, Ritter A, Dietze P, Moore T, Mazerolle L. Simdrug exploring the complexity of heroin use in Melbourne. *Drug Policy Modelling Project Monograph Series.* 2005;11.

38. Lamy F, Bossomaier T, Perez P. An ontologic agent-based model of recreational polydrug use: SimUse. *International Journal of Simulation and Process Modelling.* 2015;10:207–222.

39. Lamy F, Bossomaier T, Perez P. SimUse: simulation of recreational poly-drug use in Artificial Life (ALIFE), 2011. IEEE Symposium; 2011.
40. Dasgupta N, Funk MJ, Proescholdbell S, Hirsch A, Ribisl KM, Marshall S. Cohort study of the impact of high-dose opioid analgesics on overdose mortality. *Pain Med.* 2016;17:85–98. http://dx.doi.org/10.1111/pme.12907
41. Hoffer L, Bobashev GV. Researching a local heroin market as a complex adaptive system. *Am J Community Psychol.* 2009;44:273–286. http://dx.doi.org/10.1007/s10464-009-9268-2
42. Heard D, Bobashev GV, Morris RJ. Reducing the complexity of an agent-based local heroin market model. *PLoS One.* 2014;9:e102263.

15

Hybrid Simulation Modeling
in Population Health

SALLY C. BRAILSFORD, DAVE C. EVENDEN, AND JOE VIANA

15.1. INTRODUCTION

The term *hybrid* has many meanings in the field of modeling. Often, it is loosely used to mean applying more than one method to solve a given problem—for example, mixing qualitative and quantitative approaches or combining simulation and optimization. As with any hybrid, the aim is to compensate the weaknesses of one element by the strengths of another. However, the term *hybrid simulation* has a more specific meaning, namely, a modeling approach that combines two or more of the following three simulation methods: discrete-event simulation (DES), agent-based modeling (ABM), and system dynamics (SD). These approaches are described in Chapters 13 to 15 of this volume. Further, a review by Brailsford et al.[1] provides an in-depth introduction to hybrid simulation from an operations research perspective, while some of the findings from this review are reported in this chapter.

Hybrid simulation has rapidly grown in popularity in the academic simulation community since the early 2000s. Advances in computing power have made it possible to develop and run realistic models that exploit the strengths of the component methods. This growth in popularity has also been aided by the emergence of a commercial software tool, AnyLogic (AnyLogic Company, Oakbrook Terrace, IL, US) which, as its name suggests, allows the modeler to use any combination of simulation methods at the same time in the same modeling environment. Nevertheless, hybrid simulation remains a relatively new concept compared with the component methods, and although the number of practical applications is growing, it is still an emerging area.

Sally C. Brailsford, Dave C. Evenden, and Joe Viana, *Hybrid Simulation Modeling in Population Health* In: *Complex Systems and Population Health*. Edited by: Yorghos Apostolopoulos, Kristen Hassmiller Lich, and Michael Kenneth Lemke, Oxford University Press (2020). © Oxford University Press. DOI: 10.1093/oso/9780190880743.003.0015

Both case study examples in this chapter are UK-based but address a worldwide population health challenge: the impact of an ageing population on care delivery services. For the benefit of the non-UK reader, we first provide some brief background information about the UK health and social care systems. In the United Kingdom, healthcare is provided free at the point of delivery and is funded nationally through taxation. Inevitably, this involves an element of priority setting, since demand is constantly increasing but the budget is finite. The United Kingdom also has a small private healthcare sector. However, social care (support with activities of daily living) is means-tested and needs-assessed and hence is often co-funded by service users or provided free of charge by friends and family. The remaining costs are borne by the Local Authority, (i.e., the city or county council).

15.2. BENEFITS OF HYBRID SIMULATION FOR POPULATION HEALTH

The academic literature on health modeling contains thousands of examples of simulation models,[2,3] the vast majority of which are DES models for capacity planning and service redesign problems. SD is frequently (although not always) used at a more aggregate level where individual variability is less important and is especially useful for modeling feedback structures in complex systems. As discussed in Chapters 1 to 3 of this volume, population health systems are complex systems *par excellence*. In health, "everything affects everything," and hence a decision that appears entirely rational in one part of a system can lead to highly undesirable outcomes elsewhere, both for the individual patient and for the system as a whole. Any model that ignores this web of interconnections will only represent part of the picture, but it is obviously not possible, let alone desirable, to model the whole world in minute detail. In some cases, a limited perspective is sufficient to answer a specific narrowly-defined question (e.g., what fraction of the population should be vaccinated to prevent an influenza epidemic). However, in many cases we need to look at *both* the "big picture" and the detail. Individual variability matters—but so do the wider interconnections. Using one single simulation method can involve making unrealistic assumptions and oversimplifications, but modeling only those parts of the problem for which that method is appropriate may not be helpful either.

15.3. CONCEPTS AND FRAMEWORKS

Several frameworks to describe the ways that simulation methods can interact have been proposed in the academic literature, but that of Morgan, Howick, and Belton[4] is the most comprehensive to date. Their taxonomy considers only DES and SD, but it can easily be extended to include ABM. They identify five distinct modes of interaction, of which four can be classified as hybrid:

- **Parallel:** two or more separate models are developed, either for direct comparison or to address different aspects of the same problem. Technically, this is not hybrid simulation.

- **Sequential:** two or more independent single-method submodels are executed sequentially *but only once*, so that the output of the first becomes the input of the second.
- **Enriching:** the model uses one dominant method, but contains limited aspects of other method(s): for example, an SD model where a minor element is represented as a DES.
- **Interaction:** here, a set of distinct but equally important single-method submodels interact dynamically at runtime, either in a fixed pattern (A-B-A-B-A-B . . .) or determined "live" by the system state during the run. The former is an extension of the sequential mode.
- **Integration:** one seamless overarching model in which it is impossible to tell where one submodel ends and another begins.

Most hybrid simulation models represent the relationships between different elements of some larger system. Therefore, it is not surprising that the majority of models in the literature are of the types *interaction* or *sequential*. Of the two, interaction appears the most realistic, since the sequential method is often just a modeling choice rather than a faithful representation of information flow in the real world. The models described in Sections 15.5 and 15.6 are both examples of interaction.

True integration is the "holy grail" identified by Brailsford, Desai, and Viana[5] and is arguably unachievable. The philosophical worldviews of DES and SD modelers—the microscope and the helicopter—are totally different, which is why these methods are sometimes referred to in the simulation literature as *paradigms* rather than methods or techniques. This dichotomy of world views is discussed by Morecroft and Robinson[6] who develop separate DES and SD models for the same problem, namely, sustaining profitability in the fishing industry. Even in the AnyLogic software, there is still a clear delineation between the ABM, DES, and SD components, and the building blocks (icons) used to construct models will be familiar to users of any of these three methods.

15.4. DEVELOPING A HYBRID SIMULATION MODEL

Broadly speaking, the modeling process follows the same steps as a single-method simulation approach, but there are a few important differences, and some areas where methodological research is currently ongoing that are exciting avenues for new research. Of course, in practice these steps rarely follow the neat sequential pattern described in the following discussion, and there is almost always backwards iteration between stages. In this section, we follow the stages described by Brooks and Robinson[7] in their excellent text on (discrete-event) simulation.

15.4.1. Step 1: Problem Definition and Model Scoping

What is the purpose of the model? What question(s) does it need to answer, and what elements of the real-world problem must be included in the model to do so? Is individual variability important? Is there interaction and/or feedback between system elements? At what level of detail does the system need to be modeled? It is at this stage that the need for, or benefit of, a hybrid approach begins to emerge. If the answers to these questions are different for different aspects of the problem, it is unlikely that a single-method model will suffice.

15.4.2. Step 2: Conceptual Modeling

This is the process of developing a software-independent representation of the model[8] to ensure it is fit for purpose and will answer the question it was designed to address. DES, ABM and SD all have established methods for doing this: activity or process flow diagrams for DES, statecharts for ABM, and stock-and-flow or influence diagrams for SD. Despite the importance of the model conceptualization stage, there is as yet no recognized method or notation for representing the information or material flows between the components of a hybrid model. A variety of ad-hoc approaches can be found in the literature, but many authors do not mention this stage at all. Nevertheless, the modeler clearly needs to consider (and document) how the components will be connected and how information will pass from one to another.

15.4.3. Step 3: Data Collection

This stage, frequently glossed over in simulation textbooks, is typically the most time-consuming part of any simulation modeling project. The issues for hybrid simulation are exactly the same as for single-method models: Parameter estimation and data availability are perpetual challenges, often exacerbated by information governance constraints. The modeler is frequently reliant on estimates based on subject-matter expert opinion, combined with sensitivity analysis to assess the criticality of these estimates. Moreover, the availability, quality, and reliability of data may impact on the feasibility of modeling some aspect of the problem, and the modeler is forced to return to an earlier stage.

15.4.4. Step 4: Software Implementation

There are several ways in which the conceptual model can be implemented in computer software, in addition to using AnyLogic:

(a) linking two or more single-method software tools, either automated via some interface, or manually via the keyboard;
(b) using a single-method software tool augmented with bespoke code to implement another method;
(c) coding the model from scratch in a general programming language.

Viana et al.[9] and Chahal et al.[10] are both examples of approach (a) in which a DES submodel developed in Simul8 (Simul8 Corporation, Boston, MA, US) is linked with an SD submodel developed in Vensim (Ventana Systems, Inc., Harvard, MA, US). In the former, a model of Chlamydia infection, the linkage was automated through a Microsoft Excel interface. In the latter, a model to investigate the benefits of electronic whiteboards in emergency departments, the user has to key in parameter values after each submodel has run. Approaches (b) and (c) are now less frequently used, arguably because of the increasing popularity and user-friendliness of AnyLogic.

In summary, the choice of computer implementation is a decision for the modeler and largely depends on his or her programming skills and familiarity with—and the availability of—suitable software. However, an increasing number of published models use AnyLogic and a significant proportion of these are health-related, so there is a growing user community to provide information and support.

15.4.5. Step 5: Model Verification

This involves ensuring that the computer model is an accurate representation of the conceptual model and does not contain any coding errors. Since there is no standardized methodology for conceptual modeling in hybrid simulation, this process is often ad hoc. It is slightly easier in an integrated modeling environment (i.e. AnyLogic) that contains some debugging tools. Methods for single-method models, such as extreme value tests and dimensional consistency checks, can and should be applied where possible.

15.4.6. Step 6: Model Validation

This means checking that the computer model produces output that is consistent with real-world data not used to parameterize the model (see also Chapter 17 of this volume). Again, this is challenging for a hybrid model since it is necessary to validate the connections between submodels, as well as within the submodels themselves. In some cases, standard methods for validating single-method models (e.g., establishing face validity with domain experts, t tests for comparing means) can be applied to the whole hybrid model, but the development of generic techniques for validating hybrid models remains an active research area. Quantitative models are normally validated by "black box" methods that ignore the inner workings of the model and focus solely on the input and the output. On the other hand, the validation of qualitative models based on causal hypotheses typically involves "glass box" methods (i.e., the model must be transparent and understandable to domain experts). Agent-based models, especially those that model human behavior, are often based on hypothetical psychological rules, which may well produce aggregated results that mirror observed population-level (emergent) data but are virtually impossible to validate at the individual level.

15.4.7. Step 7: Experimentation

Stochastic models must be run multiple times for the same parameter settings to ensure that any differences between modeled scenarios are statistically significant and not just due to sampling variation. The same is true of a hybrid model that contains a stochastic submodel, but for enriching or interaction type models this may be accomplished more efficiently by performing multiple iterations of the stochastic submodel in a standalone manner and then passing the desired output from this set of iterations (e.g., the average dwelling time in some health state) to another submodel, rather than running multiple iterations of the whole model. This is one advantage of using different modeling software for the various submodels. For example, in the model of Viana et al.,[9] Simul8 was used to model a sexual health clinic, and Vensim was used to model the spread of Chlamydia infection in the community. Each month, 20 iterations of the Simul8 (DES) submodel were performed, and the output of interest—the average number of patients who left without being treated—was passed to the Vensim (SD) submodel, which then ran—just once—to generate the number of new infections. This, in turn, became the input to the DES for the following month.

15.4.8. Step 8: Real-World Model Use

This final step in the simulation modeling process, the use of the model to inform a real-world decision, is rarely reported in the academic simulation literature[2,3] although the grey literature and the health economics literature do contain examples. The same is true of hybrid simulation, although this is perhaps unsurprising as it is such a new approach. Nevertheless, the client testimonials on the AnyLogic website suggest that the AnyLogic consultancy arm is already enjoying some success.

15.5. EXAMPLE 1: A HYBRID SIMULATION MODEL FOR AGE-RELATED MACULAR DEGENERATION

Age-related macular degeneration (AMD) is a common but serious eye condition. In developed countries, it is a leading cause of vision loss in people aged over 50.[11] AMD comes in two forms: wet and dry.[12] The dry form is untreatable and disease progression is inevitable, but at the time wet AMD was managed[13] through regular monthly injections into the affected eye(s). This treatment did not cure the condition, but it did, in some cases, slow its progression. These injections had to be given monthly in a clinical setting. The introduction of this treatment, combined with the increased volume of patients due to the aging population, resulted in massively increased demand for AMD clinics.

Sight loss in older people obviously reduces their ability to live independently, and consequently increases the need for social care. If this need is not met, for example, if a partially sighted person does not have a care giver or family member who can accompany them to hospital for their injection appointment, the likelihood of missing subsequent appointments will also increase. The aim of the model was to capture some of the consequences of AMD at the individual patient level and at the system level and to illustrate the interactions between the social care and healthcare systems. The model was developed in collaboration with the Eye Unit at University Hospital Southampton as part of the larger Care

Life Cycle project.[14] The Care Life Cycle was one of four projects funded by the UK Engineering & Physical Sciences Research Council under the "Complexity Science in the Real World" scheme that sought to develop richer models than the traditional simplifications of most previous approaches.[15]

The model was developed in AnyLogic and is a hybrid of ABM, DES, and SD. Individuals with AMD are modelled as agents located in a geographical space representing the catchment area of the hospital. Each individual agent contains two SD models, one per eye, representing the level of remaining eyesight. Agents also contain basic demographic data and two types of social care information: how much care they need, and how much they actually receive. The outpatient clinic where treatment administered is modeled using DES, incorporating patient pathway information, opening times, and staffing constraints.

The elements of the hybrid model interact dynamically at runtime. A decrease in sight level in the SD component increases the agent's social care need status in the ABM component. Each month, when the time comes for an agent to visit the hospital for treatment, there is a chance of missing the appointment (determined by the agent's sight level and social care need/received status), and thus AMD may progress to a more advanced stage. Agents who do attend their appointments temporarily become entities in the DES. If the clinic is running late due to overcrowding or understaffing, wait times increase, and patients with high but unmet social care needs who are dependent on hospital transport may leave without being treated. This potentially results in disease progression, which is mapped back to the SD component when the entity exits the DES submodel and becomes an agent again. Detailed technical descriptions of the model have been published elsewhere.[16–18] The model was used to investigate the effects of different clinic staffing levels and clinic frequencies under various scenarios of social care provision.

ABM was chosen to model patients because it facilitated the spatial representation to generate the individual's chance of attending an appointment. Later (unpublished) versions of this model were integrated with a geographical information system to calculate travel times. DES was the obvious choice for the clinic. SD initially appeared a good choice for disease progression, but in fact the pair of SD eyesight models embedded in each agent led to very long runtimes for large populations. The stock-and-flow SD models were later coded separately in Java, resulting in vastly improved model performance: the runtime for a simulated year with an initial population of 500 agents was reduced from 35 minutes to 8 seconds. Validation of the individual submodels was relatively straightforward, but validating the connections between them was extremely difficult. The model was parameterized with a mixture of data from the clinical literature and synthetic data, but was never fully populated with real-world local data due to the problems of data collection.

Later, a standalone DES model of the clinic was developed address the more pragmatic operational question of how to resource the clinics.[19] At the time of the study, the clinic treated over 70,000 patients annually and relied heavily on overtime. Data on arrival patterns and service times were collected, and a patient survey conducted to investigate the impact of social care provision on patients' ability to attend. Clinics were allowed to overrun in the model, but a waiting time tolerance was included to reflect some patients' reliance on hospital transport. These behavioral parameters were derived from the data collected in the patient survey. The simulation was run for a range of realistic assumptions about growth in demand and/or the provision of extra resources. The model showed that, even in the most optimistic scenario, the clinic would still have to rely on overtime to meet demand. Moreover, referring back to the hybrid model, if social care provision was improved so that more patients could attend (and wait longer), clinic overrun time would increase even further.

15.6. EXAMPLE 2: A HYBRID SIMULATION MODEL FOR DEMENTIA

Dementia is an increasingly important global problem[20] due to a number of factors, including the aging population, the current lack of effective medical treatment, and the high costs of care, most of which are borne by families or (in the United Kingdom) the social care system. As part of a project funded by the Wessex Academic Health Science Network (wessexahsn.org), a hybrid model was developed to estimate 25-year projections of numbers of people with dementia, their level of severity of symptoms, the associated care costs, and the effect of medical treatment and lifestyle interventions, for the Wessex region in the south of England.

This model was also developed in AnyLogic and combined SD and ABM. SD is used to model population dynamics (i.e., aging), the onset of dementia, and mortality. The stocks comprise an "aging chain" of cognitively normal (CN) people in five-year age groups from 60 to 105, each with a counterpart stock of persons with dementia (PWD). Further flows between stocks (i.e., dementia incidence and the cognitively normal/PWD mortality rates) are age-related. The starting population can either be a single age group, similar to a birth cohort, or a population distributed across all age groups. The agent-based submodel represents individual patients and simulates dementia onset, progression, and death. Agents are allocated attributes representing their rate of cognitive decline (slow, medium, fast) and their potential responses to the two interventions.

There are several interfaces between the SD and ABM components, depicted schematically in Figure 15.1. Dementia onset and mortality flows are treated as discrete.[21] For each discrete arrival in the PWD stock an agent is created. Similarly, for each PWD death an agent is removed. The other important interface is the aggregation of individual results, which is managed within the SD submodel and provides population-level averages of years with dementia, quality-adjusted life years, and care costs.

Parameterization was based on a number of sources, including specialized medical literature,[22] publications on care costs,[23] national statistics,[24] and expert judgment. The agents are allocated individual attributes and parameter values by

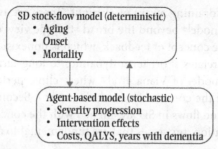

Figure 15.1 SD and ABM hybrid simulation architecture.

sampling from probability distributions derived from these sources. Verification and validation were supported by AnyLogic's in-built graphical features and by comparing model outputs with additional independent sources.[25]

The results showed that, while medication benefit can be important for people who show a delay in cognitive decline, at the population level these effects are not large. Symptom management applies to only some people, for only some symptoms, for only some of the years with dementia. Larger population-level benefits, such as lower future care costs, can accrue from improved lifestyle interventions. However, this requires a longer-term view of the intervention and its outcome.

Hybrid modeling was a useful way of combining a top–down overview with bottom–up detail. SD is a widely accepted approach for modeling at the population level, but it is deterministic and, hence, the stochastic ABM submodel provided a more realistic perspective at the individual level. Overall, the hybrid modeling approach lends itself to considerable generalizability. This includes reparameterizing for different populations, the inclusion of additional medical conditions and complications, and potentially including interactions between patients and care givers.

15.7. CONCLUSIONS

The 1960s and 1970s saw many attempts to develop simulation models containing both continuous and discrete variables. However, this early work was mainly theoretical, due largely to hardware limitations, and the topic lost popularity until the early 2000s when there was a surge of interest in combining SD and DES for practical applications. The 21st-century variant of hybrid simulation typically relates to the interplay between "micro" operational-level models and "macro" whole-system or aggregate models that take a more strategic view. The inclusion of ABM is often a response to the need to capture the cognitive and emotional aspects of decision-making and reflects the increasing interest in behavioral operations research more generally.[26]

However, it is not always the case that DES/ABS are used for the micro-aspects and SD for the macro. In the model in Section 15.5, SD is used at the very lowest level, inside the individual agents, to represent the accumulation (or, more precisely, the draining away) of eyesight. There are two reasons why SD is useful in hybrid models beyond the broad strategic view of a system. First, it explicitly models the concept of feedback, which is nonexistent in DES and tacit in ABM: Feedback relates short-term dynamics to long-term system effects, as in the Chlamydia model of Viana et al.[9] where clinic performance affects the level of infection in the community (and vice versa). Second, the fundamental concepts of stocks and flows in SD are aligned with the concept of accumulating and storing information, processes that are fundamental to agents with learning abilities.

Although its use is growing rapidly, hybrid simulation is still a relatively new methodology and there are significant overheads to its use, not the least of which is the challenge of verification and validation. It is always worth considering—at the conceptual modeling stage—whether a single-method model would be sufficient. Nevertheless, the benefits of hybrid simulation are clear and with a growing body of literature in this area and a readily available software tool in which to develop models, it is rapidly establishing its place in the modeler's toolkit.

REFERENCES

1. Brailsford S, Eldabi T, Osorio A, Kunc M, Mustafee N. Hybrid simulation modelling in operational research: A state-of-the-art review. *Eur J Oper Res.* 2019; 278:721–737. DOI: 10.1016/j.ejor.2018.10.025.
2. Katsaliaki K, Mustafee N. Applications of simulation within the healthcare context. *J Oper Res Soc.* 2011;62(8):1431–1451. doi:10.1057/jors.2010.20.
3. Brailsford SC, Harper PR, Patel B, Pitt M. An analysis of the academic literature on simulation and modelling in health care. *J Simul.* 2009;3(3):130–140. doi:10.1057/jos.2009.10.
4. Morgan JS, Howick S, Belton V. A toolkit of designs for mixing Discrete Event Simulation and System Dynamics. *Eur J Oper Res.* 2017;257(3):907–918. doi:10.1016/j.ejor.2016.08.016.
5. Brailsford SC, Desai SM, Viana J. Towards the holy grail: Combining system dynamics and discrete-event simulation in healthcare. In: Johansson B, Jain S, Montoya-Torres J, Hugan J, Yücesan E, eds. *Proceedings of the 2010 Winter Simulation Conference.* IEEE Press, Piscataway, NJ; 2010:2293–2303. doi:10.1109/WSC.2010.5678927.
6. Morecroft J, Robinson S. Comparing discrete event simulation and system dynamics: modelling a fishery. In: *Proceedings of the Operational Research Society Simulation Workshop.* OR Society; 2006:137–148.
7. Brooks R, Robinson S, Lewis C. *Simulation and Inventory Control—Texts in Operational Research.* New York: Palgrave Macmillan; 2001.
8. Robinson S. Conceptual modelling for simulation Part I: Definition and requirements. *J Oper Res Soc.* 2008;59(3):278–290. doi:10.1057/palgrave.jors.2602368.
9. Viana J, Brailsford SC, Harindra V, Harper PR. Combining discrete-event simulation and system dynamics in a healthcare setting: A composite model for Chlamydia infection. *Eur J Oper Res.* 2014;237(1):196–206. doi:10.1016/j.ejor.2014.02.052.

10. Chahal K, Eldabi T, Mandal A. Understanding the impact of whiteboard on A&E department operations using hybrid simulation. *Proc 27th Int Conf Syst Dyn Soc.* 2009;(August 2015):1–19.

11. National Eye Institute. Facts About Age-Related Macular Degeneration. https://nei.nih.gov/health/maculardegen/armd_facts. Published 2015. Accessed September 14, 2018.

12. Lim LS, Mitchell P, Seddon JM, Holz FG, Wong TY. Age-related macular degeneration. *Lancet.* 2012;379(9827):1728–1738. doi:10.1016/S0140-6736(12)60282-7.

13. Wong WL, Su X, Li X, et al. Global prevalence of age-related macular degeneration and disease burden projection for 2020 and 2040: a systematic review and meta-analysis. *Lancet Glob Heal.* 2014;2(2):e106–e116. doi:10.1016/S2214-109X(13)70145-1.

14. Care Life Cycle Project. Researching the Supply and Demand of Health and Social Care Needs. www.southampton.ac.U.K./clc/. Published 2015. Accessed September 14, 2018.

15. Edmonds B, Moss S. From KISS to KIDS—An 'Anti-simplistic' Modelling Approach. In: Davidsson P, Logan B, Takadama K, eds. Lecture Notes in Computer Science. Springer; 2005:130–144.

16. Brailsford SC, Viana J, Rossiter S, Channon AA, Lotery AJ. Hybrid Simulation for Health and Social Care: The way forward, or more trouble than it's worth? In: Pasupathy R, Kim S-H, Tolk A, Hill R, Kuhl ME, eds. *2013 Winter Simulations Conference.* IEEE Press, Piscataway, NJ; 2013:258–269. doi:10.1109/WSC.2013.6721425.

17. Viana J. Reflections on two approaches to hybrid simulation in healthcare. In: Tolk A, Diallo SY, Ryzhov IO, et al., eds. *Proceedings of the 2014 Winter Simulation Conference.* IEEE Press, Piscataway, NJ; 2014:1585–1596. doi:10.1109/WSC.2014.7020173.

18. Viana J, Rossiter S, Channon AA, et al. A multi-paradigm, whole system view of health and social care for age-related macular degeneration. In: Laroque C, Himmelspach J, Pasupathy R, Rose O, Uhrmacher AM, eds. *Proceedings of the 2012 Winter Simulation Conference.* Vol 2020. IEEE Press, Piscataway, NJ; 2012:95.

19. Brailsford SC. Hybrid simulation in healthcare: New concepts and tools. In: Yilmaz L, Chan WK V., Moon I, Roeder TMK, Macal C, Rossetti MD, eds. *Proceedings of the 2015 Winter Simulation Conference.* IEEE Press, Piscataway, NJ; 2015.

20. Prince M. *World Alzheimer Report 2016: Improving Healthcare for People Living with Dementia; Coverage, Quality and Costs Now and in the Future.* London; 2016.

21. Borshchev A, Filippov A. From System Dynamics and Discrete Event to Practical Agent Based Modeling: Reasons, Techniques, Tools. In: *The 22nd International Conference of the System Dynamics Society.* System Dynamics Society; 2004.

22. Doody RS, Pavlik V, Massman P, Rountree S, Darby E, Chan W. Predicting progression of Alzheimer's disease. *Alzheimers Res Ther.* 2010;2(4):14. doi:10.1186/alzrt38.

23. Alzheimer's Society. *Dementia U.K.: Update.* London; 2014.

24. ONS. Mortality assumptions. National population projections: 2016-based projections, methodology. https://www.ons.gov.U.K./peoplepopulationandcommunity/populationandmigration/populationprojections/compendium/nationalpopulationprojections/2016basedprojections/mortalityassumptions. Published 2017. Accessed May 4, 2018.

25. Brayne C, Gao L, Dewey M, Matthews FE. Dementia before death in ageing societies—The promise of prevention and the reality. *PLoS Med.* 2006;3(10):1922–1930. doi:10.1371/journal.pmed.0030397.

26. Franco LA, Hämäläinen RP. Behavioural operational research: Returning to the roots of the OR profession. *Eur J Oper Res.* 2016;249(3):791–795. doi:10.1016/j.ejor.2015.10.034.

16

Validation of Microsimulation Models Used for Population Health Policy

FERNANDO ALARID-ESCUDERO, ROMAN GULATI, AND
CAROLYN M. RUTTER

16.1. OVERVIEW

This chapter discusses validation of simulation models used to inform health policy. We focus on microsimulation models that simulate the life histories of individual agents in discrete time, though many considerations discussed herein apply equally to systems dynamics, agent-based, and discrete-event models. Here the term *validation* means determining whether a model is sufficiently credible, accurate, and reliable to be used for its intended applications.[1-3] In short, can we trust the model?

There is no definitive one-size-fits-all criterion to decide whether a model is validated, but confidence in a model's validity can be weaker or stronger depending on several factors. These factors include verifying whether model specifications were implemented correctly, evaluating the extent to which model-predicted results are consistent with empirical results, and examining whether model predictions are robust to alternative structural assumptions. Transparent reporting of model implementation and a greater number (and higher quality) of comparison targets increases confidence, while an opaque summary or inadequate inspection of sensitivity to a model's structural assumptions decreases confidence. In general, greater scrutiny is necessary when empirical results are not or cannot be observed and when applications involve extrapolation to new settings or over longer time horizons.

Fernando Alarid-Escudero, Roman Gulati, and Carolyn M. Rutter, *Validation of Microsimulation Models Used for Population Health Policy* In: *Complex Systems and Population Health.* Edited by: Yorghos Apostolopoulos, Kristen Hassmiller Lich, and Michael Kenneth Lemke, Oxford University Press (2020). © Oxford University Press.
DOI: 10.1093/oso/9780190880743.003.0016

A common consideration underlying the assessment of factors that determine model validity is, *Does it make sense?* Is the model structure reasonable given our understanding of the disease or the effects of an intervention? Are the empirical data used to inform the model representative of the intended population or policy setting? Are model predictions consistent with clinical expectations, including plausible magnitudes of an intervention's harms and benefits? Ultimately, having confidence in a model's validity requires acceptance of data inputs and technical implementation, rigorous interrogation of structural features, demonstrated fidelity to empirically observed outcomes, and a general coherence of the model components to give scientifically grounded results.

This chapter examines common factors and considerations that can collectively be used to gauge the extent to which a model is validated for a given application. It reviews types of validation, discusses related concepts, takes a deeper dive into cancer model validation studies, and concludes with questions that consumers of models should ask (and modelers should answer) to inform judgment about a model's fitness for purpose. Final judgments about when model results can be trusted ultimately rely on the evolving understanding of the disease and intervention effects, available data relevant to the application, and access to reporting of model validation exercises.

16.2. TYPES OF VALIDATION

16.2.1. Face Validity

Face validity refers to whether the model and model predictions "make sense." This type of validity should be considered at every stage of model development and use, including conceptualization of the model, internal design and implementation, selection of empirical data used to estimate model parameters via model calibration, calibration algorithm, evaluation of nearness of predictions to their targets, and conclusions about the degree of success of a validation for a given application. A model has face validity when it passes the proverbial "smell test" at each stage.

16.2.2. Code Validity

Code validity refers to evaluation and error-checking of model code. Code validity can be facilitated by following best practices of software design, including version control systems to manage and archive the iterative development of source code and unit testing to identify and correct unexpected effects of changes to code. While many modelers who perform validations are not software engineers by training, best practices of programming should be learned and applied. Publicly available and open source code, and code that has been made available during peer review in scientific journals, generally lends greater confidence to a model's code validity. This type of validation is often referred to as model verification.[4-6]

16.2.3. Internal Validity

Evaluating internal validity is part of the model calibration process. Model calibration is the process of estimating the parameters of a microsimulation model by identifying parameter values that result in model predictions that are sufficiently near observed clinical or epidemiological data (often called calibration targets) according to a formal distance measure. Internal validation can be thought of as the model's goodness-of-fit to calibration targets because it quantifies the performance of model predictions, using parameter values selected via calibration, relative to the calibration targets.

16.2.3.1. CALIBRATION APPROACHES

There are many approaches to model calibration. Some approaches focus on identification of a single best parameter vector (i.e., a single vector of values for unknown parameters). These methods often use hill-climbing approaches, such as the Nelder-Mead algorithm for deterministic models[7] and simulated annealing or genetic algorithms for stochastic models. A set of parameter vectors may be identified when the calibration problem has more than one solution.[8] A best set of parameter vectors can also be chosen based on a χ^2 goodness-of-fit test, where parameter vectors are selected if they are not statistically different from the calibration targets.[9] The χ^2 statistic is the squared difference between model-predicted targets and calibration targets, divided by either the model-predicted or calibration targets with degrees of freedom based on the number of independent observations associated with each target.[10] The χ^2 goodness-of-fit test can only be used when the degrees of freedom exceed the number of calibrated parameters.

Bayesian calibration approaches focus on synthesizing prior information about model parameters, including expert opinion, and empirical evidence from calibration targets.[11-18] Bayesian approaches specify prior distributions for calibrated model parameters to characterize prior knowledge and distributions for observed calibration targets to characterize the uncertainty in these targets. Bayesian calibration yields a set of simulated draws from the posterior distribution of model parameters. The posterior distribution represents the joint distribution of the model parameters given prior information, calibration targets, and the assumed distribution of calibration targets. Bayesian approaches result in an estimated posterior distribution for model parameters. When the posterior distribution is approximately symmetric and unimodal, the estimated posterior mean vector, given by the average across simulated posterior draws, can provide a good single parameter vector. Bayesian model parameter estimation is more complicated when the posterior distribution is asymmetric or multimodal.

When calibration yields a single best parameter vector, internal validation can be based on the distance between the targets and corresponding predicted values. This may be summarized by the deviance statistic, which is defined as two times the negative log-likelihood,[19] or by the χ^2 statistic. Models that more closely fit the targets have smaller distance statistics. It is less clear how to internally validate models when calibration results in a set of parameter vectors. One approach is to summarize goodness-of-fit across the set based on the average and variation of goodness-of-fit statistics. Similar issues arise when Bayesian calibration approaches are used, but because the set of simulated draws represents a sample from the posterior distribution, it can be used to estimate posterior predicted distributions of calibration targets. While overall comparisons may focus on average predicted targets, measures of variation (e.g., standard deviations, interquartile ranges) and information about the distribution of predictions (e.g., using histograms) provide additional information about model behavior and fit. A common practice uses graphical comparisons of model predicted and observed calibration targets (e.g., see Rutter and Savarino, 2010[20]).

16.2.3.2. NONIDENTIFIABILITY

Nonidentifiability is an undesirable property of some statistical models and can be a common problem for complex models. Identifiability is a statistical concept that refers to the unique mapping of model parameters to model-predicted targets. When a model is nonidentifiable, multiple unique parameter vectors result in the same model predictions, so a single best parameter vector cannot be identified.[21] When multiple unique parameter vectors result in *similar* model predictions, the model is weakly identifiable. Because microsimulation model predictions are simulated and include stochastic variation, it can be difficult to distinguish between nonidentifiable and weakly identifiable models. Models may be nonidentifiable for one set of calibration targets and identifiable or weakly identifiable for a second set of targets. In this case, the model is overspecified relative to the first set of calibration targets (i.e., there are too many calibrated parameters) and can be resolved using the second set.

Nonidentifiability can also result from functional relationships among parameters, and in this case no amount of data will resolve the identifiability problem. In this case, nonidentifiability can also be resolved by simplifying the model by fixing or removing calibrated parameters. The presence of nonidentifiability poses a problem because different distinct parameter vectors can produce the same predictions but may imply different conclusions.[21] For example, a model that simulates colorectal cancer may calibrate well to data on both prevalence of adenomas (precursor lesions) and colorectal cancer incidence with well-identified parameters describing onset of preclinical disease. However, if the model fits equally well with both short and long sojourn times (also called preclinical screen-detectable periods), this indicates that sojourn time is not identifiable from these data. In this example, sojourn times may be identified through the addition of calibration targets, such as information about which cancers were detected by screening. However, if identifiability is not resolved, the parameter vector that produces longer sojourn times will predict less benefit for more frequent screening tests. Sensitivity analysis is important for parameters that are structurally important but are nonidentifiable.

16.2.4. External Validity

External validity refers to the comparison of model predictions with validation targets not used for calibration, without "tuning" the model's calibrated parameters. When carrying out external validation, other model inputs may be deterministically changed to match predicted targets (e.g., by using demographic or risk factor distributions that are consistent with the target population). External validation provides stronger evidence of how well the model would perform when applied to policy questions *because* the model has not been tuned to predict the validation targets. External validation addresses the potential for overfitting, which can be a problem with highly parameterized models. A complex model with many calibrated parameters can be calibrated to closely reproduce targets but may not perform well when externally validated or when used to evaluate policies or interventions that deviate from those used in the calibration setting.

Examples of external validation include simulating previously conducted trials or simulating cohorts or populations with known receipt of interventions. When model calibration results in a single best parameter vector, the model can be used to simulate a trial or population using a very large sample to drive down stochastic variation. Simulating many trials of the observed sample size can be used to determine if the model reproduces the sampling variability in the validation study. In the context of Bayesian calibration, validation should reflect the way the model is used. If the model is implemented using either the estimated posterior mean parameter vector (calculated by averaging across all the simulated draws from the posterior distribution), then validation can proceed using this single parameter. However, if the model is implemented using a set of simulated draws from the posterior distribution, then validation should replicate this process, with validation targets simulated for each draw and the model prediction based on the estimated posterior mean predicted value, given by the average across these model predictions. Because microsimulation models are highly nonlinear, these two approaches may result in different predictions.

16.2.5. Predictive Validity

Predictive validity is a type of external validation in which the model predictions are generated and archived before the target results are revealed. Because the true values are not known, predictive validity tests the model in a context similar to the settings for which the model was developed and used. For this reason, predictive validity provides the strongest evidence of model reliability.[22]

Predictive validations are uncommon. Once a high-quality study demonstrates that an intervention is effective, modeling may be considered to refine and personalize the intervention,[23] and in this case, the model development typically incorporates all relevant data including data from the original study. Consequently, in addition to the general challenges of external validation, predictive validations are further restricted by opportunity.

16.2.6. Comparative Validity

Comparative validity, or collaborative modeling, refers to comparison of model predictions across multiple models to targets that are either observed (such as disease incidence) or unobservable (such as sojourn time).[24,25] Fair comparison requires that the compared targets should be used in the same way across all models (i.e., as calibration targets or external validation targets). Comparative validity can provide insight into similarities and differences across models, although, unless models are compared to empirical validation targets, comparative validity cannot determine model veracity. Even models that perform differently from each other, or with varying success in terms of matching calibration targets can be valuable for some applications and may provide insights that are not otherwise available.[26]

16.3. VALIDATION TARGETS

As previously noted, calibration targets are used for estimating the model parameters and for internal validation. Targets not used for calibration could be used for external validation. Targets are generally summary statistics that are selected to represent features of processes described by the model that the model should be able to reproduce. For example, in models describing the natural history of colorectal cancer, calibration targets can include statistics describing the prevalence of adenomas, the size of detected adenomas, and incidence and mortality rates from cancer registries before and after the introduction of screening. Targets can depend on characteristics of the entire population or of particular subgroups captured by the model, such as age, gender, and race/ethnicity. Expert opinion can be used to identify high-quality targets.

Several factors need to be considered when selecting targets. One issue is whether the targets may be subject to biases, such as population bias or transferability bias.[27] Both biases arise when the sample used to derive the targets does not represent the target population that would be subject to policy recommendations. Population bias may occur when the sample is not a representative subset of the target population; for example, due to differences in age, sex, or health status. In some cases, it is possible to address population bias when simulating targets by using the model to simulate a similar population (e.g., by matching the age and sex distribution of the sample). In other cases, this may be more difficult to address; for example, if individuals who participate in clinical trials that produce targets are systematically different from the target population and these differences cannot be easily reproduced by the model.

Transferability bias may occur when information is taken from a sample of a population that is different from the population subject to policy recommendations;

for example, using data on cervical cancer incidence from a country where there is no screening and vaccination and using it as a calibration target for a model that will be used to inform policy in a country where there is screening in place. In summary, if there is a discrepancy between the sample informing the targets and the population of interest, the targets used for either calibration or validation may be biased. If there is information about how two populations differ, targets could be bias-corrected with quantitative bias analysis techniques.[28] In addition, care must be taken when using observational studies to inform microsimulation models. Observational studies may be subject to biases that result from confounding while microsimulation models specify causal pathways. Because it is generally difficult to simulate the mechanisms that cause bias in observational studies, the most direct approach to address this issue is to use statistical approaches to estimate causal effects from observational data.[29,30]

Because calibration involves simulation of targets for a potentially large number of parameter vectors, this condition requires the ability to efficiently simulate the data generating processes within the model. Because of this, studies with complex designs or that require simulation of bias corrections may be best suited for model validation, which requires simulation of targets for a single parameter vector or a limited set of parameter vectors.

16.4. EXTENDED EXAMPLES

16.4.1. Internal Validation Example

In a recent study, a simulation model of type-specific high-risk human papillomavirus (HPV)-induced cervical carcinogenesis was used to compare the cost-effectiveness of several cervical cancer screening strategies recommended in the United States after incorporating women's preferences throughout the screening process. The model of the natural history of cervical cancer was calibrated using a Bayesian approach to type-specific HPV prevalence, cervical cancer incidence, and proportion of cancers attributable to high-risk types, all stratified by age.

The model was internally validated by simulating all calibration targets at each parameter vector drawn from the posterior distribution of the calibrated parameters and by comparing both the posterior model-predicted means and uncertainty intervals to the calibration targets. The model-predicted targets matched the calibration targets closely, especially HPV prevalence and cervical cancer incidence, and provided a good insight into the reasonable fit to the proportion of different HPV types by age.[31]

16.4.2. External Validation Example 1

In 2016, the US Preventive Services Task Force recommended biennial mammography screening for breast cancer for women aged 50 to 74 and against regular screening for women aged 40 to 49.[32] The recommendation was based in part on projections from six cancer models that found screening women aged 40 to 49 would modestly reduce mortality but substantially increase false positive tests.[33] The recommendation was controversial, with fears about rationing healthcare stoked in national media and an unprecedented intervention by the US Congress to mandate that health insurance covers annual screening beginning at age 40.[34] While the scientific validity of the model projections was not the primary concern, the model-predicted results for younger women were externally validated only recently.[35]

In their recent validation study, five of the six cancer models predicted breast cancer incidence and mortality in the United Kingdom Age trial, which screened women aged 40 to 49 annually.[35] The models replicated the participant demographics and trial protocol but did not alter their model parameters, which were estimated via a synthesis of other data sources. As shown in Figure 16.1A, all five models predicted 17-year mortality rate ratios comparing the intervention and control groups, and all predictions were within the 95% confidence limits of the observed results. Based on these graphical and numerical assessments, the authors concluded that the models successfully recapitulated the benefit of screening in younger women, and hence the models could be trusted to inform screening guidelines for these ages.

Although this validation focused on comparing each model and the model average to external targets, the consistency across models also illustrates the models' comparative validity concerning the effectiveness of mammography screening in younger women.

16.4.3. External Validation Example 2

Three models for colorectal cancer have been used to inform screening policy for the US Preventive Services Task Force and for Centers for Medicare and Medicare Services. All three models include the development of adenomas, progression from adenoma to preclinical and clinical states, and risk of cancer-specific death. However, differences in data sources and low-level implementation details led to variable predictions about distributions of relative time spent in adenoma and preclinical states—differences with potentially clinically important implications concerning the benefit of more frequent screening in the population.

In a recent study, external validity of the three models was evaluated by assessing the performance of predicted effects of a one-time flexible sigmoidoscopy screening on 10-year colorectal incidence and mortality as studied in the UK Flexible Sigmoidoscopy Screening trial.[22] In addition to these primary endpoints, secondary endpoints, including cancer stage at diagnosis, location within the colon, and the breakdown of screen versus interval detections, were examined. All three models predicted effects of the intervention that were within the trial's 95% confidence interval for effects on mortality, and, as shown in Figure 16.1B, two of three models were within the 95% confidence interval for effects on incidence. The comparisons with the primary and secondary endpoints provided valuable

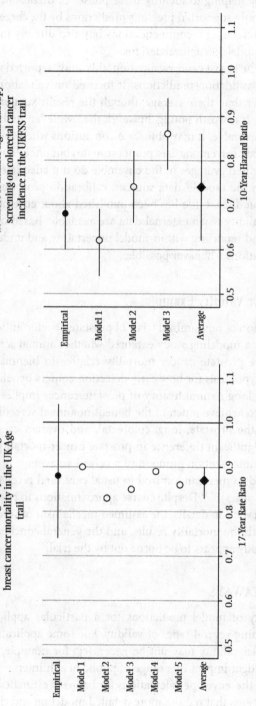

Figure 16.1 External and comparative validations of cancer interventions in microsimulation models. A: Effect of mammography screening on breast cancer mortality in the UK Age trial. B: Effect of flexible sigmoidoscopy screening on colorectal cancer incidence in the UKFSS trial.

insight into plausible distributions of the relative time spent in the adenoma and preclinical states. By helping to identify these phases of disease natural history, this validation not only supported previous predictions by the three models concerning colorectal screening recommendations but also directly indicated areas for improving the models' structural designs.

In contrast with the breast cancer validation, this study reported within-model uncertainty for the validation predictions. It focused on validation of the individual models rather than their average, though the results supported the value of model averaging. It is worth noting, however, that while "ensemble validation" may appear more favorable, it may obfuscate conclusions when there are outlier models, when comparison emphasizes point estimates but uncertainty is substantial, and when weighted averages of the ensemble do not adequately reflect variable uncertainty in the models' data sources, calibration procedures, or model parameters and structures. Little has been published about ensemble validation and comparative validity when external data are available. Based on our experience, we recommend reporting within-model uncertainty and undertaking individual model validations whenever possible.

16.4.4. Predictive Validity Example

Before the publication of randomized trials of prostate-specific antigen screening for prostate cancer, a modeling study explored whether annual screening might substantially reduce prostate cancer mortality relative to biennial screening.[36] Under a working hypothesis for how early detection confers benefit, the authors concluded that the long natural history of prostate cancer implies that biennial screening is likely to achieve much of the benefit of annual screening. A decade later, results from the prostate, lung, colorectal, and ovarian cancer screening trial reported no significant difference in prostate cancer mortality among men randomized to the intervention group (and received an average of 5.0 tests over six years) compared to men randomized to usual care (and received an average of 2.7 tests over six years).[37,38] Despite coarse approximations to population demographics and intervention details, the assumed mechanism of screening benefit was concordant with the mortality results, and the general conclusion predicted by the modeling study appears to be borne out by the trial.

16.5. KEY TAKEAWAYS

The overall validity of model predictions for a particular application can be assessed by examining several types of validity. For some applications, rigorous assessment of model validity may not be necessary; for example, an initial exploration of the budget impact of a range of public health interventions may require only back-of-the-envelope calculations for ballpark estimates. This chapter focused on applications that require more detailed modeling and rigorous model assessment; for example, clinical recommendations of an intervention with a

Table 16.1. KEY QUESTIONS THAT SHOULD BE ASKED BY CONSUMERS OF MODELS
AND ANSWERED BY MODELERS TO ASSESS VALIDITY OF A MICROSIMULATION
MODEL FOR A PARTICULAR APPLICATION

Question	Sample answers using example 1	Sample answers using example 2
What is the relevant application?	Effect of mammography screening of women aged 40–49 on long-term breast cancer mortality	Effect of flexible sigmoidoscopy on 10-year colorectal cancer incidence and mortality
What type of validation was done?	External and comparative	External and comparative
How reliable is the validation target?	High-quality randomized trial for appropriate ages and follow-up with well-documented protocol and adherence	High-quality randomized trial with well-documented protocol and adherence
How was the validation evaluated?	Numerical and graphical comparison of point estimates from each model (and their average) to empirical point estimate; of the point estimate from each model to the empirical interval estimate	Numerical and graphical comparison of point estimates from each model to empirical interval estimate; of rates in intervention and control arms; of disease stage, colon location, and mode of detection
How close was the evaluation?	Each model point estimate was within the 95% confidence interval of the empirical point estimate after 17 years	Each model point estimate was within the empirical 95% confidence interval for mortality after 10 years; 2 of 3 model point estimates were within the empirical 95% confidence interval for incidence after 10 years
What is the scope of the validation?	Validation does not necessarily extend to other patient age groups, screening modalities, clinical care settings, and follow-up horizons.	Validation does not necessarily extend to other patient populations, screening modalities, clinical care settings, and follow-up horizons.

modest net benefit that affects millions of individuals requires high confidence in
the accuracy of predictions.

Trust in results of a microsimulation model begins with face validity. Face
validity of the model design, implementation, and correspondence to outside
estimates is essential to the final assessment of model validity. If the model does

not comport with the known reality of the disease or the effects of interventions, or the results don't make sense, the model cannot be trusted for that application.

Trust in a model is further built through intensive scrutiny of model performance in settings similar to the intended application. Careful implementation—supported by best practices in programming, rigorously tested code, sensitivity analyses, and documented internal checks—is necessary but not sufficient to assess model validity for a given application. When possible, external validations that are performed using high-quality data are invaluable to demonstrating that the model adheres to empirical evidence. When external validation is not possible, such as when the outcome of interest (e.g., overdiagnosis) is not observable, comparative validation can provide insight into robustness of predicted outcomes to a range of model assumptions.

While there is no universal prescription for determining when a model has been validated for an application, it is possible to list common questions that consumers of models should ask—and that modelers should answer. These questions are given in Table 16.1 with sample answers using the external validation examples described in this chapter. At a minimum, determining answers to these questions can help consumers to identify the quality and scope of the validation. In practice, answering these questions may also help model consumers and modelers alike to identify gaps in the validation that were not addressed or discrepancies between the validation setting and the target application setting.

REFERENCES

1. Kopec JA, Fines P, Manuel DG, et al. Validation of population-based disease simulation models: a review of concepts and methods. *BMC Public Health*. 2010;10:710.
2. Eddy DM, Hollingworth W, Caro JJ, et al. Model transparency and validation: A report of the ISPOR-SMDM Modeling Good Research Practices Task Force-7. *Value Health*. 2012;15(6):843–850.
3. Vemer P, van Voom GA, Ramos IC, Krabbe PF, Al MJ, Feenstra TL. Improving model validation in health technology assessment: comments on guidelines of the ISPOR-SMDM Modeling Good Research Practices Task Force. *Value Health*. 2013;16(6):1106–1107.
4. Oberkampf WL, Trucano TG, Hirsch C. Verification, validation, and predictive capability in computational engineering and physics. *Appl Mech Rev*. 2004;57(5):345–384.
5. Oberkampf WL, Barone MF. Measures of agreement between computation and experiment: Validation metrics. *J Comput Phys*. 2006;217(1):5–36.
6. Frisch M. Calibration, validation, and confirmation. In: *Computer Simulation Validation*. Springer; 2019:981–1004.
7. Nelder J, Mead R. A simplex method for function minimization. *Comp J*. 1965;7:308–313.
8. Kong CY, McMahon PM, Gazelle GS. Calibration of disease simulation model using an engineering approach. *Value Health*. 2009;12(4):521–529.
9. Kim JJ, Kuntz KM, Stout NK, et al. Multiparameter calibration of a natural history model of cervical cancer. *Am J Epidemiol*. 2007;166(2):137–150.

10. DeGroot MH, Schervish MJ. *Probability and Statistics.* Pearson Education; 2012.

11. Rutter CM, Miglioretti DL, Savarino JE. Bayesian calibration of microsimulation models. *J Am Stat Assoc.* 2009;104(488):1338–1350.

12. Menzies NA, Soeteman DI, Pandya A, Kim JJ. Bayesian methods for calibrating health policy models: A tutorial. *Pharmacoeconomics.* 2017;35(6):613–624.

13. Whyte S, Walsh C, Chilcott J. Bayesian calibration of a natural history model with application to a population model for colorectal cancer. *Med Decis Making.* 2011;31(4):625–641.

14. Hawkins-Daarud A, Prudhomme S, van der Zee KG, Oden JT. Bayesian calibration, validation, and uncertainty quantification of diffuse interface models of tumor growth. *J Math Biol.* 2013;67(6-7):1457–1485.

15. Jackson CH, Jit M, Sharples LD, De Angelis D. Calibration of complex models through Bayesian evidence synthesis: a demonstration and tutorial. *Med Decis Making.* 2015;35(2):148–161.

16. Welton NJ, Ades A. Estimation of Markov chain transition probabilities and rates from fully and partially observed data: Uncertainty propagation, evidence synthesis, and model calibration. *Med Decis Making.* 2005;25(6):633–645.

17. Rutter C, Ozik J, DeYoreo M, Collier N. Microsimulation model calibration using incremental mixture approximate Bayesian computation. *Ann Appl Stat.* 2019; 13(4):2189–2212.

18. Bernardo JM, Smith AF. *Bayesian theory.* Volume 405 of Wiley Series in probability and Statictics. Wiley; 2009.

19. Czado C, Gneiting T, Held L. Predictive model assessment for count data. *Biometrics.* 2009;65(4):1254–1261.

20. Rutter CM, Savarino JE. An evidence-based microsimulation model for colorectal cancer: validation and application. *Cancer Epidem Biomar.* 2010;19(8):1992–2002.

21. Alarid-Escudero F, MacLehose RF, Peralta Y, Kuntz KM, Enns EA. Nonidentifiability in model calibration and implications for medical decision making. *Med Decis Making.* 2018;38(7):810–821.

22. Rutter CM, Knudsen AB, Marsh TL, et al. Validation of models used to inform colorectal cancer screening guidelines: Accuracy and implications. *Med Decis Making.* 2016;36(5):604–614.

23. Mant D. Can randomised trials inform clinical decisions about individual patients? *Lancet.* 1999;353(9154):743–746.

24. van Ballegooijen M, Rutter CM, Knudsen AB, et al. Clarifying differences in natural history between models of screening: The case of colorectal cancer. *Med Decis Making.* 2011;31(4):540–549.

25. Knudsen AB, Zauber AG, Rutter CM, et al. Estimation of benefits, burden, and harms of colorectal cancer screening strategies: Modeling study for the US Preventive Services Task Force. *JAMA.* 2016;315(23):2595–2609.

26. Kleindorfer GB, O'Neill L, Ganeshan R. Validation in simulation: Various positions in the philosophy of science. *Manage Sci.* 1998;44(8):1087–1099.

27. Turner RM, Spiegelhalter DJ, Smith GC, Thompson SG. Bias modelling in evidence synthesis. *J R Stat Soc Ser A Stat Soc.* 2009;172(1):21–47.

28. Lash TL, Fox MP, MacLehose RF, Maldonado G, McCandless LC, Greenland S. Good practices for quantitative bias analysis. *Int J Epidemiol.* 2014;43(6): 1969–1985.

29. Murray EJ, Robins JM, Seage III GR, et al. Using observational data to calibrate simulation models. *Med Decis Making.* 2018;38(2):212–224.

30. Murray EJ, Robins JM, Seage GR, Freedberg KA, Hernán MA. A comparison of agent-based models and the parametric g-formula for causal inference. *Am J Epidemiol.* 2017;186(2):131–142.

31. Sawaya GF, Sanstead E, Alarid-Escudero F, et al. Estimated quality of life and economic outcomes associated with 12 cervical cancer screening strategies: a cost-effectiveness analysis. *JAMA Intern Med.* 2019; 179(7):867–878.

32. Siu AL, Force USPST. Screening for breast cancer: U.S. Preventive Services Task Force Recommendation Statement. *Ann Intern Med.* 2016;164(4):279–296.

33. Berry DA, Cronin KA, Plevritis SK, et al. Effect of screening and adjuvant therapy on mortality from breast cancer. *N Engl J Med.* 2005;353(17):1784–1792.

34. Healy M. Breast cancer screening recommendations clarify science but muddy political waters. *Los Angeles Times.* https://www.latimes.com/science/sciencenow/la-sci-sn-breast-cancer-screening-recommendations-mammograms-20160111-story.html. Published January 11, 2016.

35. van den Broek JJ, van Ravesteyn NT, Mandelblatt JS, et al. Comparing CISNET breast cancer models using the maximum clinical incidence reduction methodology. *Med Decis Making.* 2018;38(1 Suppl):112S–125S.

36. Etzioni R, Cha R, Cowen ME. Serial prostate specific antigen screening for prostate cancer: A computer model evaluates competing strategies. *J Urol.* 1999;162:741–748.

37. Andriole GL, Crawford ED, Grubb RLr, et al. Mortality results from a randomized prostate-cancer screening trial. *N Engl J Med.* 2009;360:1310–1319.

38. Pinsky PF, Black A, Kramer BS, Miller A, Prorok PC, Berg C. Assessing contamination and compliance in the prostate component of the Prostate, Lung, Colorectal, and Ovarian (PLCO) cancer screening trial. *Clin Trials.* 2010;7(4):303–311.

17

Computational Simulation Modeling

A Tale of Five Models for Health Policy Analysis

MICHAEL C. WOLFSON

17.1. INTRODUCTION

There is an extensive and diverse literature on computer simulation models in population health and healthcare research. One way to characterize the variety is to array models along a spectrum from quite abstract, used more as a guide to intuition but with richly structured agents, to increasingly applied and "data-hungry" models focused on major real-world health policy challenges. In this chapter, I illustrate "model thinking" along this abstract to applied spectrum, with brief descriptions of five recent health simulation models.

The primary objectives of computer simulation models vary. Epstein[1] enumerates 17, of which prediction is only one and need not be the most important reason for building a model. Page[2] lists seven reasons summarized with the abbreviation REDCAPE: to reason, explain, design, communicate, act, predict, and explore some issue or phenomenon. In our sequence of illustrations, from abstract and/or relatively small (in terms of lines of code) to more detailed and intended for applied policy analysis, we describe each model's various objectives—why these models are useful.

All of the models have been developed for Canadian contexts and have been built using Statistics Canada's freely available ModGen (short for "model generator") language,[3] which, in turn, is an extension (actually a precompiler) for C++ code. They also all run using the new upward compatible open source cloud compatible successor to ModGen, openM.[4]

Michael C. Wolfson, *Computational Simulation Modeling* In: *Complex Systems and Population Health*. Edited by: Yorghos Apostolopoulos, Kristen Hassmiller Lich, and Michael Kenneth Lemke, Oxford University Press (2020).
© Oxford University Press. DOI: 10.1093/oso/9780190880743.003.0019

17.2. INCOME REDISTRIBUTION VIA PUBLICLY FUNDED HEALTH CARE

With Canada's single payer, tax-financed healthcare, one question is, How much does it redistribute income? The working age population tends to have higher incomes, pay more taxes, be healthier, and use less healthcare services than the elderly. So a careful cross-sectional calculation would likely show large amounts of redistribution when healthcare as an in-kind transfer is valued in monetary terms. But everyone, over their lifetime, passes through working age to old age (ignoring premature mortality). From a longitudinal or life-course perspective, then, healthcare can also be seen as redistributing income over an individual's life course, somewhat like a pension. From this perspective, healthcare likely redistributes income across income groups less than a cross-sectional analysis would show; the challenge was to quantify these two views of the extent of income redistribution.

To answer this question, we needed to construct a simulation model.[5,6] No model is necessary for the cross-sectional analysis, as all the required data can be obtained for a recent year. But there are no *lifetime* income, tax, and healthcare utilization data sitting on a shelf. It was necessary to simulate a set of full life-course trajectories of income, tax, and healthcare use, but with what kind of simulation model? We decided that a quite simple model would suffice –enough realism so the results have "face validity," but not so much detail that developing the model would be too costly or time-consuming.

Choosing simplifying assumptions when constructing a model is inevitably a matter of judgement, informed by intuition and experience. In this case, we looked at males and females together, divided the income range into deciles, ignored income mobility between deciles over the life course, and used the conventional period life table assumption of a steady state. At the same time, we did want to include the reality that higher income individuals live longer than poorer individuals.

Assembling the data on age- and income-specific average values of healthcare utilization and taxes involved considerable effort. Given these data, plus mortality rates by income and age, the model for lifetime redistribution could be written in fairly simple terms. Still, it was not so simple that a spreadsheet could easily have been built instead. It was simpler to "solve for" the extent of lifetime redistribution using Monte Carlo microsimulation. We randomly generated a million individuals, one-tenth in each income decile (with dollar levels varying by age group), exposed our synthetic individuals to age- and decile income-specific taxes and healthcare costs, and then mortality rates that varied by decile as well as age. In effect, the microsimulation was a numerical approximation to the implied set of integrals. The main conclusion from this modeling was that even though "healthcare redistributes from me to myself when I'm older," it still redistributes income in kind about twice as much across income deciles. This kind of result is impossible without simulation modeling.

17.3. THEORETICAL HEALTH INEQUALITY MODEL

The Theoretical Health Inequality Model (THIM)[7,8] evolved out of a special initiative funded by the US National Institutes of Health, with the growing appreciation that many problems in population health are "wicked"—involving a wide range of factors likely interacting nonlinearly, with a variety of feedbacks, and operating at many levels. This National Institutes of Health–funded "Network on Inequality, Complexity and Health" was premised on the idea that recent advances in complex systems theory could profitably be brought to bear in novel ways to understand the sources of population health inequalities and, ultimately, aid thinking about ways public policy might more effectively intervene to reduce them.

The Network brought together a diverse group of complex systems experts and social scientists, especially to use computer simulation modeling to frame and then explore various major pathways by which population health inequalities arise. Thus, in terms of Epstein's answers to "why model?" the main reason was to gain insight and understanding, to refine our intuition, and, in a word, to help "explain" the main sources of health inequalities. In terms of Page's REDCAPE, only "D = design" was not a significant objective.

Within the Network, several strands of explanation, and hence modeling, were pursued. In general, activity unfolded by a somewhat messy process of defining terms, framing a focal question or issue, and then elaborating in a kind of "box and arrow" or logic diagram manner the main constructs and their interrelationships.

In the case of THIM, the focus was on the unexplained yet remarkably different patterns for the relationship between cities' degree of income inequality and their age standardized mortality rates in Canada and the United States. In the United States, there is a clear correlation: higher city-level inequality is associated with higher mortality.[9,10] But in Canada, no corresponding correlation was observed. So, what was that different between Canada and the United States, causing such a basic relationship to disappear in Canada while being so pronounced in the United States?

One important hypothesis is that the United States has much more economic and racial segregation in its cities than Canada. But analytically, trying to probe such potential explanations for the observed differential pattern is very challenging, not least because the objects of analysis themselves, population joint distributions of income and mortality rates as well as cities and their neighborhoods, are complicated, and conceptually, there are numerous plausible causal pathways.

As a result, the best way to "think through" these complexities was to posit a set of relationships based on an "appreciation" of diverse strands of evidence, particularly a qualitative sense of the most important factors and the main causal pathways connecting them. Given this appreciation, THIM had to be dynamic to capture the co-evolution of key hypothesized factors over time. It also had to be multilevel to represent plausibly the hierarchy of relevant actors: individuals, families, neighborhoods, and cities. And it had to encompass a wide range of potential factors. Once a fairly simple set of diagrams showing these qualitative relationships was written down, it was clear that no analytically tractable mathematical model would suffice. Thus, THIM needed to be incarnated via computer simulation, though its formalization should be as simple as possible that it not be too costly to build, and to facilitate describing the model to others.

In the process of framing THIM, we ignored data availability to start. Instead, we focused on major factors where there was at least some clear empirical evidence in the literature that they mattered. As a result, the model was built on only a small number of variables or processes: parent to child transmission of educational and future income prospects, the impact of education on subsequent income, the impact of income on health and mortality, neighborhood sorting based on income, and the reciprocal effects of neighborhood income on individuals' education quality and income prospects.

Moreover, we had to allow agents to be heterogeneous. Assuming an average or "representative agent" would completely preclude any analysis of inequalities. So too would assuming that heterogeneities followed some a priori functional form. Further, and notwithstanding the small number of variables, all of which are clearly important, the individual agents needed to interact not only with each other, but hierarchically in the multiple levels of family, neighborhood, and then city. These interactions and multilevel feedbacks, plus agent heterogeneity, were all too involved to think through and derive their implications without some sort of mental help—a model.

At the same time, THIM was entering new territory since it was putting together, into a single analytical framework, dynamic relationships for which there was only fragmentary empirical evidence. This paucity of data was another reason THIM was made as simple as possible—subject to a lower limit in terms of maintaining "requisite complexity" (to adapt Hal Ashby's phrase "requisite variety" in cybernetics[11]). The model still had to include for each individual agent its education, income, health status, and location and to represent these within a hierarchy of individual, family, neighborhood, and city. THIM is therefore a semitheoretical model: abstract but informed by a fairly extensive range of empirically based "stylized facts."

Colleagues in the Network believed that the main reason for the observed difference in the inequality–mortality patterns in Canada and the United States was much greater racial segregation in the United States. As a result, much effort was spent trying to reproduce the observed Canada–US differences by exploring the parameters defining agents' income sorting across neighborhoods. However, this failed. Finally, we switched focus to the clear differences between Canada and the United States in other factors, especially Canada's significantly greater intergenerational income mobility,[12] the wider socioeconomic status gaps in US public education,[13] and the more highly fragmented governance structures in US cities. This change in perspective finally enabled THIM to succeed in reproducing the observed difference in income inequality–mortality rate correlations. Of course, it has no claims to uniqueness in this regard.

Thus, THIM has served the primary simulation modeling purpose of informing intuition and aiding explanation. In so doing, it has also generated hypotheses, but whose testing will require the collection of new data (e.g., more detailed and comparable information on neighborhoods within cities). And it has pointed to a possibly major public health intervention—municipal and school board amalgamation, which is much more extensive in Canada than in the United States—as a key but unappreciated factor in reducing population health inequalities.

17.4. HEALTHPATHS MODEL

In addition to explanation, Epstein[1] also points to computer simulation modeling as a means to challenge conventional wisdom on the relative quantitative importance of a range of competing factors. The health domain has been dominated for a century by the biomedical perspective, which has been remarkably successful in leading to treatments of infectious disease and, most recently, to deepening understanding of genetic predispositions. But the biomedical perspective generally fails to help understand the distribution of the "vernacular" burden of ill health. For example, heart disease (a biomedical construct) can range from being asymptomatic to causing pain, shortness of breath, and severe mobility impairments—vernacular or functional health status characteristics.

Another effect of the dominance of the biomedical perspective is that by far the most ubiquitous measures of population health status are based on mortality data coded by biomedically defined causes of death. It is only in the past several decades that reliable population health surveys have been fielded that collect data on functional health status (e.g., limitations in mobility, cognition, vision, and experiencing chronic pain). Correspondingly, much of modern epidemiology focuses on the major causes of death—heart disease and cancer—and their major risk factors (e.g., smoking and obesity).

But when we shift our focus from biomedically defined disease to functional health limitations, a fundamental question arises: whether we will see significant changes in the relative importance of different kinds of population health problems. For example, Manuel et al.[14] showed that when health-adjusted life expectancy (HALE; where functional limitations are considered explicitly) was used instead of simple life expectancy (LE; where variations in health status while alive are completely ignored) as the measure of population health, the most burdensome health problems for women were (generally nonfatal) musculoskeletal (e.g., arthritis), not cancer or heart disease, even though these are at the top of the cause-deleted LE league table.

To explore this question more deeply, model thinking is needed. We need an appropriate population health metric, where HALE is the obvious choice. We also need to generalize the ideas of cause-deleted life tables and attributable fractions to the explicit construction of counterfactuals—what would HALE be in the absence of health factor X? There are too many things going on to do this without mental assistance. To this end, we have been developing the HealthPaths computer simulation model.[15] The objective has been to build on and extend Manuel et al's[14] earlier analysis to provide more extensive and detailed estimates of the relative importance of factors influencing population health.

Another objective has been to transcend the conventional methods for estimating an attributable fraction. In general, it is a measure of the extent to which a disease or health problem (e.g., lung cancer) is attributable to a casual factor (e.g., smoking). However, such estimates require, albeit often implicitly, the construction of a counterfactual—for example, how much lung cancer mortality would there be in a given population if no one ever smoked? But such counterfactuals require a causal story, and typically these stories completely ignore multifactorial causal pathways and population heterogeneity.

On the other hand, with a computer simulation model, it is possible to have much richer and empirically based causal stories, and use the simulation model (rather than simplistic mathematical formulae) to construct the counterfactual explicitly. The intent with HealthPaths is to provide information of the same caliber as any high-quality observational study in epidemiology—with the main difference being that the inferences go well beyond characterizing a single relationship and the "dependent variable" is a multivariate construct, HALE for a heterogeneous population.

Achieving these objectives has entailed a different simulation modeling strategy than for THIM. HealthPaths, from a theoretical perspective, is simpler than THIM since there are no interacting agents nor multiple levels. Still both THIM and HealthPaths are "microsimulation" models, since the object of analysis or agent is the individual, rather than groups or "average" individuals. In both cases, it is critical to be able to capture agents' heterogeneity—representing explicitly the actual (joint) distributions of their characteristics or state space variables.

HealthPaths' architecture simulates one individual's full life course at a time, from birth to death, and then moves on to synthesize another individual's biography from birth to death, and so on until millions of individuals, constituting a realistic birth cohort, have been simulated—albeit without any agent interaction. Further, each simulated individual is unique in order that the full dispersion in the multivariate joint distributions of their characteristics can be realistically represented.

As a result, empirically, HealthPaths is far more detailed than THIM, though it is based on only one major longitudinal data set, Canada's National Population Health Survey (NPHS).[16]

A key feature of HealthPaths has been the tight coupling between the empirical analysis of the NPHS and the structure of the simulation model. Often in empirical health analysis, the focus is on a single dependent variable, and the statistical significance, signs, and magnitudes of the coefficients in a regression. One advantage of this approach is that it lends itself to a conventional 20-page paper that can be published as an academic journal article. For HealthPaths, however, this relatively simple approach is insufficient, since individual characteristics co-evolve. For example, the NPHS data clearly show that smoking changes not only with age, but also with educational attainment and later disease onset.

The NPHS analysis underlying the HealthPaths model therefore has involved the simultaneous joint estimation of individual-level transition probability density functions, where the dependent variable in one hazard regression is an independent variable in another. The variables estimated include both functional health status (e.g., vision, mobility, cognition, pain), conventional risk factors (e.g., smoking, obesity), psycho-social factors (e.g., Antonovsky's Sense of Coherence[17]), and socioeconomic factors (e.g., income, education, employment)—over 20 individual-level characteristics. This statistical analysis was designed from the start to feed into a simulation model. This meant that much more open and intensive regressions could be explored. As a result, HealthPaths is based on thousands of elastic net regressions (i.e., weighted averages of ridge and lasso specifications) using out-of-sample prediction errors as the objective (rather than more conventional goodness-of-fit criteria) and incorporating bootstrapping for both coefficient and specification error distributions.

The findings have indeed been provocative. In the case of smoking, HealthPaths simulations of LE and HALE indicate attributable fractions (based on the full richness of the HealthPaths estimated multifactorial causal story) both of a bit under a year of life. But for sensory (vision, hearing, speech, pain) and mental (sense of coherence, mastery, emotion, cognition) conditions, the attributable fractions shift dramatically from about one year for LE to about six years for HALE.

17.5. GENETIC MIXING MODEL

Another major objective of computer simulation modeling is to infer data that do not exist and are unlikely to be available for many years. The Genetic Mixing Model (GMM)[18] has been developed as part of a larger project to assess the prospective cost-effectiveness of changing the way breast cancer screening is organized in Canada. At present, most screening is based solely on a woman's age, typically starting at age 50. However, it has been known for many years that a woman with a family history of breast cancer will herself be at higher risk. Further, genetic mutations that greatly increase the risk of breast cancer, especially in younger women, have been known for several decades. More recently, a large number of smaller genetic variations (single nucleotide polymorphisms [SNPs]) have been discovered. These SNPs, individually, increase a woman's risk of breast cancer only slightly. But when dozens or hundreds of SNPs are combined into a polygenic risk core (PRS), this aspect of a woman's genotype becomes much more reliably predictive of her breast cancer risk.[19]

To assess whether it would be cost-effective to shift public health programs in Canada from primarily age-based to risk-based breast cancer screening, it is necessary to build a computer simulation model. Fortunately, the Canadian Partnership Against Cancer has already led the development of the OncoSim-BC breast cancer model.[20] However, this model had no capacity for assessing policy scenarios where breast cancer screening programs would be based on women's genetic risk profiles. The GMM has been designed and built to meet this need.

To stratify women for breast cancer screening conditional on their individual level of risk, it is necessary to have data on the multivariate joint distribution of genotypes and family history for a representative population sample. However, no such data exist, nor are they likely to exist in the near to medium term, as it would be far too expensive (and intrusive) to collect such data. GMM was therefore designed and built to infer, as best as possible, the needed multivariate joint distribution.

To accomplish this inference, GMM is an interacting agent model, like THIM, but empirically grounded like HealthPaths. In this case, the agents are men and women who conceive and give birth to offspring who are, in turn, followed over multiple generations. GMM starts with a population of millions of individuals who are initially randomly assigned sex and age in a way that represents the current population. These individuals in the starting sample are also given an initial independent random distribution of genotypes—both for rare variant mutations and the PRS. In this area, the data are limited since they come from collections of dozens of clinical and research studies, where none of the studies' samples were necessarily population representative.

GMM then simulates individuals forming unions and giving birth to children based on detailed demographic data on union formation and dissolution transition probabilities and on age- and parity-specific fertility rates, where the children's genetic endowments are based on those of their parents' using standard genetics including well-known Mendelian inheritance. Further, based on age- and genotype-specific risks, women are simulated to have incident breast cancers.

The result, after 200+ years (albeit with a steady-state assumption for all the demographic dynamics), is a population sample where it is possible (since the simulation model retains pointers to all biological relatives) to construct full first- and second-degree family histories of breast cancer for each woman in the simulated population. GMM has therefore constructed (inferred) an approximately representative population sample of a biologically reasonable trivariate joint distribution of rare genetic variants, polygenic risk scores, and family histories.

GMM is being incorporated into the broader OncoSim-BC model to assess the comparative cost-effectiveness of various scenarios for risk- rather than age-based breast cancer screening. These evaluations involve many questions. For example, at what age should risk be assessed? And above what threshold of risk should more intensive breast cancer screening be provided? Preliminary results suggest that for population health policy (as compared to individual clinical assessments), knowing the PRS is much more valuable than knowing the patient's family history, or whether she has a rare genetic mutation.

17.6. LIFEPATHS MODEL

LifePaths,[21-26] like GMM, is a policy-oriented computer simulation model, focused on income security-related policies.

In terms of its design and architecture, along the abstract to applied spectrum noted at the outset, LifePaths is very much at the applied end. It uses mostly a noninteracting agent approach, like HealthPaths. The only interactions among agents are that for each "core" individual in a simulation, spouses (there may be more than one) and children are also simulated in order to have information on the complete nuclear family structure at each moment over an individual's full life course.

LifePaths goes beyond HealthPaths in its breadth. It simulates multiple birth cohorts, extending back to the 1890s, to ensure that today's elderly are included. It also includes a much wider range of variables in each individual's biography— education, labor market participation, incomes, savings, home ownership, private pensions, disability, public pensions, income and payroll taxes, and utilization of long-term care (LTC).

The main reasons for this breadth of variables are first that they are all important components of the main results of interest, such as what the standard of living of the future elderly will be, how will it be distributed by various socio-economic characteristics (e.g., family type, education, and disability), and how it compares to their standards of living before retirement during their working years (the "net replacement rate").

Second, this range of variables is necessary for the model to be empirically reasonable. For example, one-at-a-time longitudinal statistical analysis shows clearly that educational attainment depends on fertility history and labor market experience, while at the same time another statistical analysis shows that labor market experience depends on educational attainment, fertility history, and nuptiality. As in the HealthPaths model, there is ample evidence that these characteristics co-evolve at the individual level.

The LifePaths microsimulation model also serves as an extensible modeling platform. Its demographic core and earnings module provide the foundation for the previously discussed OncoSim-BC breast cancer model. Most recently, LifePaths is being used for a major policy-oriented study of the implications of population aging on the future needs for LTC (both nursing homes and home care). For this analysis, it is necessary to encompass both economics (e.g., affordability), health status (disability severity), and public policy options for the provision of LTC. This extension of LifePaths has been developed to project the government budgets needed to fund the publicly paid portions of LTC, as well as the distributions of individual-level costs and informal care hours for the privately borne portions.

17.7. GENERAL LESSONS

There is a tremendous amount of art and judgment embodied in the construction of a simulation model. All the models discussed in this chapter are dynamic; there is a time dimension and the agents' histories unfold over simulated time. These dynamics are essential given the reasons for the development of all the models.

But a model cannot do everything; to be feasible, simplifying assumptions are essential. The main question is where to simplify or abstract away from something, versus where to retain the requisite complexity. For example, sex is ignored completely in the first two models. THIM is the most elaborate of the models in terms of its multiple levels, but this was essential given the question it was designed to address.

Many economists would consider the omission in LifePaths of a macroeconomy level with feedbacks in areas like the labor market a serious concern. Such joint micro/macro models have been built, and development in this direction may be worthwhile. In this case, though, the choice of direction should be dependent on the amount of resources available, and judgments as to the areas of greatest remaining weakness regarding the reasons for which the model was built. For LifePaths, many of these macroeconomic concerns can be addressed by sensitivity analysis to the macroeconomic assumptions.[27]

How behavior is represented in these simulation models raises perhaps the most interesting questions. Some economists have criticized LifePaths-type models for their omission of "behavioral response." However, the multivariate transition probability density functions underlying individual-level dynamics, especially in HealthPaths and LifePaths, are empirical distillations of observed dynamic behavioral response patterns. For example, as educational attainment changes, smoking may change in HealthPaths, and labor market behavior may change in LifePaths. Still, agents in all the models described do not behave in ways determined by either neoclassical economics-style utility maximization or by more realistic satisficing represented by rules of thumb. Adding these kinds of behavioral response capabilities is an area for future research.

In sum, we have illustrated a range of "model thinking" by relating it to the varying objectives of five different simulation models, starting with a comparison of the cross-section versus lifecycle redistributive impact of Canada's universal healthcare. For THIM, the objective is a deeper understanding of the sources of differences in health inequalities between Canada and the United States via explicit and quantitatively plausible theorizing. GMM is an example of using model thinking to fill in a major gap in the available data by inferring the multivariate joint distribution of genetic profiles. The modeling objective with HealthPaths has been shedding new light on the relative importance of different vernacular health determinants and, indeed, upsetting the conventional wisdom that puts heart disease and cancer at the top of the league table of health problems. Finally, LifePaths illustrates how modeling can be central to supporting applied public policy analysis of retirement income adequacy and provision of LTC.

REFERENCES

1. Epstein JM. Why model? *J Artif Society Soc Simul.* 2008;11(4):12–16.
2. Page SE. *The Model Thinker.* New York, NY: Basic Books; 2018.
3. Statistics Canada. Modgen (Model generator). https://www.statcan.gc.ca/eng/microsimulation/modgen/modgen. Published 2017. Accessed August 12, 2019.
4. OpenM++: open source microsimulation platform. https://ompp.sourceforge.io/wiki/index.php/Main_Page. Published 2019. Accessed August 12, 2019.
5. Wolfson M, Corscadden L. Does public health care redistribute from me to you, or just to myself when I'm old? On the Lifetime Redistributive Impact of Publicly Financed Health Care in Canada. Biennial Meeting of the International Association for Research in Income and Wealth; 2014; Rotterdam, Netherlands.

6. Corscadden L, Allin S, Wolfson M, Grignon M. Publicly financed healthcare and income inequality in Canada. *Healthc Q.* 2014;17(2):7–10.

7. Wolfson MC, Beall RF. Contingent inequalities: An exploration of health inequalities in the United States and Canada. In: Kaplan GA, Diez Roux AV, Simon CP, Galea S, eds. *Growing Inequality: Bridging Complex Systems, Population Health, and Health Disparities.* Washington, DC: Westphalia Press; 2017.

8. Wolfson M, Gribble S, Beall R. Exploring contingent inequalities: Building the theoretical health inequality model. In: van Bavel J, Grow A, eds. *Agent-Based Modelling in Population Studies.* New York NY: Springer; 2017:487–513.

9. Wolfson M, Kaplan G, Lynch J, et al. Relation between income inequality and mortality: Empirical demonstration *BMJ.* 1999;319(7215):953–957.

10. Ross NA, Dorling D, Dunn JR, et al. Metropolitan scale relationship between income inequality and mortality in five countries using comparable data. *J Urban Health.* 2005;82:101–110.

11. Ashby WR. Requisite variety and its implications for the control of complex systems. *Cybernetica.* 1991;1(2):83–99.

12. Corak M. Income inequality, equality of opportunity, and intergenerational mobility. *J Econ Perspect.* 2013;27(3):79–102.

13. Programme for International Student Assessment. Data base—PISA. https://www.oecd.org/pisa/data/pisa2012database-downloadabledata.htm. Published 2012. Accessed August 12, 2019.

14. Manuel DG, Luo W, Ugnat A-M, Mao Y. Cause-deleted health-adjusted life expectancy of Canadians with selected chronic conditions. *Chronic Dis Inj Can.* 2003;24(4):108.

15. Wolfson MC, Rowe G. The relative importance of socioeconomic status and other major factors for population health: Estimates using the Healthpaths agen-tbased microsimulation model. In: Kaplan GA, Diez Roux AV, Simon CP, Galea S, eds. *Growing Inequality: Bridging Complex Systems, Population Health, and Health Disparities.* Washington, D.C.: Westphalia Press; 2017.

16. Statistics Canada. National Population Health Survey Overview, 1996/7. https://www150.statcan.gc.ca/n1/pub/82-567-x/82-567-x1997001-eng.pdf. Published 1998. Accessed February 14, 2012.

17. Antonovsky A. The structure and properties of the sense of coherence scale. *Soc Sci Med.* 1993;36(6):725–733.

18. Wolfson M, Gribble S, Pashayan N, et al. Potential of polygenic risk scores for improving population estimates of breast cancer genetic risks. Under review.

19. Mavaddat N, Michailidou K, Dennis J, et al. Polygenic risk scores for prediction of breast cancer and breast cancer subtypes. *Am J Human Genet.* 2019;104(1):21–34.

20. Gauvreau CL, Fitzgerald NR, Memon S, et al. The OncoSim model: Development and use for better decision-making in Canadian cancer control. *Curr Oncol.* 2017;24(6):401–406.

21. Wolfson M. Sketching LifePaths: A new framework for socio-economic statistics. In: Conte R, Hegselmann R, Terna P, eds. *Simulating Social Phenomena.* New York, NY: Springer; 1997:521–527.

22. Fellegi I, Wolfson M. Towards systems of social statistics: Some principles and their application in Statistics Canada. *J Official Statist.* 1999;15(3):373–393.

23. Wolfson M. Not-so-modest options for expanding the CPP/QPP. Montreal, QC: Institute for Research on Public Policy; 2013.

24. Wolfson M, Rowe G. Perspectives on working time over the life cycle. In: Houseman S, Nakamura A, eds. *Working Time in Comparative Perspective: Volume II—Life-Cycle Working Time and Nonstandard Work*. Kalamazoo, MI: Upjohn Press; 2001:43–71.

25. MacDonald B-J, Moore KD, Chen H, Brown RL. The Canadian National Retirement Risk Index: Employing statistics Canada's LifePaths to measure the financial security of future Canadian seniors. Can Pub Pol. 2011;37(Suppl 1):S73–S94.

26. Légaré J, Décarie Y. Using Statistics Canada LifePaths microsimulation model to project the disability status of Canadian elderly. *Int J Microsimul*. 2011;4(3):48–56.

27. Wolfson M, Rowe G. Aging and inter-generational fairness: A Canadian analysis. In: Lambert PJ, ed. *Equity Research on Economic Inequality*. Bingley, UK: Emerald Group; 2007:197–231.

Physical Sciences for Nonphysical Problems

Understanding and Controlling Human Disease

LAZAROS K. GALLOS

18.1. INTRODUCTION: USING STATISTICAL PHYSICS TOOLS TO STUDY HUMAN DISEASE

Noncommunicable diseases (NCDs), such as heart disease, stroke, diabetes, and cancer, are responsible for the death of 41 million people each year, corresponding to 71% of all deaths globally.[1] The lack of infectious agents makes NCDs seem a highly individual and atom-centric problem, since there is no obvious mechanism to transfer these diseases between two people—with the exception of genetic inheritance. On the contrary, many of these diseases are considered largely preventable by appropriate personal or societal choices and actions, such as healthier eating, lower environmental pollution, or less stressful work environments. A naïve approach would then classify this as a problem of personal and social accountability where individuals and societies are responsible for their actions and decisions in vacuum.

How then can we explain the numerous observations that NCDs do not appear uniformly across a population, but follow patterns that are strongly reminiscent of infectious diseases? The obvious answer is the existence of many external factors that directly or indirectly influence choices and actions related to NCDs. For example, peer pressure through social networks, environmental global effects, and marketing systems that influence decisions can all significantly affect the probability that an individual is exposed to NCD risks. In broad terms, the main drivers of NCDs can be seen as a combination of personal traits, interpersonal influences, and global forces acting upon entire populations. This system of individuals with

Lazaros K. Gallos, *Physical Sciences for Nonphysical Problems* In: *Complex Systems and Population Health*. Edited by: Yorghos Apostolopoulos, Kristen Hassmiller Lich, and Michael Kenneth Lemke, Oxford University Press (2020).

complicated internal interactions and external influences is a typical example of a *complex system* in statistical physics (see also Chapters 2 and 3 of this volume).

An obvious objection to using physics methods for population health problems is that matter is always bound by physical laws, but people can think and act according to their own volition. For example, any family can decide whether or not to vaccinate their kids. This may feel like a strictly personal choice, but in practice this decision was based on input from friends, media, the Internet, etc. Many other people receive similar information (which already includes interaction with a large number of people), and they have to make similar decisions. At the population level, the actions of one individual will have little to no impact, but collectively these events will shape the global behavior. The individuality is still incorporated in the majority of the complex system models via probabilistic rather than deterministic actions. In other words, even if we know that, for example, 30% of the population are smokers, we cannot predict with certainty if any single individual is a smoker.

In this view, to begin understanding NCDs in a population, we need to understand how people are connected to each other, how they interact with each other, and if there are external influences. In other words, we need to consider a complex system that includes, among others, social interactions, opinion dynamic processes, personal preferences, and external global influences such as state policies or advertising campaigns, cognitive processes, etc. Each of these processes can be studied as separate complex systems on their own,[2] so it is a big challenge to consider the simultaneous action of all of these forces.

The traditional approach in studying NCDs is based on statistical methods that attempt to isolate one macroscopic factor and use statistical analysis to determine if there is a measurable effect on a quantity of interest. For example, the dietary patterns in a sample of people with diabetes will be compared to the dietary patterns in a sample of healthy people. In practice, these approaches can only detect interactions among macroscopic variables and not among individuals, and any correlations that are found between variables may not be easily translated into causal mechanisms. Additionally, the population itself is considered as one body without any local structure. For example, social connectivity is not taken into account and as a result there are no discernible paths of social influence. Under this light, the problem with traditional methods is mainly conceptual and not methodological. If we hope to understand how global behavior emerges from interactions at the individual level, we need a paradigm shift to where NCDs in a population represent the result of emergent behavior in a complex system.

We can translate a wide variety of problems related to NCDs in statistical physics language. There are four main questions to consider when building such a model system:

    (a) What is the basic unit of the system? Given the abundance of data today, in most cases the basic unit is an individual, but it can also be local neighborhoods, organizations, countries, etc.

(b) How are the units connected with each other? The assumption is that individuals can only be connected with a limited fraction of the population. These connections may represent their neighbors, their relatives, people they come in proximity during the day in mass transportation, people with similar ideas, or any other type of connection that can be relevant for the given study.

(c) What is the form of interactions between the units? These interactions only act along existing connections, and the exact mechanism is defined according to the problem studied. A simple rule, for example, is "pass any new information you acquire to half of your connections." More than one type of interaction may be acting at the same time.

(d) What are the external influences? These are external forces that can impact a large portion of the population at the same time. Typical examples are news or advertisements broadcasted in mass media that can influence many individuals, independently of interpersonal interactions or government policies, and, ultimately, affect population consumption and health. This approach allows for a direct study of various social mechanisms and can also be used to examine many intervention scenarios, such as how different policies targeting specific parts of the population may modify the global response.

This chapter reviews many of the fundamental concepts and methods in statistical physics that can be readily applied to population health research. The reader does not need any prior knowledge of complex systems, and there is no mathematical background required to follow the text. However, given the concise character of the chapter most ideas are presented in a simplified way. The interested reader should consult the Resources for Further Reading at the end of this section of the book and the broader literature for further information.

18.2. PHASE TRANSITIONS

A *phase transition* in physics is the change of state in a system. How is this physical process relevant to understanding NCDs? We can treat changes in obesity prevalence as a complex system undergoing a transition from a "healthy" state to an "unhealthy" state, or vice versa. This idea can describe how processes evolve in social, political, or economic settings, to mention just a few.

There are two main quantities needed to characterize a phase transition (see also Chapter 5 of this volume): the *control parameter*, which we can tune at will, and the *order parameter*, which provides a measure of order/disorder. In a social system, the control parameter may refer to incentives, such as the expected reward for a given action, while the order parameter characterizes the overall state of the system for a given value of the control parameter, such as obesity prevalence.

The change in the system occurs when the control parameter reaches *a critical value* or *critical threshold*. If this change is permanent and irreversible then this point is called a *tipping point*.

There are two main transition types, *first-order* (abrupt transitions) and *second-order* (continuous transitions). It is important to know the type of transition because they have different properties and they require a different approach for control. In practice, most transitions are second-order.

Phase transitions are of paramount importance in complex systems. If we know the critical threshold and the type of transition, we can potentially understand the necessary conditions that can drive a population system from low disease prevalence to high disease prevalence. If we are convinced that such a system undergoes a first-order transition, then it may be difficult to determine early signals that the system moves toward that direction and protection may be more difficult compared to the gradual increase observed in second-order transitions.

18.3. PERCOLATION

Percolation is a process that can model phase transitions and provides an intuitive way to understand key underlying mechanisms. There are numerous studies where percolation is used in different contexts to interpret social or physical phenomena, among others, and it can be useful to build models of how diseases evolve or how opinions spread in a given population.

Consider an empty square lattice, such as a checkerboard, where every site connects to its four immediate neighbors. Each node in this site can be in one of two states, "blue" or "red," and initially all nodes are in the blue state. We select a random percentage, p, of these nodes and switch them to the red state. If p is large enough then some of the red nodes will be next to each other, and they will start forming clusters. Our main question is whether the largest cluster formed by red nodes at a given p value "percolates"—that is, if we can reach one side of the lattice from the other side by staying on red nodes only. Intuitively, if p is very small (e.g., 1%), then there are very few red nodes, and they are spread all over the lattice so that the largest cluster is negligible (*subcritical* phase). On the contrary, a large fraction of nodes (e.g., 90%) would guarantee that the largest cluster percolates (*supercritical* phase). It is natural then that at some intermediate point in this interval (the approximate percolation threshold in this case has been shown to be 59%) the system undergoes a phase transition from small size clusters to one spanning cluster that absorbs all the smallest ones (*critical* phase). This process describes a phase transition where our control parameter, the fraction of red nodes p, controls our order parameter, which is the size of the largest cluster—or, more accurately, the percentage of existing red nodes that belong to the largest cluster.

In the subcritical phase, only small and localized red islands exist. As the percentage of red nodes increases, these islands start growing in size but still remain isolated. At exactly the critical point, the majority of these islands merge into one large component, which then absorbs almost all red nodes for higher values of p in the supercritical phase.

The importance of percolation for practical applications can be seen through the following example. If the lattice nodes correspond to individuals in a population, then the lattice connections represent personal contacts that allow infectious disease spreading. Initially, all nodes are susceptible to the disease (blue state). When a node is immunized it can no longer be infected, so it turns to the red state. What percentage of the population needs to be immunized to guarantee immunity? Using the critical percolation value, we know that, if we immunize at least 59% of the population, there is a spanning cluster that covers the entire population. Viruses can travel only through blue (unvaccinated) areas, which means that any outbreaks will remain localized in the population of the small blue islands, surrounded by red areas where the virus cannot penetrate.

There is an enormous number of variations on this idea, such as opinion spreading, message passing, monetary transactions, exchange of goods or rumors, etc. A percolating state would indicate that there is a prevalent opinion while the opposite opinion is largely suppressed, but when a system is on or close to criticality, then the evolution of the system becomes largely unpredictable.

Percolation processes are markedly different in inhomogeneous structures, such as scale-free networks, compared to homogeneous structures, such as lattices.

18.4. NETWORKS

In the late 1990s, large-scale data started becoming available on how people are connected to each other. Analysis of the data indicated that the connectivity patterns in a population differ significantly from random networks. Their *scale-free* character indicates that most nodes have very few connections while a few nodes, the hubs, are extremely well-connected. This heterogeneity was shown to be true for a large number of networks and in diverse contexts. These similarities, in turn, pointed to common underlying mechanisms, such as *preferential attachment*, where nodes with many connections tend to attract even more nodes.[3]

There are many ways to characterize properties of individual nodes in a network, mainly through centralities such as *degree centrality, betweenness centrality, coreness centrality*, etc. These quantities can identify nodes with specific features and allow for more realistic interventions. For example, there is a lot of research on how to identify the most influential nodes in a network, and it can be shown that these are not necessarily the most connected nodes.[4] At a larger scale, there is a lot of effort on efficient detection of *modules*, which represent groups of nodes with significantly more connections within the group compared to connections outside the group. The degree of *modularity* in a network is important in identifying whether the network is well-mixed or if separate communities have been formed, with significant implications on the efficiency of spreading and influence.

Of particular importance is the recent extension to *multilayer networks*, where a number of networks are connected to each other.[5] This can describe, for example, different types of simultaneous interactions among individuals, such as online interactions, phone conversations, personal contacts, etc.

Building a network is one of the most important tasks for data analysis of large populations. Transforming raw data into a network form provides the immediate benefit of numerous tools to analyze the system, predict the outcome of dynamic processes, and potentially design efficient intervention strategies. There is not a unique network for a given group of individuals, since their connections will depend on the application. For example, weak social ties may inform but may not persuade, and acquiring the same information from two friends is redundant while getting the same advice from two friends is not. The specific research questions or hypotheses studied will eventually determine the basic features of the network model.

If nodes are removed randomly in a scale-free network, then under most circumstances the percolation threshold is close to 1 (i.e., the surviving nodes are always connected in one giant cluster), and we need to remove almost all nodes before destroying the connected cluster. On the contrary, if we target and remove the most connected nodes, then the percolation threshold is close to zero (i.e., the long-range connectivity of the network is destroyed very quickly). The identification of the hubs becomes an obvious priority, but in real situations this may be a very difficult task. Advances in percolation and network theory have provided efficient ways to reach the hubs, even with limited additional information, using methods such as *acquaintance immunization*.[6] Under this scheme, random people are selected and nominate one of their connections. This simple approach dramatically reduces the percolation threshold to roughly 10% to 20%. This strategy has been successfully tested in rural Honduras[7] where two public health interventions, chlorine for water purification and multivitamins, were adopted by the population at significantly higher numbers using the nomination strategy, compared to random or targeted selections.

Christakis, Fowler, and collaborators[8] have published a series of papers analyzing data from the Framingham Heart Study by employing network science ideas. The Framingham study is a longitudinal survey that started in 1948 and follows the medical history, physical examination results, and social factors for thousands of adult participants, their children, and their grandchildren. These data allowed the formation of different networks, for example, by connecting individuals who were friends with each other or by connecting family members. A large number of attributes were examined, such as smoking patterns, obesity, reported happiness, etc. The analysis showed the existence of network modules within which friends had similar levels in each of these attributes. Moreover, analysis of networks at different times showed that people quit smoking together with their friends in large groups. As smoking was going out of fashion, the smokers would also be pushed toward the periphery of their social network, while in earlier years they were largely in the core of it. These findings would be very difficult to demonstrate quantitatively without performing a network analysis. This work provided direct quantitative evidence that many habits, emotions, ideas, behaviors, and NCDs can be attributed to social networking, and these attributes are contagious between friends in a social network. Interestingly, this influence is much stronger between friends, even when they are geographically apart, compared to, for instance, influence from spouse or family. These findings attracted a lot of attention, including some controversy on their interpretation (e.g., for criticism, see Shalizi and Thomas,[9] and for extended response, Christakis and Fowler[10]).

Network-mediated influence has been shown to be more effective on health-related behavior when it is based on homophily. Homophily refers to the tendency of creating ties with people of similar interests. In an experimental demonstration,[11] a new website was created to build an Internet-based health community. The website fixed the "health buddies" of the participants so that these could not be changed by the user. The researchers could thus create two networks where the only difference was in the connection patterns. Initially, one person suggested to his buddies to register in a health-related website, and the study could follow the users who were convinced and registered in that website. The results clearly demonstrated that the adoption rate was significantly higher and faster in a social network where people connected with users who had similar profiles with them rather than in the other network. In a similar experiment, people would start keeping a "diet diary" in a homophily-based social network, but not in a random network.

18.5. SPATIAL CORRELATIONS

Correlation is a frequently used statistical measure of association between two variables. Typically, a correlation coefficient quantifies whether two variables are independent or have a linear dependence on each other. For example, analysis of population data may show that there is a strong, weak, or nonexisting dependence between exercise and cardiovascular health. There is a large body of literature on the interpretation of such correlations, but unless there is a controlled environment, it is difficult to reliably detect the underlying mechanisms or causation behind those variables.

In statistical physics, the concept of correlation is expressed mainly through the *correlation function, $C(r)$*. This function describes how a variable co-varies with distance (or how two variables co-vary with each other) and quantifies the range over which order extends in a system. For example, if we are located on a red site in percolation, what is the probability that the first neighbors will also be red, and more generally, what is the probability to find a red node at a distance r? This function decays from a value of $C(0) = 1$ at $r = 0$ to a value of $C(\xi) = 0$ at a given distance, ξ, which is called the *correlation length*. The correlation length is the distance after which the two variables are completely independent. The correlation function and the correlation length are important quantities in describing spatial effects and can be used to detect local or global influence. In particular, the correlation length diverges in a system at criticality, which means that this length is of the order of the system size. As a result, in criticality, local influences can spread over the entire system. Mathematically, in the vicinity of criticality, many quantities scale as *power laws*, and this fact is typically used as a hallmark of criticality.

An interesting analogy can be made with the telephone game, where people in a line whisper a phrase to their neighbor. Parts of the phrase may be transmitted incorrectly so that after, for example, seven neighbors the phrase is completely distorted. In physics terms, the interactions extend over distance 1 since players can only directly communicate with their neighbors. The correlation length, though, will be 7, which means that what a player whispers to their neighbor can influence what the others transmit up to a distance of seven from the originator of the message. From this point of view, correlation is the expression of indirect information transfer mediated by the direct interaction between individuals.[12]

Large values of ξ correspond to a higher degree of order in the system, but the correlation length cannot reveal the origin of order. Order may be the result of centralized action, where the system units respond almost exclusively to external forces. This is the case, for example, for a marching group of soldiers who always follow the directions of their group leader without interacting with each other. This system is strongly ordered, since everyone moves in the same direction. On the contrary, *self-organized order* is an emergent phenomenon where there is no central authority and the soldiers move following the general direction of their neighbors, which under many conditions also leads to an ordered system. The two cases can be distinguished by the *collective response* of the group to external perturbations. If a small part of the group is disturbed (e.g., attacked by adversaries), the collective response in the centralized case will be very poor: Everyone will continue moving to the same direction unless the leader provides different instructions. In self-organized order, this perturbation will transfer through the mutual local interactions and end up influencing a much larger part of the group than the one that was directly affected. Behavioral correlations are well-suited to describe how a group responds collectively to its environment and to changes in this environment, and they can be a very useful concept in population health research.

There is strong evidence that obesity levels have been increasing in the United States since the 1970s. The fact that the entire country follows similar trends indicates that this may be an example of *collective behavior*. Using data from the Centers for Disease Control and Prevention at the county level, a recent study calculated the obesity correlation function.[13] This is a measure of how probable it is for two counties to have obesity rates that behave similarly when they are at a distance r. Weak spatial correlations would result to a random distribution of obesity—that is, distance would not be important and correlations would drop fast. Surprisingly, the correlation length for obesity was found to be of the order of 1,000 miles. In contrast, correlations in population density are much weaker, with a correlation length of the order of a few hundred miles. In other words, obesity trends behave similarly within large-scale "islands" that extend over a large part of the country and cannot be explained by the spatial distribution of the population. In the telephone game analogy, if the participants were the 50 states, the influence of the population would reach two states away, while in obesity it would influence roughly 15 of them. The findings in that study were largely described via power laws. As previously mentioned, this suggests that the system is close to criticality. In this case, the entire system is self-organized so that any small change may be suppressed fast, but if it survives its early steps then it can spread over the whole system. The importance of this finding is that, in a system at criticality, details of individual behavior are no longer important (e.g., local cuisine, socio-cultural environments, etc.) and act simply as local moderators. Similar results were found for other human activities and NCDs. Of particular importance is the case of cancer mortality, where stronger spatial correlations in the 1970s gave way to much weaker correlations by 2000, with the notable exception of lung cancer mortality, where correlations remained strong, as shown in the same study.[13]

From a complex systems view, obesity and other NCDs are the result of people responding to the environments they find themselves in and are largely influenced by social interactions. The work by Christakis et al.[8,10] provided a mechanism of interactions at the personal level, while the study of obesity correlations at the population level demonstrates the macroscopic effect of these interactions.

18.6. CASCADES

Cascades in complex systems are one of the main mechanisms behind abrupt transitions, and typically they proceed, or are the main cause, for first-order transitions. A cascade is induced when one part of the system, usually small and localized in space, fails or switches state. This seemingly small change can lead to a much broader change and reach global proportions. A system may seem stable and this may create a false sense of security. The impact of cascades in a complex system can be severe, and because they evolve rapidly, they are not easy to mitigate. Understanding whether the system is close to criticality is the key to finding whether cascades are probable.

Not all nodes are equally probable to cause a cascade.[14] If cascades are possible, then we want to know how to enable or prevent them. This leads to a search for influential spreaders, as previously mentioned. A node is considered influential when a new process is initiated by it and it reaches a large part of the network. In general, it is possible to locate such influential spreaders according to their network centralities.[4]

The triggering and evolution of cascades have been analyzed in numerous empirical situations, such as rumor spreading.[15] Lately, cascades have been shown to play a central role in the study of spreading and failures in multilayer networks,[5] where small failures in one layer may lead to global failures in the entire system.

18.7. CONTROL THEORY

Linear control theory has been used in the study of dynamical systems to determine if and if so, how a system can be brought to a desirable final state. In population health, similar methods can be useful in determining whether the state of a population can be reverted (e.g., from high prevalence to low prevalence) by intervening at specific locations. These analytical techniques can be useful in determining the extent of intervention in populations. An evolving system, if left without external influence, reaches an equilibrium state. The basic question behind control theory in networks is if it is possible to move the system to a different—and desirable—state, when we have the ability to influence a certain fraction of nodes. Additionally, we want to be able to locate these driver nodes (i.e., identify a small subset of nodes), which we can adjust to fully control the network state at any given time.

The "state" of a system in control theory is a set of inputs, outputs, and internal state variables. Assume that every individual has a given opinion on dietary habits, which is the result of interactions among the node and its neighbors. The set of these opinions represent the *internal state* of the system. The *output state* is a quantity that can be measured experimentally on each node (e.g., the weight of each individual). If it is possible to influence the opinion of individuals, then this influence represents the *input* variables, which enables control of the system. A system is defined to be controllable when it is possible to reach any final state from any initial state in finite time, and the evolution of the system is described mathematically via a set of differential equations.

An important concept of control theory is the feedback mechanism. This is used to tune the system response toward the desired output, by calibrating changes in the input. These changes can be in the form of selecting different input nodes or modifying the extent of influence. Recently, this topic has received considerable interest in network science, as a possible method to relate network generation mechanisms and topological features with network functionality.[16]

18.8. CONCLUSIONS

Statistical physics theory and methods offer an arsenal of tools to analyze and interpret the increasing volume of available data on NCDs. These tools allow the study of complex mechanisms that drive similar phenomena and they can additionally suggest novel intervention strategies. The few applications that were mentioned in this chapter only scratch the surface of the extensive ongoing research in the field.

REFERENCES

1. World Health Organization. *World health statistics 2018: Monitoring health for the SDGs, sustainable development goals*. Geneva; 2018.
2. Castellano C, Fortunato S, Loreto V. Statistical physics of social dynamics. *Rev Mod Phys*. 2009;81:591–646.
3. Barabási A-L. *Network Science*. Cambridge University Press; 2016.
4. Kitsak M, Gallos LK, Havlin S, et al. Identification of influential spreaders in complex networks. *Nat Phys*. 2010;6:888–893.
5. Boccaletti S, Bianconi G, Criado R, et al. The structure and dynamics of multilayer networks. *Phys Rep*. 2014;544:1–122.
6. Cohen R, Havlin S, Ben-Avraham D. Efficient immunization strategies for computer networks and populations. *Phys Rev Lett*. 2003;91:247901.

7. Kim DA, Hwong AR, Stafford D, et al. A randomized controlled trial of social network targeting to maximize population behavior change. *Lancet*. 2015;386:145–153.
8. Christakis NA, Fowler JH. The spread of obesity in a large social network over 32 years. *N Engl J Med*. 2007;357:370–379.
9. Shalizi CR, Thomas AC. Homophily and contagion are generically confounded in observational social network studies. *Sociol Methods Res*. 2011;40:211–239.
10. Christakis NA, Fowler JH. Social contagion theory: examining dynamic social networks and human behavior. *Stat Med*. 2013;32:556–577.
11. Centolla D. The Spread of Behavior in an Online Social Network Experiment. *Science*. 2010;329:1194–1197.
12. Cavagna A, Cimarelli A, Giardina I, et al. Scale-free correlations in starling flocks. *Proc Natl Acad Sci U S A*. 2010;107:11865–11870.
13. Gallos LK, Barttfeld P, Havlin S, Sigman M, Makse HA. Collective behavior in the spatial spreading of obesity. *Sci Rep*. 2012;2:454.
14. Pastor-Satorras R, Castellano C, Van Mieghem P, Vespignani A. Epidemic processes in complex networks. *Rev Mod Phys*. 2015;87:925–979.
15. Friggeri A, Adamic L, Eckles D, Cheng J. Rumor cascades. In: *Eighth International AAAI Conference on Weblogs and Social Media*. https://www.aaai.org/ocs/index.php/ICWSM/ICWSM14/paper/view/8122/8110. Published May 16, 2014.
16. Liu Y-Y, Barabási A-L. Control principles of complex systems. *Rev Mod Phys*. 2016;88:035006.

TAKE-HOME MESSAGES

The complex systems science analytical armamentarium is quite large and continues to grow. The depth and breadth of past applications of these approaches in population health point to their potential to transform diverse population health research and practice-based initiatives. However, similar to the choice of research approach (as described in Part II of this book), the choice of analytical method is contingent on our motivating questions and the underlying complexity it sits within. Different analytical approaches have their own strengths and weaknesses; further, the costs can vary greatly between approaches. For example, we might choose to prioritize generalizability, precision, parsimony, or the ability to support rapid cycles of learning, testing, and acting based on improving understanding—and the analytical approaches we select are likely to change with our priorities.

While we must appreciate research and practice budgets when deciding on an approach, we should also consider downstream implications of inadequately investing in foundational research. For example, if interventions are developed based on an incomplete understanding of the inherent complexity of the problem, they are unlikely to be as effective as they could be, if they are indeed effective at all (e.g., due to policy resistance). Finding this out only after an intervention is implemented and evaluated is likely more costly than investing in complex systems science in the first place.

While the analytical approaches presented in this part of the book are varied, they actually have more in common than different—particularly in their quest to represent and test representations and implications of aspects of complexity within decision support models. Further, models are not crystal balls—they are tools that help us to understand. Instead of focusing exclusively on the knowledge gleaned from analysis results, the modeling process itself can be—and we would argue that it needs to be structured to be—a greatly beneficial part of analysis. Finally, having some explicit model—even one that is incomplete—is usually better than having no model at all in representing knowledge and guiding action. As articulated in Chapter 8, we always have a model, but it is not always *explicit*—that is, it is not always disclosed, discussed, and tested. Because population health phenomena are complex, analysis needs to accommodate that complexity. Failing to do so relegates complexity to our mental models—which is no better than an imperfect but explicit model that makes underlying assumptions transparent. Ultimately, the choice of analytical approach, as well as the detail within the end model or the analytical objectives, should be carefully deliberated, with the motivating questions, the available resources, the state of extant theory and evidence, and the structure of the available data in mind.

Because many of these analytical approaches are relatively young, they are continually evolving and have a great deal of untapped potential. For example, many configurations of hybrid modeling remain unexplored, such as incorporating other aspects or approaches from traditional or complex systems science. Model replication—analogous to replicating results for an experimental study—remains relatively rare. And for many models, they are never "finished"—as is the case with the "Rethink Health" model; they can always be improved or extended as new evidence and theories emerge, new data require questioning and iterating assumptions or different motivating objectives require modifications. While the innovativeness of these approaches provides exciting opportunities for innovation, there are downsides to this level change. For example, there are not always best analytical practices to follow—requiring innovation and more extensive methodological exposition than is always allowed in traditional population health journals and creating a steep learning curve. Attempts to create such guidelines can bound potential use or lead to fragmentation in analytical approaches and application domains. Despite these challenges, complex systems-grounded analytical approaches are often the only way to sufficiently investigate complex systems in population health.

RESOURCES FOR FURTHER READING

Arnold KF, Harrison WJ, Heppenstall AJ, Gilthorpe MS. DAG-informed regression modelling, agent-based modelling and microsimulation modelling: A critical comparison of methods for causal inference. *Int J Epidemiol.* 2018;48(1):243–253.

Barabási A-L. *Network Science.* Cambridge, UK: Cambridge University Press; 2016.

Brailsford SC, Harper PR, Patel B, Pitt M. An analysis of the academic literature on simulation and modelling in health care. *J Simul.* 2009;3(3):130–140.

Castellano C, Fortunato S, Loreto V. Statistical physics of social dynamics. *Rev Mod Physics.* 2009;81(2):1–58.

Cioffi-Revilla C. Computational social science. *Wiley Interdis Rev Comput Statist.* 2010;2(3):259–271.

Epstein JM. *Generative Social Science: Studies in Agent-Based Computational Modeling.* Princeton, NJ: Princeton University Press; 2006.

Ford A. *Modeling the Environment: An Introduction to System Dynamics Models of Environmental Systems.* Washington, DC: Island Press; 2010.

Hamid TKA. *Thinking in Circles about Obesity: Applying Systems Thinking to Weight Management.* New York, NY: Springer; 2012.

Hassmiller Lich K, Minyard K, Niles R, Dave G, Gillen EM. System dynamics and community health. In: *Methods for Community Public Health Research: Integrated and Engaged Approaches.* New York, NY: Springer; 2014:129–170.

Homer J, Milstein B, Labarthe D, et al. Simulating and evaluating local interventions to improve cardiovascular health. *Prev Chronic Dis.* 2010;7(1):1–11.

Hoppensteadt FC, Peskin CS. *Mathematics in Medicine and the Life Sciences.* New York, NY: Springer Science & Business Media; 2013.

Kopec JA, Finès P, Manuel DG, et al. Validation of population-based disease simulation models: A review of concepts and methods. *BMC Public Health.* 2010;10(1):710.

Liu Y-Y, Barabási A-L. Control principles of complex systems. *Rev Mod Physics.* 2016;88(3):1–61.

Luke DA, Stamatakis KA. Systems science methods in public health: Dynamics, networks, and agents. *Annu Rev Public Health.* 2012;33:357–376.

Maglio PP, Mabry PL. Agent-based models and systems science approaches to public health. *Am J Prev Med.* 2011;40(3):392–394.

Maglio PP, Sepulveda M-J, Mabry PL. Mainstreaming modeling and simulation to accelerate public health innovation. *Am J Public Health.* 2014;104(7):1181–1186.

Marshall DA, Burgos-Liz L, IJzerman MJ, et al. Applying dynamic simulation modeling methods in health care delivery research—the simulate checklist: Report of the ISPOR Simulation Modeling Emerging Good Practices Task Force. *Value Health.* 2015;18(1):5–16.

Marshall D, Burgos-Liz L, Ijzerman MJ, et al. Selecting a dynamic simulation modeling method for health care delivery research—Part 2: Report of the ISPOR Dynamic Simulation Modeling Emerging Good Practices Task Force. *Value Health.* 2015;18(2):147–160.

Marshall B, Galea S. Formalizing the role of agent-based modeling in causal inference and epidemiology. *Am J Epidemiol.* 2015;181(2):92–99.

Ottensen JT, Olufsen MS, Larsen JK. *Applied Mathematical Models in Human Physiology.* Philadelphia, PA: Society for Industrial and Applied Mathematics; 2004.

Railsback SF, Grimm V. *Agent-Based and Individual-Based Modeling: A Practical Introduction.* Princeton, NJ: Princeton University Press; 2011.

Senge PM. *The Fifth Discipline: The Art & Practice of the Learning Organization.* New York, NY: Random House; 2006.

Sturmberg JP, Martin C. *Handbook of Systems and Complexity in Health.* New York, NY: Springer; 2013.

Wilensky U, Rand W. *An Introduction to Agent-Based Modeling: Modeling Natural, Social, and Engineered Complex Systems with NetLogo.* Cambridge, MA: MIT Press; 2015.

PART V

Toward a New Population Health Science

19

Making the Global Complexity Turn in Population Health

BRIAN CASTELLANI

19.1. POPULATION HEALTH: A STORY OF SUCCESS?

Nuances aside, the intertwined histories of population and public health throughout the world are ultimately a story of significant accomplishment.[1-2] As proof, a short list is sufficient: clean drinking water, sanitation, food safety, air quality, vaccines and preventable diseases, tobacco control, family planning and so forth.[1-2] And these accomplishments have extended themselves well into the globalized era in which we presently live.[3]

Still, despite these accomplishments, population health in the 21st century faces a "crisis of complexity."[4] And the major culprits, it appears (in addition to more localized factors) are the same economic, political, cultural, and technological forces of globalization that have, in many ways, purportedly made the world a better place.[5-7] In short, the crisis is one of global complexity.[5-7] For example, while our collective well-being, as a planet, has improved overall,[8-9] the more nuanced reality is that population health—broken down by country or region or community—is far too complex, nonlinear, and multiple in its path dependencies to be evolving along a singular path of "getting better" or "getting worse." Also, "getting better" is not the same as "doing great!" As such, claims of improvement need to be modified such that they are more context-dependent, trend-specific, temporally sensitive, and short-term predictive.[10]

Relative to this point, as Szreter[11] outlined in *The Population Health Approach in Historical Perspective*, it appears that, as with most major socioeconomic and scientific-technical advances—albeit with certain exceptions—globalization's economic growth often produces as much harm as good, particularly amongst the

Brian Castellani, *Making the Global Complexity Turn in Population Health* In: *Complex Systems and Population Health*. Edited by: Yorghos Apostolopoulos, Kristen Hassmiller Lich, and Michael Kenneth Lemke, Oxford University Press (2020). © Oxford University Press. DOI: 10.1093/oso/9780190880743.003.0019 poor and most vulnerable. It is for this reason that Szreter[11p421] states, "The origin of the population health approach is a historic debate over the relationship between economic growth and human development." And, more to the point, it is not, therefore, simply the neoliberal view of growing the economy that leads to a concomitant linear increase in health and well-being.[10-12] Nor is such a "constant growth" solution to health, circa 2020, sustainable.[4-7] Consider, for example, if India or China, to obtain higher levels of health, lived at the consumption level of the United States.

In short, we need more complex ways of thinking to handle the current complex "globalized" problems of population health. We need the *complexity sciences*.[13-16]

19.2. ADOPTING A COMPLEX POPULATION HEALTH PERSPECTIVE

As outlined by a growing network of complexity scholars, it is mainly through the complex, corrective actions of civil society—of which public health is a major part—that the deleterious and corrosive effects of globalization on population health can be assuaged.[2,5,13,17,18] Or, alternatively, it is through global civil society that the positive dimensions of globalization can be harnessed to improve population health the world over. Either way, the point is the same: Improving population health involves a civil society-based array of complex ecological, geographical, socioeconomic, political, psychological, and medical-technical factors, all of which combine to form the complex systems in which population health is situated and with which the health of populations is interdependent.

As illustration of this difference, consider, for example, the distinction between the following two research questions. The first is reductionist and ignores the complex systems in which population health is situated. Here the question is, How do we help poor people deal with their health vulnerabilities? In contrast is the complex systems question, which asks, How do we fix the communities and social institutions and socio-ecological systems in which people live (of which the economy is a part) so that poverty is not a vulnerability to population health?

Still, adopting a complex-systems view of population health, while both necessary and useful, is not always a guarantee for success—no matter what the approach, everything has its limitations. Nor is it true that the current methodological, theoretical, and practical conventions of population health are not still incredibly important—because they are. The better question, then, is how can a *complex systems view* be used to improve how we engage in the science and practice of population health sufficient to better manage the crisis of complexity it currently faces, particularly vis-à-vis the challenges of globalization and global health? All of which brings us to the purpose of the current chapter. We will use a *complex systems perspective* to critically review how the current conventions of population health—from policy and interventions to research design and methods to accepted standards of practice and education—can be advanced to more effectively deal with its crisis of complexity. Our review will take the form of a "top 10" list of critiques.

19.3. MAKING THE GLOBAL COMPLEXITY TURN: A "TOP 10" LIST

19.3.1. Theorizing Global Health as Complex

Of the various conventions that need to be overcome, the first—which we have already suggested—is probably the most important: Population health needs to accelerate its current trend toward a complex global health framework, from research and practice to policy and academic training.[17,18] More specifically, the field needs to theoretically embrace, as a basis for its models, a *complex global systems* view of population health—that is, one grounded in the understanding that population health, the world over, is self-organizing, emergent, nonlinear, dynamic, path dependent, network-like in structure, and so forth, resulting in a world-wide system of interdependent and interconnected systems—albeit even if these systems are only partially connected in fragmented ways.[7]

Getting population health to embrace this view, however, will most likely prove difficult. Part of the problem is the larger socio-political context in which such a *complex global systems* view approach is situated, including populist debates over the value of science and expertise in policy[3]; as well as the neoliberal tendency—as discussed earlier—of international policy to focus too narrowly on growing the economy of "developing" countries to improve population health.[6]

Relative to this point is the mindset amongst many western societies that global health is a foreign problem. As Frenk, et al.[18p94] state, "in the media, in lay and scientific literature, and in major initiatives, global health is still identified with problems supposedly characteristic of developing countries, and global cooperation in health with a sort of paternalistic philanthropy that is armed with the technological developments of developed countries." What is ironic about this approach is that the real essence of globalization, in truth, is that the health of any given population, including western countries, is often tied in highly complex and nuanced ways to the well-being of others. Which we have recently seen, for example, with the coronavirus pandemic. Frenk et al.[18p94] ask, "How should global health be understood in an era marked by the rising burden of non-communicable diseases (NCDs), climate change and other environmental crises, integrated chains of production and consumption, a power shift towards emerging economies, intensified migration, and instant information transmission?" Their answer: "Global health should be reconceptualized as the health of the global population, with a focus on the dense relationships of interdependence across nations and sectors that have arisen with globalization."[18p94] And the reason for doing so, they argue, is that it will help to ensure that the health of any one population is "duly protected and promoted, not only in the post-2015 development agenda but also in the many other global governance processes—such as trade, investment, environment, and security—that can profoundly affect health."[18p94]

19.3.2. Definitional Struggles

In addition to embracing a *complex global systems* view, scholars and practitioners alike need to resist the temptation to reduce population health to the purview of cost control or bureaucratic management. The first, as outlined by Sharfstein,[19] is the extent to which controlling costs should ultimately dictate the goals of population health. For example, seeing air pollution prevention in strictly economic terms often pushes policies to be more reactive and policy-cycle focused. Such an approach also tends to devalue, reduce, or remove more long-term but important services, particularly large-scale population-based preventive measures, which are in a better position to embrace a complex-systems view of the problem being addressed. An example would be reducing exposure to $PM_{2.5}$ by improving the built environment for vulnerable groups in urban environments.

The second mindset (which is more of a western society issue among globally northern countries) is the degree to which a population should be limited to the patients, employees, or members of an insurance plan or, in turn, the degree to which a population is confined to a specific health issue or a clinical group.[19-21] The result, as Diez Roux[12] explains, is one of the current challenges for the population health movement: Despite its best attempts to treat populations across scientific and bureaucratic categories, the complexity of this concept is regularly appropriated in the service of the more focused goals of health finance, healthcare management or research.[1,2,4,12] Examples include such neologisms as *population health strategy* (i.e., enrolling as many people as possible in a healthcare plan) and *population health solutions* (i.e., offering healthcare members and providers such options as wellness programs and surgical device management).[19-21]

19.3.3. The Methodological Problem of Organized Complexity

The third is the need for a *complex global systems* view of population health to see complexity as organized.[22] In 1948, Warren Weaver[23] published an article titled, *Science and Complexity*, that addressed what he saw as the future problem of all research, including the burgeoning fields of population health and policy evaluation. According to Weaver, the basic problems of science can be organized, historically speaking, into three main phases. The first phase focused on *simple systems*, comprised of a few variables and amenable to near-complete mathematical descriptions. The second phase, which was the birth of statistical mechanics, focused on *disorganized complex systems*, where the unpredictable microscopic behavior of a very large number of variables makes them highly resistant to simple formulas. Hence, this phase was the golden age of statistics.

Finally, there was the forthcoming third phase (*ca.* 1948), based on the challenges of *organized complex systems*. Here, the focus is on how the qualitative interactions amongst a profile of variables and the (equally important) emergent, self-organizing, aggregate system they create come together to determine their complexity. For Weaver, examples of such systems cut across the health and social sciences, including population health.[10,13–15,24,26] The problem, however, is that such systems cannot be effectively modelled using the conventional statistics of disorganized complexity. Needed, therefore, was a methodological revolution, grounded in the forthcoming age of the computer, which Weaver presciently saw on the horizon.

So that was 1948. What has happened since then? As we know, the computational modeling revolution took place, along with the sweeping development of the complexity sciences, all of which changed (and are presently changing) the world.[22] Meanwhile, public health has basically kept calm and carried on, continuing to develop the same repertoire of conventional quantitative methods and treating populations as disorganized complex systems of aggregate individuals and households. The result, circa 2020, is that most population health experts are woefully unequipped to effectively model the global complexity that has thrown the field into crisis.

19.3.4. Data Mining Big Health Data

Related to the crisis of complexity is that of big data. As outlined elsewhere,[24–27] the globalized world(s) in which we now live, including the complex health systems in which population health is grounded, have become massively digital—from diagnostic software and geospatial disease-tracking systems to nudgewear and the big-data health-informatics databases upon which population health increasingly depends. In terms of big health data, the challenges revolve around what are called the Six Vs. First, there is *volume*: Big health data often exceed current capacity for storage. Second is *variety*: Big health data come in a wide array of types and formats and at multiple levels of scale, including inconsistencies in how a factor or variable is defined or measured, as in the case of a disease or health condition. Third is *velocity*: In our big data world, the issue is not just the speed at which health data are being generated, but also the speed at which they often need to be acquired. Also, there is a significant amount of health data that need to be understood in real time (e.g., flu season trends), which speeds up the decision-making process, forcing population health officials to make decisions, often times, in a matter of days or weeks. Fourth is *variability*: While the velocity and volume of health data appear constant, in actuality they are rather variable, with inconsistencies in their flow, as in the case of a sudden Twitter trend or online searches in response to a disease outbreak. Fifth is *veracity*: Big health data are often not in a format that makes them easily explored or linked together. Consider, for example, the massively unstructured and inconsistent formats in which health data are currently available. Sixth is *vulnerability*, which exists in two major forms: (a) hardware or software breakdown and (b) hacking, cybersecurity, and privacy issues.

As a result of these six major challenges, the critics of big data warn that, for all of its potential, it cannot fully deliver on its promise, as there is a major difference between lots of data and high quality information.[26] Correct or not, the problem is that big data are not going away, particularly in terms of the massive increase in health data (ranging from smart phones and health apps to government gathered public health data). The more important focus, therefore—as argued in the new field of digital sociology[27]—is for public health experts (along with the public) to engage in a critical dialogue about how best to deal with big health data.[24-27] Getting such a critical interdisciplinary debate to happen, however, is particularly difficult, given that such changes are as much about changing culture and getting population health experts out of their comfort zones, as they are about advancing institutional bureaucracy and undergraduate and postgraduate curriculum to better educate the next generation of population health experts.[28]

19.3.5. Overcoming Simplicity

In addition to embracing an organized complexity view of population health, experts also need to overcome the entrenched view that the best models are the simplest. Consider, for example, the way most health research (or policy) is done. As outlined elsewhere,[25,28] the brilliance of reductionist modeling is as follows: (1) population health is treated as a form of disorganized complexity, (2) which is best studied using statistics, (3) where the goal is to explain majority (aggregate) behavior in terms of probability theory and the macroscopic laws of averages, (4) which is done by developing simple linear models, as in the case of conventional epidemiology or randomized clinical trials, (5) and in which variables are treated as "rigorously real" measures of health outcomes. (6) Then, model-in-hand, the goal is to identify, measure, describe (or remove control or manage, as in randomized clinical trials) how certain independent variables impact one or more dependent variables of concern. (7) And, if done right, these models will lead to reasonably generalizable explanations of why health outcomes happen the way they do, (8) which, in turn, will lead to relatively straightforward population health policy recommendations for what to do about them.

Such a review is not to suggest, however, that this approach is not useful. In fact, as I stated earlier, quite the opposite: The problem is that it has been almost too successful! In fact, as Andersson et al.,[29] explain, there are times when viewing complex systems as simple remains crucial. However, many of the population health problems we currently face demand a different approach. All of which takes us to the importance of cases.

19.3.6. Cases versus Variables

As we all learn in our first courses on the history of population health, the field was born of the *case*. That is, the "science" of population health emerged from experts using case-comparative observation to understand why, for example, one part of a city got sick while other parts did not. Eventually, however, as population health moved along into the 1950s, the study of cases was replaced with survey research and, in turn, during the 1970s and 1980s, powerful variable-based statistical software. And, in the process, case-comparison went to the wayside. Or, at least, it did so in the health sciences.

In other areas, such as field research and qualitative method, as well as the data mining and the computational and complexity sciences, the case remained the primary focus.[24,28,30] In other words, despite their significant technical differences, all of these "other" methods focus on modeling, exploring, clustering, or cataloguing cases, based on key characteristics or etiological differences. For example, smart machines can be used to identify tumor or disease types; predictive analytics can explore public policies and their multiple outcomes; artificial intelligence can identify reliable community health opportunities; genetic algorithms can detect subtle changes in an epidemic; agent-based modelling can be used to explore simulated interventions into disease-outbreak patterns; and network analyses can find the fastest route through a health informatics network to get from a healthcare question to the best answer.

And—in terms of the issue of health complexity—all of them (albeit to varying degrees) can be counted as an improvement on conventional statistics, mainly because they avoid aggregate-based, one-size-fits-all solutions; instead, they focus on identifying multiple case-based trends, which, in turn, they catalogue and examine based on differences in their respective profile of key factors and variables. In short, all of these techniques treat the topics they study as evolving sets of complex cases, which is a very effective way of "decomplexifying" complex data by breaking it down into multiple and much smaller groupings (i.e., trends, models), while at the same time holding on to the complexity of the topic being studied.[28,30-32]

19.3.7. Changing Journal Publishing Culture

The other needed shift is a change in journal culture. For example, while the academic book publishing industry has been steadily advancing the cause of complexity, the population health journals have yet to make the *complexity turn* in any meaningful way. Even more problematic is that, even when editors are sympathetic to the complexity sciences, their reviewers are not. Case in point is the strategy many of my colleagues and I use to get published. We start by sending our study to a health journal or two (my best score so far is five rejections!), it gets rejected, and then, given the need to move on, we publish it (with almost no problems) in a complexity science or computational modeling journal, which often then means it does not get read by population health experts. If population health is truly going to make the *complexity turn*, which it desperately needs to do, this sort of approach to publishing needs to change.

19.3.8. Opening the Social Sciences

Related, population health—as an academic discipline tied to department and schools—needs to be "opened up" into some type of complexity-based, postdisciplinary applied science. And, unfortunately, this is not a new point: Weaver made it in 1948; Talcott Parsons did the same with the Department of Social Relations in 1946 at Harvard, and so did the Gulbenkian Report[33] and, more recently, Nicholas Christakis.[34] The key here is that population health scholars and practitioners need to work more directly (via curriculum, funding, research and institutional and departmental arrangements) with computational and complexity scientists. However, this requires two additional advances, which have as much to do with the complexity sciences as they do population health. And so, we turn to these two advances now.

19.3.9. Grounding Computational Modelling in Social Theory

While the first eight points on my top 10 list focused on population health experts, the last two address the complexity (and computational) sciences. Here the main issue is that, while complexity and computational scientists are heavily trained in systems thinking and computational methods, they do not have a background in population health or, more widely, the social and health sciences upon which population health is based. For example, as Duncan Watts (the theoretical physicist famous for developing the small-world hypothesis) pointed out regarding the field of complex network analysis:

> Physicists [and complexity scientists] may be marvelous technicians, but they are mediocre sociologists. Thus, if the science of networks is to live up to its early promise, then the other disciplines—sociology in particular—must offer guidance in, for example, the interpretation of empirical and theoretical findings, particularly in the context of policy applications, and also in suggesting measures and models that are increasingly relevant to the important problems at hand.[35p264]

And so, complexity scientists need to be just as open-minded and thoughtful about their own theoretical and substantive limits as they are of the limits of others—which takes me to my final point.

19.3.10. Facilitating the Complexity Turn

To effectively foster the global complexity turn, population health scholars need to engage in a much more rigorous and critical engagement with the complexity sciences. For example, while a growing network of population health researchers have made the complexity turn, it has been of a limited nature. Case in point is Chughtai and Blanchet's[36] *Systems Thinking in Population Health: A Bibliographic Contribution to a Meta-Narrative Review*, which found that, while there has been, since 2010, a significant and positive advance in the population health literature's usage of complexity science, the articles ($N = 557$) they examined nonetheless left room for significant improvement.

I agree with their assessment. For example, population health scholars employing the tools of complexity science tend to cluster into what Chughtai and Blanchet[36p588] identify as "distinct citation and co-authorship groups homophilous by common geography, research focus, inspiration or institutional affiliation." As Sturmberg et al.[14,15] point out in their edited two volumes on complexity in health and healthcare research, this insularity is potentially problematic, as it means scholars are regularly ignoring the work of others involved in the intersection of population health and the complexity sciences or, worse, reinventing ideas already developed.

Chughtai and Blanchet's[36] review also found that some of the complexity science literature in population health tends to be highly abstract and less clearly empirical; what one could call *metaphorical complexity*. Also, given the tendency of this approach to draw from the managerial sciences literature, there is a tendency to uncritically apply key concepts from the complexity sciences—as in the case of self-organization, emergence, chaos, and nonlinearity—to the study of health systems and population health, the results being that, while the insights of this approach are not entirely wrong, are also potentially not right.

The other major issue is a tendency amongst population health researchers toward what Morin[37] and others[28,30,33] call *restrictive complexity*. For Morin,[37] the problem with the restrictive approach is that, while it has certainly made for some of the most important discoveries that established the field in the 1980s, it is trapped in the epistemological limitations of classical science insomuch as it (a) continues to look for the fundamental laws governing all complex systems (or, alternatively, complex networks); (b) treats complexity as an extension of, rather than a critical response to conventional science; (c) noncritically approaches the observation of complex systems and networks as objective and real; and (d) attempts to "decomplexify" the global-temporal behavior of complex systems by reducing them to their smaller microscopic interactions and by ignoring macroscopic factors. Given the critical role that differences in health outcomes and sociopolitical and economic context play in population health, such an approach is rather problematic. And that is not the end of it. A restrictive approach to complexity is also problematic for population health, as it rarely deals with power relations, structured inequality, and, generally speaking, lacks a sociological imagination.[3,5,10,13,25,28] It also tends to assume that mathematical and computational modeling is superior to qualitative analysis, and that all such computational methods work equally well for any topic.[28]

Given these concerns, Chughtai and Blanchet[36p593] concluded as follows:

Based on our review, we argue a need to balance adapted theory with empirical study beyond unidisciplinary mathematical modelling or network analysis and encourage scientists to conduct further interdisciplinary studies in order to acquaint themselves with unfamiliar methods and combinations. We advise a greater emphasis on synthesizing higher order mental constructs with high-quality empirical evidence in order to refine existing definitions and adapted models to population health systems.

I completely agree with these recommendations. All of which brings me to my conclusion.

19.4. CONCLUSION

As my top 10 list has hopefully made clear, while population health faces a rather significant set of challenges relative to its crisis of complexity, it is necessary for the field to make the *global complexity turn* and adopt many of the latest advances in the complexity and computational sciences. Equally important is to ground these advances in a *complex global systems* view of population health—particularly one that is as critical of the new ideas coming out of the complexity sciences as it is of the conventions of population health research and practice.

REFERENCES

1. Rosen, G. (2015). *A History of Population Health*. JHU Press.
2. Baum, F. (2016). *The new Population Health*. 4th ed. Oxford University Press.
3. Fidler, D. P. (2001). The globalization of population health: The first 100 years of international health diplomacy. *Bulletin of the World Health Organization, 79,* 842–849.
4. Armstrong-Mensah, E. (2017). *Global Health: Issues, Challenges, and Global Action.* Wiley-Blackwell.
5. Walby, S. (2009). *Globalization and Inequalities: Complexity and Contested Modernities*. SAGE.
6. Castellani, B. (2018). *The Defiance of Global Commitment: A Complex Social Psychology*. Routledge.
7. Ritzer, G., & Dean, P. (2015). *Globalization: A Basic Text*. 2nd ed. Wiley.
8. Pinker, S. (2018). *Enlightenment Now: The Case for Reason, Science, Humanism, and Progress*. Penguin.
9. Rosling, H., Rönnlund, A. R., & Rosling, O. (2018). *Factfulness: Ten Reasons We're Wrong about the World—And Why Things are Better Than You Think*. Flatiron Books.
10. Castellani, B., Rajaram, R., Buckwalter, J. G., Ball, M., & Hafferty, F. (2015). *Place and health as Complex Systems: A Case Study and Empirical Test*. Springer.
11. Szreter, S. (2003). The population health approach in historical perspective. *American Journal of Population Health, 93*(3), 421–431.
12. Diez Roux, A. V. (2016). On the distinction—or lack of distinction—between population health and population health. *American Journal of Population Health, 106*(4), 619.
13. Capra, F., & Luisi, P. L. (2014). *The Systems View of Life: A UNIFYING vision*. Cambridge University Press.
14. Sturmberg, J. P. (2016). *The Value of Systems and Complexity Sciences for Healthcare*. Springer.
15. Sturmberg, J. P., & Martin, C. M. (2013). *Handbook of Systems and Complexity in Health*. Springer.
16. CECAN. [Home page]. https://www.cecan.ac.uk/.

17. Brown, T. M., Cueto, M., & Fee, E. (2006). The World Health Organization and the transition from "international" to "global" population health. *American Journal of Population Health, 96*(1), 62–72.

18. Frenk, J., Gómez-Dantés, O., & Moon, S. (2014). From sovereignty to solidarity: A renewed concept of global health for an era of complex interdependence. *The Lancet, 383*(9911), 94–97.

19. Sharfstein, J. M. (2014). The strange journey of population health. *The Milbank Quarterly, 92*(4), 640–643.

20. Kindig, D., & Stoddart, G. (2003). What is population health? *American Journal of Population Health, 93*(3), 380–383.

21. Labonte, R., Polanyi, M., Muhajarine, N., Mcintosh, T., & Williams, A. (2005). Beyond the divides: Towards critical population health research. *Critical Population Health, 15*(1), 5–17.

22. Hafferty, F. W., & Castellani, B. (2010). The increasing complexities of professionalism. *Academic Medicine, 85*(2), 288–301.

23. Weaver, W. (1991). Science and complexity. In *Facets of Systems Science* (pp. 449–456). Springer.

24. Castellani, B., & Rajaram, R (2020). *Data Mining Big Data: A Complexity and Critical Approach.* SAGE Quantitative Methods Kit. Sage. Forthcoming.

25. Bar-Yam, Y. (2006). Improving the effectiveness of health care and population health: A multiscale complex systems analysis. *American Journal of Population Health, 96*(3), 459–466.

26. Bar-Yam, Y. (2016). From big data to important information. *Complexity, 21*(S2):73–98.

27. Lupton, D. (2014). Digital sociology. Routledge.

28. Byrne, D., & Callaghan, G. (2013). *Complexity Theory and the Social Sciences: The State of the Art.* Routledge.

29. Andersson, C., Törnberg, A., and Törnberg, P. (2014). Societal systems–complex or worse? *Futures,* 63:145–157.

30. Byrne, D., & Ragin, C. C. (2009). *The Sage Handbook of Case-Based Methods.* SAGE.

31. Complex-It. (n.d.). Durham University. https://www.dur.ac.uk/sociology/research/health/complex-it/

32. Castellani, B., Rajaram, R., Gunn, J., & Griffiths, F. (2016). Cases, clusters, densities: Modeling the nonlinear dynamics of complex health trajectories. *Complexity, 21*(S1), 160–180.

33. Gulbenkian Commission on the Restructuring of the Social Sciences. (1996). *Open the Social Sciences: Report of the Gulbenkian Commission on the Restructuring of the Social Sciences.* Stanford University Press.

34. Christakis, N. A. (2013, July 19). Let's shake up the social sciences. *The New York Times, 21.*

35. Watts, D. J. (2004). The "new" science of networks. *Annual Review of Sociology, 30,* 243–270.

36. Chughtai, S., & Blanchet, K. (2017). Systems thinking in population health: A bibliographic contribution to a meta-narrative review. *Health Policy and Planning, 32*(4), 585–594.

37. Morin, E. (2007). Restricted complexity, general complexity. In *Worldviews, Science and Us: Philosophy and Complexity* (pp. 1–25). Singapore: World Scientific.

Harnessing Complex Systems

An Emerging Paradigm for a New Population Health Science

YORGHOS APOSTOLOPOULOS

> *Only those who will risk going too far can possibly find out how far one can go.*
> —Thomas S. Elliot, excerpt from Preface,
> "Transit of Venus: Poems" (Harry Crosby, 1931)

20.1. POPULATION HEALTH SCIENCE AT A TIPPING POINT

The advent of institutionalized public health has made great contributions to the betterment of population health around the world. Progress, however, has been compromised by the inadequacy of current population health science to fully address preventable excess disease burden and especially its uneven distribution along socioeconomic, racial/ethnic, and geographic lines.[1] While most pressing population health priorities of our time operate as complex systems or are embedded in larger complex systems (see Chapter 1 of this volume), the prevailing paradigm—mainly entrenched in linearity, analytical reductionism, and causal inference—continues to drive population health science. The chasm between prevalent science and the ubiquitous dynamic complexity of population health has sustained an overall inconsequential prevention context (see Chapter 1 of this volume), thereby maintaining the ongoing evaluation of the prescribed epistemological monopoly.[2] As a result, this conundrum has invoked the belated and limited discourse focusing on how interacting parts of population health

Yorghos Apostolopoulos, *Harnessing Complex Systems* In: *Complex Systems and Population Health*. Edited by: Yorghos Apostolopoulos, Kristen Hassmiller Lich, and Michael Kenneth Lemke, Oxford University Press (2020). © Oxford University Press. DOI: 10.1093/oso/9780190880743.003.0020 can produce, often undesirable, aggregate behavior over time and how it can be curtailed.

Amid this epistemological flux and unprecedented advances in the computational and physical sciences, I advocate an *epistemological overhaul in population health science*. The logic is simple: *Population health challenges that operate as or are determined by complex systems should be studied as such.* The proposed overhaul is predicated on the development, refinement, and validation of a *new, theory-grounded, science-driven, and model-centered unifying paradigm in population health science*. It is founded on a fundamental shift in thinking: from a quest for causes and accurate predictions to control population health problems—that we have not fully addressed because of both unsuitable science and sheer uncontrollability of complex problems—to knowledge generation based on complex-systems-science–grounded theories and analytical methods to fully understand, anticipate, curtail, and manage these pressing problems, by way of *harnessing their complexity* or designing solutions that are aligned with the complexity causing problems. Because both current and proposed epistemologies represent models of simpler and complex problems, respectively, appropriate use of each under a unifying paradigm can only strengthen population health science. The current paradigm can only take us so far[3]; therefore, its continuing dominance only delays our ability to engage with new scientific frontiers and, in turn, effectively influence policies that can improve people's health.

The proliferation of this emerging paradigm is poised to unleash groundbreaking ideas that can eventually lead to the emergence of a *new population health science* to shed light on those complex and dynamic causal structures that have driven disease burden over time and eventually to advance policy planning and action. In the following discussion, I delve briefly into the known as well as the possible and still unknown. Some ideas are grounded in long-standing scientific evidence, while others are of an emerging nature; some are testable, others are partially tested, and still others remain untested fantasies about how to contend with intractable population health challenges.[a]

20.2. QUEST FOR METHODOLOGICAL INNOVATION

Social network analysis[5] and mathematical modeling[6]—both grounded in complex systems principles—have long been implicated in mainly infectious disease prevention. It was not until the 1990s, however, when US academia and federal health agencies initiated a discourse on the potential value of broader complex-systems *methods* in research and policy planning. This was mainly driven by stalemates in cancer and obesity-driven comorbidity prevention research,[7] recognition of the importance of social determinants in health inequalities,[8] and breakthroughs in health-related research drawing on complexity.[9] As a result, there was increasing attention on whether and how *complex-systems approaches* can *complement* the prevailing science, which not only signified an emphasis on

---

a. Building on Miller's and Page's views on complex-systems grounded social sciences.[4]

analytical methods but also denoted their implicit *secondary role*. At the same time the need for more integrative approaches was emphasized, indicating the relevance of using these new tools within extant epistemology to strengthen our grasp of intractable population health problems.

Along these lines, while immersed in established socioecological[10] and emerging syndemic frameworks,[11] a series of multifaceted initiatives have generated a new landscape in population health research. Key among these were National Institutes of Health's (NIH) Cancer Intervention and Surveillance Modeling Network[12] and Systems Thinking in Tobacco Control program[13]; Centers for Disease Control and Prevention's Syndemics Prevention Network[14] and HealthBound Policy Simulation Game[15]; NIH's Institute on Systems Science and Health initiatives[16]; and NIH/ Centers for Disease Control and Prevention/Robert Wood Johnson Foundation/ US Department of Agriculture's National Collaborative on Childhood Obesity Research Envision project.[17] As a result, sought-after methodological innovation came about in the form of primarily mathematical and simulation modeling and, secondarily, somewhat timid conceptualization of distal socioeconomic domains as part of causal frameworks, which supplemented the existing armory to advance what at the time was an overall well-resourced but inadequate epistemology and policy planning.

Over these nearly 25 years, a growing number of research projects and manuscripts has contained complex systems science jargon and rationale and, in some cases, novel computational modeling applications. While overall there has been impressive and sustained progress, the vast majority continues to lack a critical underpinning in comprehensive complex-systems-science–grounded theoretical and methodological epistemology. As it has been the case with many population health areas, case studies, and applications, complex-systems-science– grounded works in population health research have been overall unsystematic and rather haphazard.[18] Slow growth in these methods was partially due to the reluctance of the population health community to meaningfully engage with novel scientific advancements and partially due to resistance, despite mostly unfounded rationale—evidenced by federal and private funding agency reviews of proposals grounded in complex systems science methods. This has slowed down efforts to fully introduce complex systems science *methods* (as per original intent) to population health research. This void is corroborated by a scant review of academic curricula and doctoral dissertations originating from diverse, English-language-based, public and population health schools, and presentations at the American and European Public Health Association and Interdisciplinary Association for Population Health Science meetings, as well as funded projects.

While, as part of this method-based innovation run, there have been several programmatic calls for more comprehensive "complex systems approaches,"[19] most are based on computational simulation modeling applications—adopting a rather utilitarian perspective. This has included, primarily, publications on collaborative model-building methodologies,[20] system dynamics,[21] and agent-based modeling[22] and, secondarily, discrete event simulation,[23] microsimulation,[24] and hybrid modeling.[25] Other, more novel and rigorous analytical methods, such as mathematical modeling,[26] Bayesian networks,[27] and machine learning methodologies[28] have played only a minor role. Newer, more innovative theories and analytical methods originating from the physical, natural, network, data, and engineering sciences have been overall negligible or have been originating outside population health science.[29]

While these efforts have revealed the capabilities of mainly computational modeling in both understanding intractable population health challenges and illuminating more effective interventions, they have only inspired a limited paradigmatic, curricular, research, or policy transformation, and limited *methodological innovation alone does not suffice*.[30] Ultimately, not only has this approach hindered substantive engagement of population health science with the scientific frontier, but it has also abstracted opportunities for more widespread novel research and ultimately more effective health policy. These efforts, while well-intended, have in fact been a disservice because of their narrow perspective, because many graduate students or researchers perceive them as only providing the techniques to bring about better outcomes—something akin to an auxiliary "silver-bullet" for the prevailing paradigm. Finally, while complex systems science is still in its infancy in population health science, other scientific domains (e.g., operations research, industrial and systems engineering)[31] are employing these methodological frameworks in their engagement with disease and injury prevention as well as health services research.[32]

20.3. A ROAD MAP FOR A COMPLEX SYSTEMS SCIENCE EPISTEMOLOGY

Lessons from this quest for methodological innovation point to a different engagement with foregoing scientific advances grounded in a well-planned road map that can lead to a more comprehensive and ultimately more pertinent integration of complex systems science into population health science. Such a road map would be fueled by (1) substantive inclusion of sociostructural determinants of population health in both theoretical and methodological causal frameworks, as failure to tackle social inequalities continues to exacerbate health inequalities[33]; (2) what emerges from the nexus of social, health, mathematical, physical, computational, engineering, data, and network sciences with current population health science epistemologies at the leading edge of the scientific frontier; and (3) the intelligent exploitation of diverse forms of massive available data. While this road map is in its infancy, the following sections provide a description of fundamental, key working pillars.

20.3.1. Pillar 1: Establishing That Population Health Problems Are or Determined by Complex Systems

In view of ongoing relevant developments in diverse scientific domains, including health sciences,[34-36] and grounded in the foregoing rationale, population health operates as a complex and adaptive dynamical system of systems (CADSoS).[2,31,37,38] It is a stochastic multiagent, multinetwork, multisystem, multiscale, hierarchically organized mega-system, the properties of which cannot be understood by adding together the sum of the properties of its components. It includes a plethora of social, physical, technical, and biological systems (smaller or larger, regional or national), the interaction of which can generate emergent behaviors that are difficult to explain or predict—often not linear and certainly not independent. We can influence smaller- and larger-scale population health challenges to the extent we can uncover and understand their structure and organization. While the study of large complex systems is relatively unattainable because of their intractability, the following paragraphs discuss one among various ways of conceptualizing the architecture of CADSoS with an emphasis on components, properties, and relationships.

Population health (of different scales) includes numerous heterogeneous and interacting components (i.e., agents, networks, systems) that form an integrated whole, performing a collective function. Exogenous and endogenous forces that influence health outcomes are clustered within four key nested scales (*government bodies; corporate and business organizations; living and work environments*; and *population health and well-being*) and are embedded within global, national, or regional socioeconomic environments. These clusters interact across varying temporal and topological scales according to known rules, exchanging information, data, and processes. Clusters and components exhibit bidirectional exchanges where interdependent parts within each cluster and component influence other agents, networks, or systems within and across other clusters and scales over time and space. This architecture is exemplified by adaptive interactions and nonlinear feedback processes as well as the generation of self-organizing, time-delayed, nonreductive phase transitions and emergent macroscopic outcomes. These properties arise from relationships among system components, with type and degree of connectivity, hetero-/homogeneity of components, and topology being capable of determining how population health outcomes respond to changing conditions.

Because the study of population health problems as CADSoS can be overwhelming, diligence is required in scoping boundaries around research questions, where system elements that most affect undesirable outcomes under investigation lie. Maps and models of complex systems are designed to represent and communicate hypotheses about how systemic structures of CADSoS produce outcomes, which is also a natural way to build theory and test its generalizability.

20.3.2. Pillar 2: Explicating Fundamental Properties of Population Health Problems

To meaningfully explore the extent to which we can understand and possibly influence the dynamic complexity of population health problems, *emergence, phase transitions,* and *resilience* comprise three unique properties (see Chapters 2 and 5 of this volume). Not only can they provide useful information about shifts from desired to undesired health states, but they can also offer opportunities to be harnessed and transformed into positive influences.

First, *emergence* exemplifies what parts of a complex system can do together that they would not be able to do alone.[39] The challenge for decision makers is to influence emergence in a way that it facilitates mainly desirable outcomes. Second, *phase transition* is a sudden or gradual shift in the macro-level state of complex systems when they approach a threshold that can be triggered by small perturbations, when it may be impossible to return to their initial state.[40] Detection, anticipation, and influence of transitions can be challenging in population health. Third, *resilience* is the ability of complex systems to adapt and respond to disturbances, by ultimately remaining functional.[41] Making population health states more resilient, or, conversely, more fragile when we seek to interrupt unwanted outcomes remains a significant challenge. These properties—present in all population health problems—are interlinked, not always distinct, and at times overlapping[42] and offer unique opportunities for interventions.

Along these lines, *self-organized criticality*—another fundamental property in population health research and policy—depicts how interacting agents self-organize into spatial and temporal micro-states, which, in turn, produce large events (e.g., epileptic seizure attacks).[43] The distribution of these events, on the one hand, resembles power laws (see Chapter 10 of this volume) and, on the other, shares similarities with critical phase transitions (see Chapter 5 of this volume). But, unlike physical or technical systems that are dominated by their physics and exogenous influences, population health outcomes are more likely to depend on, for example, public and private policies driven by diverse endogenous forces that could definitely accelerate or undermine criticality (e.g., those passing legislation have their own incentives to alter policies in ways that might change key mechanisms and determinants of criticality).

Finally, understanding whether and how we can exert some type of "control" over intractable population health challenges would be critical in curbing undesirable outcomes. While improving our grasp over some form of control remains quite challenging in all complex systems, evidence shows that it *might* be possible if we identify critical system components and how they are connected.[44] As with other complex systems, the delineation of the controllability of population health problems can possibly improve our chances to understand key laws governing their behavior. This evidence reveals that we can increase our chances for *some* control, if we establish[44,45] (a) a reliable map of interactions among key components—briefly described in Section 20.3.1; (b) a mathematical description of dynamical laws governing the temporal behavior of system components; and (c) the ability to influence their state and temporal behavior. While promising, these principles remain underdeveloped in population health science. To address the control principles of population health problems, as with other complex systems,[44] we need to explore the interplay between network topology and dynamical laws and then marry pertinent results with empirical findings and applications.

Uncovering control principles will help us to understand the fundamental laws governing the behavior of population health problems.

20.3.3. Pillar 3: Grounding Population Health Theory in Complex Systems Science

In the process of organically integrating complex systems science into population health science, the previous two pillars can comprise two foundational blocks toward the development of new theory appropriate for understanding population health challenges. As it has been the case with other social, ecological, technical, and natural systems,[3,42,46] a new theory base in population health science must also be developed, expanded, refined, and tested over time. From a mainly social psychological and secondarily organizational behavior and, typically, linear theory in population health, we need a transition to a theory base that encapsulates the complex systems properties of population health problems. This new theory needs to be grounded in diverse schools of thought from the social, population health, natural, and physical sciences. An indicative framework can be ascertained from these schools of thought:

1. *Theory from public and population health sciences:* aside from traditional theories that explain facts from diverse aspects of population health,[47] additional theories will originate from macrosocial and structural perspectives and domains such as syndemics, ecosocial, exposome, social determinants, political economy, and other population health schools of though[48–56];

2. *Theory from complex-systems-science–grounded advances in population health and other health sciences*[2,37,57];

3. *Theory from complex-systems-science advances in the social sciences*[3,4, 58–61];

4. *Theory from network and complex systems sciences*[62–67]; and

5. *Theory from complex systems engineering.*[46,68]

Population health science needs new theory to provide valid explanations of complex, adaptive, and dynamic phenomena in diverse behavior, disease, and injury states. It is anticipated that the process of theory development will pave the way for questioning the boundaries of current theories, reframing old and new problems, and ultimately building, expanding, testing, and validating a contemporary theory base applicable to diverse population health contexts (see Chapter 6 of this volume).

20.3.4. Pillar 4: Grounding Research Designs and Analytical Methods in Complex Systems Science

New robust methodologies, research designs, and analytical techniques grounded in network and complex systems sciences, and adapted to population health, must also be developed, tested, and validated. Current analytical, computational, and experimental methods in complex systems science can help researchers and practitioners adapt and produce powerful tools for tackling intractable population health problems as well as for validating theoretical assumptions. Stubborn population health challenges require methodological frameworks designed to help us delineate relationships among multilevel factors, across varying temporal and topological scales, to track state changes and interaction events, as well as to understand, identify, and characterize mechanisms that drive unwanted outcomes and, ultimately, try to *harness* complex systems in ways that benefit everyone.

Firmly placed within networks and complex systems, new methodologies will be grounded in the nexus of mathematical, physical, computational, and data sciences. They will be predicated on currently unexploited strengths of *model thinking* and *multiple rigorous models*. While model thinking and model development can greatly improve our ability to "reason, explain, design, communicate, act, predict, and explore" dynamically complex problems,[60p15] they are missing from core education and training competencies and have not played a central role in scholarship and policy planning in population health science. Especially the development of multiple models can greatly elevate our inadequate understanding of population health problems, as different models can extenuate different causal forces, thus providing deeper insights into persistent problems.[60] Along these lines, qualitative—stakeholder and community-based—modeling can provide invaluable insights.

This type of methodological thinking and accompanying analytical techniques can challenge established notions of causality, by expanding prevailing counterfactual causal inference perspectives.[69] The very nature of population health—grounded in mutual interdependencies of distributed systems of causation, context-/time-dependence, and emergence—suggests that intervention targets might not be for simply a few causes because there exist multiple intervention targets and configurations to facilitate optimal system changes. While key causal-inference methods, such as directed acyclic graphs or Bayesian causal nets, have been valuable in addressing causality,[70] stringent adherence might restrict us from finding lasting remedies to persisting challenges.[71] The appropriate use of these or otherwise expanded, or even new causal-inference, frameworks that address dynamic complexity would improve the efficiency of disease burden prevention (e.g., using multiple systems/models as counterfactuals can be powerful in delineating problems and identifying solutions).[72] Furthermore, causal triangulation by using different research designs and testing different hypotheses over time with different populations can help to examine whether our findings are robust to the confounding structures we have encountered and the analytical methods we have used—ultimately strengthening both explanation and causal inference.[30,73]

Because pressing population health problems are subject to fat-tailed and other nonnormal distributions (see Chapter 10 of this volume), as it is the case with many other complex systems,[74] the following categories of relevant methodologies, especially adapted for and integrated into population health science, can literally metamorphosize the methodological and analytical landscape.

1. More traditional modeling methodologies, including *mathematical modeling*—covering mainly graph, game, and network theories; Markov and Monte Carlo modeling; stochastic dynamical systems; bifurcations; and chaotic attractors[75]—and *computational simulation modeling*—with an emphasis on dynamic modeling, including mainly agent-based, system dynamics, discrete-event, and hybrid modeling.[76,77]

2. *Statistical physics and mechanics*, grounded in probability theory, statistics, and classical/quantum mechanics to delineate a variety of complex problems, and including nonlinear dynamical systems, control theory, stability and bifurcation of attractors, phase transitions, and thermodynamics.[78] Among the most promising advances in science, statistical physics and mechanics can revolutionize population health research and policy.

3. *Machine learning and data mining* can make momentous contributions to population health research, as methods of data analysis that automate analytical model building, on the one hand, and a branch of artificial intelligence based on the understanding that systems can learn from data, identify patterns and make decisions with minimal human intervention, on the other.[79]

The organic nexus of these four working pillars can provoke unprecedented methodological innovation with potential for actual discovery in population health science. Because it should not be the analytical methods that drive our quest for solutions in persisting problems, the foregoing ideas are based on the view that problematic health situations should be the drivers of epistemological frameworks, by reconciling and interweaving diverse theories and methods, as needed,[80] or even discovering new or more appropriate theories and methods, in the pursuit of answers. Emerging unifying theoretical, methodological, and analytical frameworks are expected to provide a renewed dynamic in population health science. Because essential data to address pressing problems remain hard to assemble, the revolution of massive and passive, big and small data can change the scientific landscape in population health. This can improve our currently inadequate and fragmented data, facilitate causal triangulation in diverse areas, help in connecting theory and data as well as in collecting new data grounded in newly developed theories and adapted to emerging needs, and even produce better and more useful models with practical benefits for larger and more diverse population segments.

20.4. AN EMERGING PARADIGM, A NEW POPULATION HEALTH SCIENCE

The intersection of dynamic complexity of population health with the capabilities of complex systems science provides an endless grist for our cognitive mills. This largely unexploited in-between space in the scientific landscape, where all pressing population health problems lie, opens boundless opportunities for paradigmatic innovation. But as the current paradigm presumes that it provides all necessary tools to help us understand the dynamics of and identify remedies for intractable population health challenges, it has, thus far, suppressed any quest for fundamental novelty outside its realm.

Predicated on accumulated evidence from other sciences, with wide population health applicability, as well as the foregoing discussion, *several key and mostly untested working assumptions* can corroborate the necessity for and reinforce the feasibility of an epistemological transition in population health science. They are as follows: (1) Many complex systems share "universal" properties that govern their structure, operation, and behavior, and, as a result, display comparable behavioral patterns; (2) population health problems—despite thematic, temporal, topological, scalar, structural, or other variation—operate as CADSoS and adhere to analogous principles, dynamics, and behaviors; (3) population health problems should be studied as complex systems, however crudely it might have to be done, because of scale of complexity and current state of population health science, as this is how we can begin to understand their dynamics and aggregate behavior; (4) only the understanding of the behavior of population health problems as wholes (complex systems) can possibly reveal sources of their intractability; (5) studying population health problems as complex systems can help to map foundational drivers, mechanisms, interactions, organization, topologies, temporalities, and causal structures—each invaluable for explaining unpredictable and intractable outcomes; and (6) complex-systems-science–grounded study of population health problems can enhance efforts to better understand them by trying to harness their complexity or design solutions that are aligned with the complexity of the systems creating them.

Within these emerging assumptions, the confluence of (a) complex-systems-science–grounded breakthroughs in various scientific and applied fronts; (b) a slow-moving, covert crisis[b] in population health science that has hindered progress; and (c) a long-overdue recognition of the importance of addressing deep-rooted socioeconomic and racial/ethnic inequalities that drive population health inequalities, provides a unique opportunity to advance population health science. The road ahead is neither to *untie* (by imperfectly complementing prevailing science with complex systems *methods*—current status quo) nor *cut* (by building a bottom–up complex-systems-science–based epistemology) the *Gordian knot* (the current epistemological conundrum). The proposed unifying paradigm will emerge from a *synthesis* of current and ongoing efforts and advancements from other sciences, grounded in the foregoing assumptions. Currently used qualitative, quantitative, and experimental frameworks[c]—as they can only enhance

b. Prominent population health scientists have asserted that population health science stands at a crossroads, juncture, or inflection point.[81]

c. For example, though linearity is an illogical assumption for many dynamically complex population health problems, linear models can be useful for taking a first cut at data, enabling the identification of magnitude and significance of variables, thus guiding the development of more intricate nonlinear models.[60]

understanding of the irreplaceable behavior of the whole, by providing context, scale, direction, detail, or measurable evidence—can be integrated within a newly developed, population-health adapted, epistemology in the *emerging unifying paradigm*.

The proposed paradigm is diametrically different than that of current population health science, where limited complex systems science *methods* are being used within prevailing general linear reality, proximal risk-factor epidemiology, and restrictive counterfactual causal inference. For instance, complex systems science theory that can fundamentally change how we conceptualize population health problems and ask research questions, thus altering research designs and types of data collected, is totally missing from current research frameworks. At best, the emergent implications of complex-systems-science–grounded conceptual study frameworks have been misunderstood, underestimated, and ultimately ignored.

The systematic development, validation, and proliferation of this emerging paradigm will eventually shake up the status quo, leading to the gradual emergence of a *new population health science*, realigning it in such a way that gradually moves the field further along to the scientific frontier. Not only is the new population health science expected to show us different and possibly more effective ways of getting a handle on persistent population health challenges to our benefit by minimizing negative emergent behaviors, but it can also reveal how complex-systems properties can generate positive emergent behaviors out of simpler system components. This, by itself, can comprise a sufficient condition that can open up astonishing new avenues in population health research and policy.

Such developments can catalyze the acceleration of a sweeping overhaul of academic education leading to different student training and therefore better prepared future scholars and practitioners, who understand and treat dynamic complexity for what it really is and does for population health problems and how it defines our policies. New academic curricula will, in turn, invigorate transdisciplinary research and scholarship that actually views problems as real wholes and not disconnected components. We will start asking different research questions and devise research designs that delve into the interactions and mechanisms of persisting population health outcomes over time. This will also enrich funding streams with far-reaching implications for advancing scholarship and science. Finally, production of new theoretical and applied scholarship will better inform and dramatically influence both public and private policy as well as action.

While it has become clear that population health problems operate as complex systems, failing to accommodate this dynamic complexity in research and policy planning has perpetuated undesirable outcomes, with limited prevention resources being used inefficiently and ineffectively. This direction can provide much more than a crude look at the whole of population health challenges, because even coarse-grained, simplified models of complex problems can be quite revealing. Because innate interdependencies and feedbacks in complex systems make searching these systems for solutions extremely hard, we cannot hope to literally control complex population health problems through interventions. Therefore, it would be best to learn how to appreciate and harness complexity.

20.5. THINKING ABOUT THE FUTURE

Pressing population health challenges have eluded scientists, policymakers, and practitioners for years because of misunderstanding or mismanagement of complexity. Now, however, we have the knowledge to surpass our currently inefficient use of complex systems science methods entrenched in inadequate theory, linearity, reductionism, and causal inference and can start building a unifying, forward-looking paradigm to *harness the ubiquitous complexity of population health*. Flourishing breakthroughs in other sciences have already planted their seed in population health research and scholarship. The time is now ripe to extend, cultivate, and transform accumulated knowledge into a comprehensive epistemology to impact population health policy and action. In his *No Man Is an Island* poem, John Donne eloquently articulated the ubiquity of interconnectedness in life; in similar fashion, it is time for population health scientists to reach a fundamental consensus on which to build their new science: *All* pressing population health problems operate as or are determined by complex systems and, therefore, should be studied as such to understand the irreplaceable behavior of the whole. It is my utmost hope that these evolving ideas will trigger a programmatic discourse that will lead to the development and proliferation of a new unifying paradigm and the eventual development of a new population health science. Foregoing assumptions are not written in stone. They represent *emerging* ideas to enrich the ongoing conversation so that we can exploit the scientific frontier and improve population health. Without a population health science that adheres to complex systems science, we have little chance to improve the health of the people most in need in our global village. Herein, my objective has been not to validate the enduring and comfortable delusion of prevailing, and ultimately inadequate, epistemology but rather to challenge us all toward the essential journey of comprehensively transforming population health science, thus making it more useful for more people.

REFERENCES

1. Sepulveda, J. and C. Murray (2014). The state of global health in 2014. *Science*, 345, 1275–1278.
2. El-Sayed, A.M. and S. Galea (eds.) (2017). *Systems Science and Population Health*. Oxford University Press.
1. Miller, J.H. (2015). *A Crude Look at the Whole*. Basic Books.
2. Miller, J.H., and S.E. Page. (2007). *Complex Adaptive Systems*. Princeton University Press.
3. Klovdahl, A.S. (1985). Social networks and the spread of infectious disease: The AIDS example. *Social Science and Medicine*, 21, 1203–1216.
4. Siettos, K. and L. Russo (2013). Mathematical modeling if infectious disease dynamics. *Virulence*, 4, 295–306.
5. Popkin, B.M. (2002). An overview of the nutrition transition and its health implications: The Bellagio meeting. *Public Health Nutrition*, 5, 93–103.

6. Marmot, M. (2005). Social determinants of health inequalities. *Lancet*, 365, 1099–1104.

7. Michor, F., J. Liphardt, M. Ferrari, and J. Widom (2011). What does physics have to do with cancer? *Nature Reviews Cancer*, 11, 657–670.

8. Stokols, D. (1992). Establishing and maintaining healthy environments: Toward a social ecology of health promotion. *American Psychologist*, 47, 6–22.

9. Singer, M. and S. Clair (2003). Syndemics and public health: Reconceptualizing disease in a biosocial context. *Medical Anthropology Quarterly*, 17, 423–441.

10. Cancer Intervention and Surveillance Modeling Network. Modeling to guide public health research and priorities. Retrieved from https://cisnet.cancer.gov/, May 27, 2019.

11. Best, A., P.I. Clark, S.J. Leischow, and W.M.K. Trochim (2007). *Greater than the sum: Systems thinking in tobacco control.* Retrieved from https://cancercontrol. cancer.gov/brp/tcrb/monographs/18/m18_complete.pdf, June 12, 2019.

12. Milstein B. (2002). *Hygeia's constellation.* Centers for Disease Control and Prevention. Retrieved from http://www.cdc.gov/syndemics/monograph/index.htm, June 25, 2019.

13. Milstein, B., J. Homer, and G. Hirsch (2009). The HealthBound policy simulation game: An adventure in U.S. health reform. International System Dynamics Conference, Albuquerque, New Mexico, July 26–30.

14. Mabry, P.L. and R.M. Kaplan (2013). Systems science: A good investment for the public's health. *Health Education & Behavior*, 40(IS), 9S–12S.

15. National Collaborative on Childhood Obesity Research. [Home page]. Collaborative Obesity Modeling Network, National Institutes of Health, Robert Wood Johnson Foundation, Centers for Disease Control and Prevention, and US Department of Agriculture. Retrieved from https://www.nccor.org/, June 27, 2019.

16. Apostolopoulos, Y., K. Hassmiller Lich, M.K. Lemke, and A.E. Barry (2018). A complex-systems paradigm can lead to evidence-based policymaking and impactful action in substance misuse prevention—A rejoinder to Purshouse et al. (2018). *Addiction*, 113, 1155–1156.

19. Chughtai, S. and K. Blanchet (2017). Systems thinking in public health: A bibliographic contribution to a meta-narrative review. *Health Policy and Planning*, 32, 585–594.

20. Williams, F., G.A. Golditz, P. Hovmand, and S. Gehlert (2018). Combining community-engaged research with group model building to address racial disparities in breast cancer mortality and treatment. *Journal of Health Disparities Research and Practice*, 11, 160–178.

21. Loyo, H.K., C. Batcher, K. Wile, et al. (2013). From model to action: Using a system dynamics model of chronic disease risks to align community action. *Health Promotion Practice*, 14, 53–61.

22. Tracy, M., M. Cerda, and K.M. Keyes (2018). Agent-based modeling in public health: Current applications and future directions. *Annual Review of Public Health*, 39, 77–94.

23. Glover, M.J., E. Jones, K.L. Masconi, et al. (2018). Discrete event simulation for decision modeling in healthcare: Lessons from abdominal aortic aneurysm screening. *Medical Decision Making*, 38, 439–451.

24. Rutter, C.M., A. Zaslavsky, and E. Feuer (2011). Dynamic microsimulation models for health outcomes: A review. *Medical Decision Making*, 31, 10–18.

25. Tejada, J.J., J. Ivy, J. Wilson, et al. (2015). Combined DES/SD model of breast cancer screening for older women, I: Natural history simulation. *IIE Transactions*, 47, 600–619.

26. Pawlus, W., J.E. Nielsen, H.R. Karimi, and K.G. Robbersmyr (2010). Development of mathematical models for analysis of a vehicle crash. *WSEAS Transactions on Applied and Theoretical Mechanics*, 5, 156–165.

27. Zou, X. and W.L. Yue (2017). A Bayesian network approach to causation analysis of road accidents. *Journal of Advanced Transportation*, doi.org/10.1155/2017/2525481.

28. Ashrafian, H. and A. Darzi (2018). Transforming health policy through machine learning. *PLoS Medicine*, 15, doi.org/10.1371/journal.pmed.1002692.

29. Lahti, L., J. Salojärvi, A. Salonen, et al (2014). Tipping elements in the human intestinal ecosystem. *Nature Communications*, 5. doi:10.1038/ncomms5344.

30. Keyes, K. and S. Galea (2017). The limits of risk factors revisited: Is it time for a causal architecture approach? *Epidemiology*, 28, 1–5.

31. Moore, T.W., P.D. Finley, J.M. Linebarger, et al. (2011). Public healthcare as a complex adaptive system of systems. Sandia National Laboratories, Albuquerque, New Mexico. https://www.sandia.gov/CasosEngineering/_assets/documents/ICCS_Public%20Health%20Care%20As%20CASoS_2011-3188%20C.pdf, June 23, 2019.

32. Greenhalgh, T. and C. Papoutsi (2018). Studying complexity in health services research: Desperately seeking an overdue paradigm shift. *BMC Medicine*, 16, doi.org/10.1186/s12916-018-1089-4.

33. Galea, S. (2018). *Healthier*. Oxford University Press.

34. Cramer, A.O.J., C.D. van Borkulo, E.J. Giltay, et al. (2016). Major depression as a complex dynamic system. *PLoS ONE*, 11, doi:10.1371/journal.pone.0167490.

35. Trefois, C., P.M.A. Antony, J. Goncalves, et al. (2015). Critical transitions in chronic disease: Transferring concepts from ecology to systems medicine. *Current Opinion in Biotechnology*, 34, 48–55.

36. Olde Rikkert, M.G.M., V. Dakos, T.G. Buchman, et al. (2016). Slowing down of recovery as generic risk marker for acute severity transitions in chronic diseases. *Critical Care Medicine*, 44, 601–606.

37. Kaplan, G.A., A.V. Diez Roux, C.P. Simon, and S. Galea (eds.) (2017). *Growing Inequality: Bridging Complex Systems, Population Health, and Health Disparities*. Westphalia Press.

38. Rutter, H., N. Sanova, K. Glonti, et al. (2017) The need for a complex systems model of evidence for public health. *Lancet*, 390, 2602–2604.

39. Holland, J.H. (1999). *Emergence: From Chaos to Order*. Helix Books.

40. Scheffer, M. (2009). *Critical Transitions in Nature and Society*. Princeton University Press.

41. Deffuant, G. and N. Gilbert (eds.). (2011). *Viability and Resilience of Complex Systems*. Springer.

42. Netherlands Organization for Scientific Research. (2014) *Grip on Complexity*. Retrieved from https://www.nwo.nl/en/about-nwo/media/publications/ew/paper-grip-on-complexity.html, February 25, 2019.

43. Bak, P., C. Tang, and K. Wiesenfeld (1987). Self-organized criticality: An explanation of 1/f noise. *Physical Review Letters*, 59, 381–384.

44. Liu, Y.Y. and A.L. Barabási (2016). Control principles of complex systems. *Review of Modern Physics*, 88, doi:10.1103/RevModPhys.88.035006.
45. Pósfai, M., J. Gao, S.P. Cornelius, et al. Controllability of multiplex, multi-scale networks. *Physical Review E*, 94, doi:10.1103/PhysRevE.94.032316.
46. Glass, R.J., A.L. Ames, T.J. Brown, et al. (2011). Complex adaptive systems of systems (CASoS) engineering: Mapping aspirations to problem solutions. Retrieved from https://www.sandia.gov/CasosEngineering/_assets/documents/ICCS_Mapping_Aspirations_2011-3354.pdf, April 29, 2019.
47. Glanz, K., B.K. Rimer, and K. Viswanath (eds.) (2008). *Health Behavior and Health Education: Theory, Research, and Practice*. Jossey-Bass.
48. Krieger, N. (2011). *Epidemiology and the People's Health: Theory and Context*. Oxford University Press.
49. Singer, M., M. Bulled, B. Ostrach, and E. Mendenhall (2017). Syndemics and the biosocial conception of health. *Lancet*, 389, 941–950.
50. Stokols, D., R.P. Lejano, and J. Hipp (2013). Enhancing the resilience of human-environment systems: A social ecological perspective. *Ecology and Society*, 18, dx.doi.org/10.5751/ES-05301-180107.
51. Benach, J., C. Muntaner, V. Santana, et al. (2007). *Employment Conditions and Health Inequalities*. EMCONET. Retrieved from https://www.who.int/social_determinants/resources/articles/emconet_who_report.pdf, March 21, 2019.
52. Galea, S. (ed.) (2007). *Macrosocial Determinants of Population Health*. Springer.
53. Keyes, K.M. and S. Galea (2016). *Population Health Science*. Oxford University Press.
54. Marmot, M. (2015). The health gap: The challenge of an unequal world. *Lancet*, 386, 2442–2444.
55. Raphael, D. (2016). *Social Determinants of Health: Canadian Perspectives*. Canadian Scholars' Press.
56. Smith, K.E., S. Hill, and C. Bambra (eds.) (2016). *Health Inequalities, Critical Perspectives*. Oxford University Press.
57. Sturmberg, J.P. and C. Martin (eds.) (2013). *Handbook of Systems and Complexity in Health*. Springer.
58. Byrne, D. and G. Callaghan (2014). *Complexity Theory and Social Sciences*. Routledge.
59. Castellani, B. and F.W. Hafferty (2009). *Sociology and Complexity Science: A New Field of Inquiry*. Springer.
60. Page, S.E. (2018). *The Model Thinker*. Basic Books.
61. Urry, J. (2003). *Global Complexity*. Blackwell.
62. Barabási, A.L. and M. Pósfai (2016). *Network Science*. Cambridge University Press.
63. Holland, J.H. (2014). *Complexity*. Oxford University Press.
64. Meadows, D.H. (2008). *Thinking in Systems: A Primer*. Chelsea Green Publishing.
65. Mitchell, M. (2009). *Complexity: A Guided Tour*. Oxford University Press.
66. Newman, M.E.J. (2010). *Networks: An Introduction*. Oxford University Press.
67. Thurner, S., R. Hanel, and P. Klimek (2018). *Introduction to the Theory of Complex Systems*. Oxford University Press.
68. Leveson, N.G. (2012). *Engineering a Safer World*. MIT Press.
69. Aiello, A.E. and L.W. Green (2019). Introduction to the symposium: Causal inference and public health. *Annual Review of Public Health*, 40, 1–5.

70. Vandenbroucke, J.P., A. Broadbent, and N. Pearce (2016). Causality and causal inference in epidemiology: The need for a pluralistic approach. *International Journal of Epidemiology*, 45, 1776–1786.

71. Krieger, N. and G. Davey Smith (2016). The tale wagged by the DAG: Broadening the scope of causal inference and explanation for epidemiology. *International Journal of Epidemiology*, 45, 1787–1708.

72. Hernan, M.A. (2015). The C-word: Scientific euphemisms do not improve causal inference from observational data (with discussion). *American Journal of Public Health*, 108, 616–619.

73. Naimi, A.I. (2017). On wagging tales about causal inference. *International Journal of Epidemiology*, 46, 1340–1342.

74. Newman, M.E.J. (2005). Power laws, Pareto distributions, and Zipf's law. *Contemporary Physics*, 46, 323–351.

75. Bender, E.A. (2000). *An Introduction to Mathematical Modeling*. Wiley.

76. Sterman J.D. (2000). *Business Dynamics*. Irwin/McGraw-Hill.

77. Wilensky, U. and W. Rand (2013). *An Introduction to Agent-Based Modeling: Modeling Natural, Social, and Engineered Complex Systems with NetLogo*. MIT Press.

78. Cowan, J.D., J. Neuman, B. Kiewiet, and W. van Drongelen (2013). Self-organized criticality in a network of interacting neurons. *Journal of Statistical Mechanics: Theory and Experiment*, 2013. doi:10.1088/1742-5468/2013/04/P04030.

79. Kavakiotis I., O. Tsave, A. Salifoglou, et al. (2017). Machine learning and data mining methods in diabetes research. *Computational and Structural Biotechnology*, 15, 104–116.

80. Ip, E.H., H. Rahmandad, D.A. Shoham, et al. (2013). Reconciling statistical and systems science approaches to public health. *Health Education and Behavior*, 40(1 Suppl), 123S–131S.

81. Galea, S. and K.M. Keyes (2018). What matters, when, for whom? Three questions to guide population health scholarship. *Injury Prevention*, 24, i3–i6.

GLOSSARY OF TERMS

Adaptation—The mechanisms by which individuals (or other agents) change their behaviors in response to interactions with other individuals (agents) and their environments as they pursue their goals.

Agent—A representation of an individual or other (e.g., organizational) autonomous entity in an agent-based model. Agents have defined static and dynamic characteristics. Dynamic characteristics change through specified rules as agents interact with each other and their environments.

Agent-Based Model—A bottom–up computational modeling approach that simulates macro-level outcomes based on micro-level within agent dynamics and agent–agent and agent–environment interactions among populations of individual agents.

Attractor—Specific system states that complex systems tend to settle at or periodically oscillate between.

Basin of Attraction—The point at which a complex system will transition to the system state of an attractor.

Bifurcation—A sudden change of the properties of a dynamical system.

Cellular Automata—The earliest form of agent-based modeling in which entities in discrete cells change from one time step to the next based on mathematical rules and characteristics of their environment, typically a function of nearby entities.

Co-Evolution—The mechanisms by which elements in a system, or systems themselves, change over time based on their interactions with other elements and with their environments.

Complex Adaptive System—A system that consists of diverse, interacting and adaptive entities, whose aggregated behaviors result in emergent, system-level patterns and functionalities.

Complex Adaptive Systems of Systems (CADSoS)—A collection of multiple connected and complex systems.

Complex Network—A network with properties that are not found in regular lattices or random networks but are often seen in real-world networks.

Complex System—A system consisting of interconnected elements that has characteristics of complexity (e.g., interactions and interdependencies in the system, interconnected web of determinants, nonlinear relationships, heterogeneity, and feedback loops).

Complexity—A characteristic of a system where the interactions and interdependencies among elements in the system, rather than just the number and characteristics of elements that constitute the system, are most important in determining system structure and behavior. Complexity often indicates the presence of an interconnected web of determinants, nonlinear relationships, dynamics, heterogeneity, and feedback loops that makes causality hard to intuit.

Complicated—A characteristic of a system where the number and attributes of elements that constitute the system, rather than the interactions and interdependencies among elements in the system, are most important in determining system structure and behavior.

Computational (Simulation) Modeling—An approach to modeling that allows for the creation and use of digital (computer-based) representations of real-world, complex phenomena to understand influences on population health outcomes and evaluate how different intervention and policy choices could influence outcomes. Computational modeling is particularly useful when closed-form solutions (mathematical equations) characterizing system steady states or optimal values cannot be obtained or when analysis focuses on understanding system dynamics.

Connectionism—A network model approach that focuses on how macro-level behaviors can be understood through understanding the interactions of micro-level networks of nodes. These micro-level networks of nodes are either uniform or simple.

Critical Slowing Down—The tendency of the recovery rate after an external disturbance slows down when systems are close to a tipping point.

Critical Transition—The change that occurs when a system exceeds a tipping point threshold, causing the system to transfer from one stable state to another.

Detail Complexity—A characteristic of a system where system outcomes arise from a large number of variables.

Dynamic—A characteristic of a system, where components of the system change over time.

Dynamic complexity—A characteristic of a system, where the interactions and interdependencies among elements in the system exhibit dynamics (change over time) and other characteristics of complexity including feedback loops, accumulations, and nonlinear relationships, making cause and effect unclear and the system impossible to study by breaking it into its component parts.

Dynamical Disease—A disease that occurs in an intact physiological control system operating in a wide range of control parameters that leads to abnormal dynamics. Dynamical diseases have two or more stable states or attractors.

Dynamical System—A system that is described by temporal change of a point in a state space; at any given time, the system is in a particular state in its space, and it evolves according to rules that describe how it changes its state over time. There are many types of dynamical systems, including continuous, discrete, stochastic, and deterministic that are best described using different approaches.

Emergence—The process by which micro rules (e.g., adaptation, based on interactions among micro-level entities, or micro-level entities and their environments) produce macro-level patterns that are novel and separate from what could have been predicted by summing each micro-level change.

Equilibrium—The description of a system in which processes of change have stabilized and steady state is realized.

Feedback Loops (Positive, Negative)—Mechanisms within a system, where two or more variables mutually influence each other over time (e.g., a change in X triggers a change in Y, which triggers further change in X over time). Positive feedback loops are also called reinforcing feedback loops because they amplify change within a system and result in the system moving away from its current state. Negative feedback loops are also called balancing feedback loops because they work to maintain stability by counteracting changes that move the system away from its current state.

Flow—A term typically associated with system dynamics modeling; in- and outflows change the level of a stock (accumulation) over time.

Frailty—A state of increased vulnerability of a system (e.g., patients or organs) to poor resolution of homeostasis following a stress, which increases the risk of change to another set point. In medicine, frailty often refers to an adverse outcome for patients such as seizures, falls, syncope, and depression (opposite of resilience).

Graph Theory—A foundational theory in network science. Grounded in mathematics, graph theory employs graphs, consisting of edges (links) connecting nodes (elements in a system) to study the properties of networks or webs of connections.

Group Model Building—A facilitated participatory process that actively engages decision-makers, subject-matter experts, and other relevant stakeholders to build, evaluate, and use qualitative and quantitative system models for learning and action planning.

Heterogeneity——Diversity among characteristics, behaviors, or other properties among system elements or outcomes.

Hybrid Modeling—Modeling approaches that combine two or more modeling techniques to compensate for the weaknesses of each specific approach with the strengths of another.

Interaction—A characteristic of complexity that refers to mutual influence among elements in a system that may occur across multiple scales or socioeconomic levels.

Interdependence—A characteristic of complexity that refers to the interconnections among two or more system elements, often across multiple scales, that are marked by mutual dependence.

Long-Tailed Distribution—A distribution defined by a skewed, or slowly decaying, tail consisting of extreme values; these distributions are sometimes characterized by power laws.

Markov Chain—A stochastic model comprised of various system states and the possible transitions among them over time, in which the probability(ies) of an event(s) depend only the most current state. Higher order Markov chains retain more historical memory, where an ith order Markov chain predicts state based on i most recent states.

Markov Chain Monte Carlo—A class of algorithms for sampling from a probability distribution that are primarily used for calculating numerical approximations of multidimensional integrals.

Mathematical Modeling—The use of mathematical notation and techniques to describe, represent, and/or analyze real-world phenomena.

Mental Model—An implicit, internal, and nonformal model that is a simplified representation of a real-world phenomenon.

Microsimulation—A computational modeling approach that focuses on large numbers of independent agents with observable states.

Model—A simplified version of something in the real world that is purposeful and allows us to better understand the world around us.

Modeling—The act of creating a model.

Model Thinking—A world view that emphasizes the necessity of models and modeling to make sense of the world and act effectively upon it.

Network—A collection of elements consisting of edges and links.

Newtonian Science (see Reductionism)

Noise—System behaviors that are considered to obscure clarity or understanding in the context to the paradigmatic approach being brought to bear or research questions being considered.

Nonlinearity—A characteristic of complexity; describes nonproportional cause and effect relationships.

Normal Distribution—Also known as a bell-shaped or Gaussian distribution. A normal distribution represents random variables that are independent and identically distributed.

Organized Complexity—A characteristic of a system where interdependencies exist between variables.

Paradigm—A world view. In science, a paradigm is a framework that defines a scientific discipline, including all the commonly accepted views on the discipline and how research should be conducted, at a certain point in time.

Path Dependence—A characteristic of complex systems, where small historical events can become durable effects within the greater system, and once on this path it can be difficult, if not impossible, to switch to a new path.

Phase Transition (see Critical Transition)

Policy Resistance—The scenario where our inadequate understanding of a complex system we are trying to act on leads to solutions that are either ineffective or make things worse, creating what we see as "side effects" and leading to frustration and helplessness.

Population Health—The study of health outcomes within and across populations, as well as the study of determinants and mechanisms that shape health outcomes within and across populations.

Post-Newtonian Science—A paradigmatic approach to studying real-world phenomena using complex systems approaches.

Power Law—A functional relationship between two variables, where a small change in one variable can lead to a large change in another.

Randomness—A characteristic often attributed to complex systems; unpredictability, uncertainty, or irregularity in the behaviors of elements in a system or system outcomes.

Random Network—A type of network, where the likelihood of any two edges in a system being connected in completely random.

Recovery—The total process of readaptation after the initial decline in health after a stressor or acute disease or intervention, until the person reaches a new equilibrium.

Reductionism—A scientific paradigm that posits that phenomena are best understood by reducing them down into component parts, studying those component parts independently, and aggregating what is learned about those parts.

Resilience—Ability of a system to bounce back to its steady state after a perturbation.

Robustness (see Resilience)

Scaling—The degree of aggregation employed in the development of a model.

Scale-Free Network—A type of network that is more hierarchical in structure than a random network and follows power laws.

Self-Organization—The creation of global-level coordination out of local-level interactions among agents, as opposed to a central controller.

Self-Organized Criticality—Describes when system's components that are independent or weakly interdependent over small distances under a normal state become globally interdependent at critical transitions. This is related to critical transitions.

Simulation Modeling (see Computational Simulation Modeling)

Small-World Network—A type of scale-free network, where the presence of major hubs reduces the average path length between edges.

Stable State—System states that are defined by relative constancy of state variables over time. In equilibrium states, state variables will approximate a Gaussian distribution.

Stakeholders—People or organizations that have an interest in, and a critical role (for better or worse) in affecting, population health outcomes.

State Variables—Variables that captures the state of a system.

Statistical Mechanics—An approach that focuses on explaining how macro-level behaviors of a system emerge from the statistical properties of the large numbers of micro-level components that make up the system.

Steady State (see Stable State)

Stochastic—Exhibits randomness over time.

Stock—A term typically associated with System Dynamics Modeling. A stock represents accumulations of elements in a system over time.

System—An array of interconnected elements, bounded in space and time, that form a collective whole.

System Dynamics Modeling—A computational modeling approach that emphasizes uncovering the structure of dynamically complex systems and determining how to leverage this understanding of system structure to create desirable change in outcomes.

Systems Thinking—A world view that emphasizes seeing the world as consisting of systems.

Tipping Point—Critical threshold that marks the border of an equilibrium state. Exceeding the tipping point results in an abrupt change from the current state to another state.

Validation—One aspect of model testing, in which efforts are taken to ensure that the model is a good representation of the world.

Verification—One aspect of model testing, in which efforts are taken to ensure that the model represents intended system structure.

INDEX

Tables and figures are indicated by *t* and *f* following the page number
For the benefit of digital users, indexed terms that span two pages (e.g., 52–53) may, on occasion, appear on only one of those pages.